Durability and reliability of medical polymers

Related titles:

Biocompatibility and performance of medical devices
(ISBN 978-0-85709-070-6)
Implant and device manufacturers are increasingly being faced with the challenge of proving that their implants or devices are safe/biocompatible and perform as expected. This book describes and explains the factors that influence the biocompatibility of materials and medical devices, the methods to predict or screen biocompatibility, how to build a biological safety evaluation plan for medical devices, strategies and tactics in biocompatibility and biological performance evaluation of medical devices. It also provides insights into recent changes in regulations and standards, standards interpretation and worldwide health authorities' expectations with regard to the biocompatibility and performance of new products.

Biomaterials in plastic surgery: Breast implants
(ISBN 978-1-84569-799-0)
Breast implants are one of the most regularly used prostheses (both for cosmetic and reconstructive purposes) in plastic surgery. Unfortunately, they are also one of the most controversial implants available and some types of breast implants have gained a reputation for being unreliable and in some cases dangerous. This book discusses the history of this lucrative field and how it is developing. Chapters in Part I explore a wide range of breast implants whilst chapters in Part II review important safety issues.

Joining and assembly of medical materials and devices
(ISBN 978-1-84569-577-4)
Medical devices are becoming more intricate with the use of a wide range of materials and components that must be joined effectively and safely. *Joining and assembly of medical materials and devices* provides a comprehensive analysis of the practical techniques that can be used to join and assemble medical materials. Part I reviews issues such as adhesive selection, testing and modelling. Part II discusses processes, materials and applications whilst the final set of chapters reviews safety and regulatory considerations.

Details of these and other Woodhead Publishing books can be obtained by:

- visiting our website at www.woodheadpublishing.com
- contacting Customer Services (e-mail: sales@woodheadpublishing.com; fax: +44 (0) 1223 832819; tel.: +44 (0) 1223 499140 ext. 130; address: Woodhead Publishing Limited, 80 High Street, Sawston, Cambridge CB22 3HJ, UK)
- contacting our US office (e-mail: usmarketing@woodheadpublishing.com; tel. (215) 928 9112; address: Woodhead Publishing, 1518 Walnut Street, Suite 1100, Philadelphia, PA 19102-3406, USA)

If you would like e-versions of our content, please visit our online platform: www.woodheadpublishingonline.com. Please recommend it to your librarian so that everyone in your institution can benefit from the wealth of content on the site.

Woodhead Publishing Series in Biomaterials: Number 44

Durability and reliability of medical polymers

Edited by

Mike Jenkins and Artemis Stamboulis

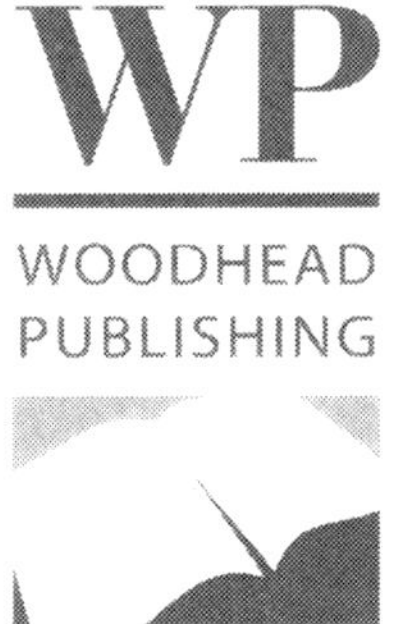

Oxford Cambridge Philadelphia New Delhi

Published by Woodhead Publishing Limited,
80 High Street, Sawston, Cambridge CB22 3HJ, UK
www.woodheadpublishing.com
www.woodheadpublishingonline.com

Woodhead Publishing, 1518 Walnut Street, Suite 1100, Philadelphia, PA 19102-3406, USA

Woodhead Publishing India Private Limited, G-2, Vardaan House, 7/28 Ansari Road, Daryaganj, New Delhi – 110002, India
www.woodheadpublishingindia.com

First published 2012, Woodhead Publishing Limited

British Library Cataloguing in Publication Data
A catalogue record for this book is available from the British Library.

Library of Congress Control Number: 2012939821

ISBN 978-1-84569-929-1 (print)
ISBN 978-0-85709-651-7 (online)
ISSN 2049-9485 Woodhead Publishing Series in Biomaterials (print)
ISSN 2049-9493 Woodhead Publishing Series in Biomaterials (online)

The publisher's policy is to use permanent paper from mills that operate a sustainable forestry policy, and which has been manufactured from pulp which is processed using acid-free and elemental chlorine-free practices. Furthermore, the publisher ensures that the text paper and cover board used have met acceptable environmental accreditation standards.

Typeset by Replika Press Pvt Ltd, India
Printed by TJ International Ltd, Padstow, Cornwall, UK

Contents

Contributor contact details

(* = main contact)

Editors

Mike Jenkins* and Artemis Stamboulis
School of Metallurgy and Materials
University of Birmingham
Edgbaston
Birmingham
UK
B15 2TT

E-mail: m.j.jenkins@bham.ac.uk; A.Stamboulis@bham.ac.uk

Chapters 1 and 3

Tommaso Casalini and Giuseppe Perale*
Politecnico di Milano
Department of Chemistry, Materials and Chemical Engineering 'Giulio Natta'
Via Mancinelli 7, 20131 Milan
Italy

E-mail: tommaso.casalini@mail.polimi.it; giuseppe.perale@polimi.it

Chapter 2

Dr Gianni Pertici
Industrie Biomediche Insubri SA
via Cantonale CH-6805
Mezzovico
Switzerland

E-mail: gianni@ibi-sa.com

Chapter 4

Filippo Rossi* and Giuseppe Perale
Politecnico di Milano
Department of Chemistry, Materials and Chemical Engineering 'Giulio Natta'
Via Mancinelli 7, 20131 Milan
Italy

E-mail: filippo.rossi@mail.polimi.it; giuseppe.perale@polimi.it

Chapter 5

R. E. Cameron*
Department of Materials Science and Metallurgy
University of Cambridge
Pembroke Street
Cambridge
CB2 3QZ
UK

E-mail: rec11@cam.ac.uk

A. Kamvari-Moghaddam
Biocompatibles UK Ltd
Chapman House
Farnham Business Park
Weydon Lane
Farnham
Surrey
GU9 8QL
UK

Chapter 6

Marco Santoro
Politecnico di Milano
Department of Chemistry, Materials and Chemical Engineering 'Giulio Natta'
Via Mancinelli 7
20131 Milan
Italy

E-mail: msantoro@chem.polimi.it

Giuseppe Perale*
Industrie Biomediche Insubri SA
via Cantonale
CH-6805, Mezzovico
Switzerland

E-mail: giuseppe@ibi-sa.com

Chapter 7

Dr D. E. T. Shepherd* and Dr K. D. Dearn
School of Mechanical Engineering
University of Birmingham
Edgbaston
Birmingham
B15 2TT
UK

E-mail: D.E.Shepherd@bham.ac.uk; k.d.dearn@bham.ac.uk

Chapter 8

Dr Aziza Mahomed
Research Fellow
School of Mechanical Engineering
Biomedical Engineering
University of Birmingham
Edgbaston
Birmingham
B15 2TT
UK

E-mail: a.mahomed@bham.ac.uk; aziza.mahomed@gmail.com

Chapters 9 and 10

Dr Peter R. Lewis
Reader in Forensic Engineering
Materials Engineering
The Open University
Walton Hall
Milton Keynes
MK7 6AA
UK

E-mail: petelewisr@gmail.com; p.r.lewis@open.ac.uk

Woodhead Publishing Series in Biomaterials

1 **Sterilisation of tissues using ionising radiations**
Edited by J. F. Kennedy, G. O. Phillips and P. A. Williams

2 **Surfaces and interfaces for biomaterials**
Edited by P. Vadgama

3 **Molecular interfacial phenomena of polymers and biopolymers**
Edited by C. Chen

4 **Biomaterials, artificial organs and tissue engineering**
Edited by L. Hench and J. Jones

5 **Medical modelling**
R. Bibb

6 **Artificial cells, cell engineering and therapy**
Edited by S. Prakash

7 **Biomedical polymers**
Edited by M. Jenkins

8 **Tissue engineering using ceramics and polymers**
Edited by A. R. Boccaccini and J. Gough

9 **Bioceramics and their clinical applications**
Edited by T. Kokubo

10 **Dental biomaterials**
Edited by R. V. Curtis and T. F. Watson

11 **Joint replacement technology**
Edited by P. A. Revell

12 **Natural-based polymers for biomedical applications**
Edited by R. L. Reiss et al

13 **Degradation rate of bioresorbable materials**
Edited by F. J. Buchanan

14 **Orthopaedic bone cements**
Edited by S. Deb

15 **Shape memory alloys for biomedical applications**
Edited by T. Yoneyama and S. Miyazaki

16 **Cellular response to biomaterials**
Edited by L. Di Silvio

17 **Biomaterials for treating skin loss**
Edited by D. P. Orgill and C. Blanco

18 **Biomaterials and tissue engineering in urology**
Edited by J. Denstedt and A. Atala

19 **Materials science for dentistry**
B. W. Darvell

20 **Bone repair biomaterials**
Edited by J. A. Planell, S. M. Best, D. Lacroix and A. Merolli

21 **Biomedical composites**
Edited by L. Ambrosio

22 **Drug-device combination products**
Edited by A. Lewis

23 **Biomaterials and regenerative medicine in ophthalmology**
Edited by T. V. Chirila

24 **Regenerative medicine and biomaterials for the repair of connective tissues**
Edited by C. Archer and J. Ralphs

25 **Metals for biomedical devices**
Edited by M. Ninomi

26 **Biointegration of medical implant materials: science and design**
Edited by C. P. Sharma

27 **Biomaterials and devices for the circulatory system**
Edited by T. Gourlay and R. Black

28 **Surface modification of biomaterials: methods analysis and applications**
Edited by R. Williams

29 **Biomaterials for artificial organs**
Edited by M. Lysaght and T. Webster

30 **Injectable biomaterials: science and applications**
Edited by B. Vernon

31 **Biomedical hydrogels: biochemistry, manufacture and medical applications**
Edited by S. Rimmer

32 **Preprosthetic and maxillofacial surgery: biomaterials, bone grafting and tissue engineering**
Edited by J. Ferri and E. Hunziker

33 **Bioactive materials in medicine: design and applications**
Edited by X. Zhao, J. M. Courtney and H. Qian

34 **Advanced wound repair therapies**
Edited by D. Farrar

35 **Electrospinning for tissue regeneration**
Edited by L. Bosworth and S. Downes

36 **Bioactive glasses: materials, properties and applications**
Edited by H. O. Ylänen

37 **Coatings for biomedical applications**
Edited by M. Driver

38 **Progenitor and stem cell technologies and therapies**
Edited by A. Atala

39 **Biomaterials for spinal surgery**
Edited by L. Ambrosio and E. Tanner

40 **Minimized cardiopulmonary bypass techniques and technologies**
Edited by T. Gourlay and S. Gunaydin

41 **Wear of orthopaedic implants and artificial joints**
Edited by S. Affatato

42 **Biomaterials in plastic surgery: breast implants**
Edited by W. Peters, H. Brandon, K. L. Jerina, C. Wolf and V. L. Young

43 **MEMS for biomedical applications**
Edited by S. Bhansali and A. Vasudev

44 **Durability and reliability of medical polymers**
Edited by M. Jenkins and A. Stamboulis

45 **Biosensors for medical applications**
Edited by S. Higson

46 **Sterilisation of biomaterials and medical devices**
Edited by S. Lerouge and A. Simmons

47 **The hip resurfacing handbook: a practical guide for the use and management of modern hip resurfacings**
Edited by K. De Smet, P. Campbell and C. Van Der Straeten

48 **Developments in tissue engineered and regenerative medicine products**
J. Basu and J. W. Ludlow

49 **Nanomedicine: technologies and applications**
Edited by M. Webster

50 **Biocompatibility and performance of medical devices**
Edited by J-P. Boutrand

51 **Medical robotics**
Edited by P. Gomes

52 **Implantable sensor systems for medical applications**
Edited by A. Inmann and D. Hodgins

53 **Non-metallic biomaterials for tooth repair and replacement**
Edited by P. Vallittu

54 **Joining and assembly of medical materials and devices**
Edited by Y. N. Zhou and M. D. Breyen

55 **Diamond based materials for biomedical applications**
Edited by R. Narayan

56 **Nanomaterials in tissue engineering: characherization, fabrication and applications**
Edited by A. K. Gaharwar, S. Sant, M. J. Hancock and S. A. Hacking

57 **Biomimetic biomaterials: structure and applications**
Edited by A. Ruys

58 **Standardisation in cell and tissue engineering: methods and protocols**
Edited by V. Salih

59 **Inhaler devices: fundamentals, design and drug delivery**
Edited by P. Prokopovich

60 **Bio-tribocorrosion in biomaterials and medical implants**
Edited by Y. Yan

61 **Microfluidics for biomedical applications**
Edited by X-J. J. Li and Y. Zhou

62 **Decontamination in hospitals and healthcare**
Edited by J. T. Walker

63 **Biomedical imaging: applications and advances**
Edited by P. Morris

64 **Characterisation of biomaterials**
Edited by M. Jaffe, W. Hammond, P. Tolias and T. Arinzeh

Part I

Types and properties of bioresorbable medical polymers

1 Types of bioresorbable polymers for medical applications

T. CASALINI and G. PERALE, Politecnico di Milano, Italy

Abstract: A review is presented of the main types of bioresorbable or bioabsorbable materials used in medical applications such as drug delivery. Groups discussed include aliphatic polyesters, polyanhydrides, poly(ortho esters) (POE), polyphosphazenes, poly(amino acids) and 'pseudo' poly(amino acids), polyalkylcyanoacrylates, poly(propylene fumarate) (PPF), poloxamers, poly(*p*-dioxanone) (PPDO) and polyvinyl alcohol (PVA).

Key words: bioresorbable medical polymers, aliphatic polyesters, polyanhydrides, poly(ortho esters), polyphosphazenes, poly(amino acids), polyalkylcyanoacrylates, poly(propylene fumarate), poloxamers, poly(*p*-dioxanone), polyvinyl alcohol.

1.1 Introduction

The growth in polymer-made biomedical devices has in part been made possible thanks to the discovery of a new class of materials: bioresorbable polymers. The term 'bioresorbable' has become a common expression, used in order to qualify this type of macromolecules. A scientifically accepted definition for such materials is the following: 'a material for which the degradation is mediated, at least partly, from a biological system' (Ottenbright and Scott, 1992). This statement shows one of the most important features of these materials. Devices made of bioresorbable polymers are subjected to degradation in the human body which means they do not need to be removed.

The degradation process involves polymer long chains, which are reduced to shorter segments that can be absorbed by the cells. In a physiological system (i.e., the human body), degradation follows a two-phase mechanism:

- First of all, fission of long chains takes place because of hydrolysis and/or enzymatic attack (this phase can be both biotic and abiotic).
- During the second biotic phase, smaller fragments are dissolved in extracellular fluids, where they are destroyed by phagocytes or metabolized by the cells.

This phenomenon is related to another interesting feature of bioresorbable polymers. Degradation products are removed by the cells themselves in order to achieve a complete degradation of the implanted device. As an example, degradation of poly-L-lactic acid produces L-lactic acid, a compound involved in the Krebs' cycle for aerobic living systems, which is metabolized by the cells by enzymatic degradation. In this way a biodegradable or bioresorbable device can degrade entirely into an organism. To be more precise, it is more correct to talk of biodegradability in environmental terms and bioresorption or bioabsorption in physiological terms, even if these words are used as synonyms.

The degradation of these materials into the human body combined with their biocompatibility has made bio-absorbable polymers suitable for biomedical applications. A good understanding of the phenomena involved in degradation kinetics has contributed to their utilization. Indeed, the knowledge of properties which influence the degradation dynamics makes it possible to modify the chemical and mechanical properties of the material and thus its degradation rate. As an example, if a rapid degradation is desired, then a hydrophilic polymer with a low crystallinity degree is chosen. If slow degradation is required, a crystalline and hydrophobic polymer is used. It is possible to obtain a polymeric matrix which disappears, say, in two weeks or in six months according to the specific application.

In the field of biomedical devices, bioresorbable polymers can be used for several purposes. Suture threads represent an established example of a bioabsorbable device. They were introduced for the first time during the early 1970s. They were first made of poly(glycolic acid). Threads made of poly(lactic acid) and polydioxanone appeared later in 1981. Currently there is a wide variety of types of commercial suture thread (monofilament or polyfilament) depending on requirements such as degradation time and mechanical behavior.

Another important and widely studied application is devices for drug delivery. Polymeric matrices made of a bioresorbable material can be loaded with drugs (as well as proteins, growth factors and genes) which are released during device degradation. It is generally accepted that drug release dynamics depends both on device degradation and drug diffusion in the polymeric matrix. Modifying degradation dynamics makes it possible to tune drug delivery, e.g. to obtain a burst or a slow release depending on circumstances. Suture threads can, for example, be loaded with an analgesic or antibacterial drug in order to improve wound healing or patient well-being (Zurita *et al.*, 2006a, Zurita *et al.*, 2006b, Perale *et al.*, 2010). Polymeric nanoparticles can also be loaded with drugs and then injected into the body.

Drug release rate is affected by many factors, such as polymer composition, molecular weight, and particles size. Polymers such as poly(lactic acid), poly(glycolic acid), poly(lactic-co-glycolic acid), and polyalkylcyanoacrylates have been tested for this purpose (Batycky *et al.*, 1997, Liggins and Burt, 2001, Siepmann *et al.*, 2002, Park, 1995, Dossi *et al.*, 2010, Freiberg and Zhu, 2004). However, devices can also be film-shaped or disc-shaped

(Woo *et al.*, 2006, Kim *et al.*, 2005, Loo *et al.*, 2009, Wang *et al.*, 2005, Mochizuki, 2005). Another interesting application of bioresorbable polymers is the synthesis of hydrogels, i.e. heterogeneous, strongly hydrophylic and crosslinked polymeric matrices (Peppas, 1986). Hydrogels can be loaded with drugs or with drug-containing nanoparticles, in order to perform a release at a certain rate.

1.2 Aliphatic polyesters

Aliphatic polyesters have a chemical structure characterized by the presence of ester groups along the chains. They can be classified according to their preparation method (Albertsson and Varma, 2005) in four main categories:

- naturally-occurring polyesters;
- microbial polyesters;
- condensation polyesters; and
- polyesters from ring-opening polymerization (ROP).

The most representative naturally-occurring polyester is 'shellac', a resin secreted by female lac bugs in India and Thailand. Shellac is a complex mixture of monoesters and polyesters, whose backbone is mainly formed of terpenic acids, aleuritic acid and several minor fatty acids (Wang *et al.*, 1999). This is therefore a non-homogeneous material from a chemical point of view, because it contains isolated and conjugated double bonds, and aldehydic and primary alcoholic groups, that make shellac a polyfunctional resin (Fig. 1.1).

Examples of microbial polyesters are the so-called polyhydroxyalkanoates (PHA), which are produced by bacterial fermentation of sugars and lipid, in order to store carbon and energy. There are about 100 different monomers that had been included into PHA polymers (Rehm and Steinbuchel, 2005); this list comprises hydroxyalkanoate units with a substituted group (alkyl, aryl, alkenyl, halogen, cyano, epoxy, ether, acyl, ester, and acid groups) (Fig. 1.2).

However, PHA polymers are also classified according to monomers carbon units. Short-chain-length (SCL) PHAs consist of 3–5 carbon units monomers, whilst medium-chain-length (MCL) PHAs have 6–14 carbon units monomers (Lee and Park, 2005). The most representative polymer belonging to this family is poly-3-hydroxybutyrate (P3HB), whose main component is *R*-3-hydroxybutanoic acid, a metabolite found also in human blood (Fig. 1.3).

The PH3B homopolymer is a stiff, brittle and rigid material with a Young modulus similar to that of polypropylene (Abe and Doi, 2005) and with a high melting temperature, around 170 °C; this implies a difficult processability (Satkowski *et al.*, 2005) because the polymer degrades during processing.

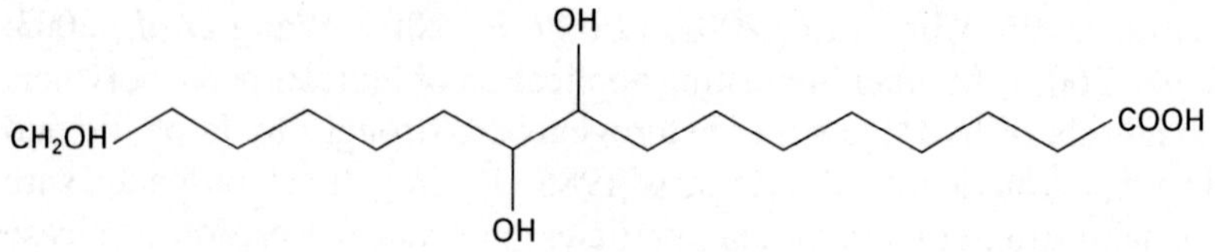

1.1 Shellac main components: (a) aleuritic acid and (b) terpenic acids (R = COOH, CH_2OH, CHO, R′ = CH_3, CH_2OH).

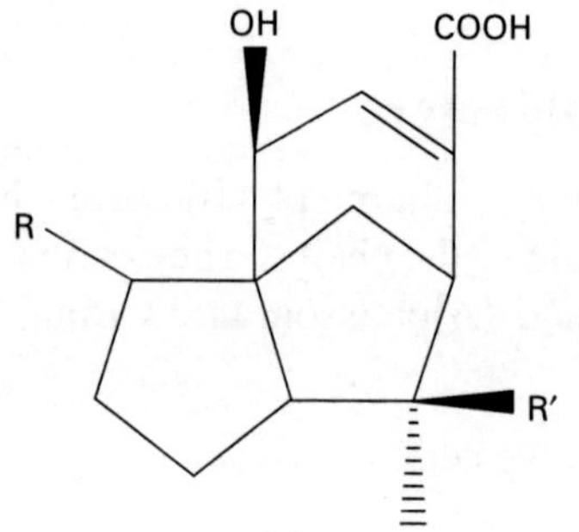

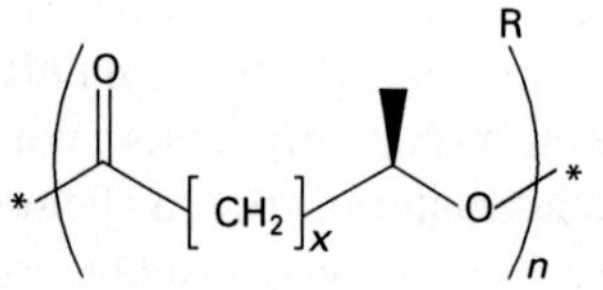

1.2 Structure of polyhydroxyalkanoate.

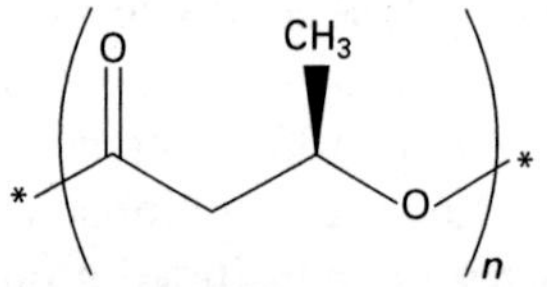

1.3 Structure of poly-3-hydroxybutyrate.

Moreover, P3HB shows a crystalline structure because of its stereoregularity similarity to isotactic polypropylene. In order to improve mechanical properties and processability, and thus to obtain a more flexible material, P3HB copolymers are nowadays used. The first attempt to synthesize a random copolymer is a blend of 3-hydroxybutanoic acid and 3-hydroxyvaleric acid, obtaining poly(3-hydroxybutyrate-co-3-hydroxyvalerate) P(3HB-co-3HV) copolymer. Other blends are obtained using, for example, hydroxyhexanoic acid, 4-hydroxybutanoic acid, and hydroxyoctanoic acid. Physical and mechanical properties of these copolymers have been reported (Lee and Park, 2005, Marchessault and Yu, 2005, Williams and Martin, 2005) as well as examples of production processes. PHAs homopolymers and copolymers were first introduced in the 1980s by ICI under the name of Biopol (Williams and Martin, 2005), and were used as an alternative to petroleum-based plastic. However, the production cost was too high and interest in PHAs faded rapidly. Recently, PHAs polymers have gained an important role in the field of biomedical devices and tissue engineering because of their low toxicity and bioresorbability properties.

Condensation polymers are materials obtained through a polycondensation reaction (which follows a step growth polymerization mechanism) involving one or more different monomers. The most representative materials of this category are the poly-alpha-hydroxy-acids such as the poly(lactic acid) (PLA) and poly(glycolic acid) (PGA) which were first introduced during the 1950s. PGA is the simplest linear aliphatic polyester, obtained through polycondensation of glycolic acid; it has a high crystalline ratio, a high melting point, and it is insoluble in water and in almost all common organic solvents. PGA degrades mainly because of hydrolysis, producing glycolic acid, which is a natural metabolite and thus recognized by human body (Figs 1.4 and 1.5).

PGA was used to produce the first example of bioabsorbable synthetic suture threads under the commercial name of Dexon, although the mechanical strength of such devices decreased in a short period of time (2–4 weeks) (Ratner, 2004), limiting the application of this polymer. In order to improve PGA mechanical characteristics, PGA and PLA copolymers were realized; PLA is hydrophobic and limits water uptake, slowing the hydrolysis mechanism

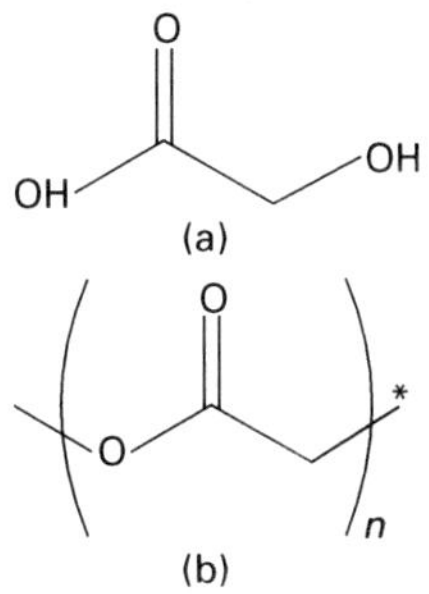

O
OH
OH
(a)
O
O
*
n
(b)

1.4 (a) Glycolic acid and (b) polyglycolic acid.

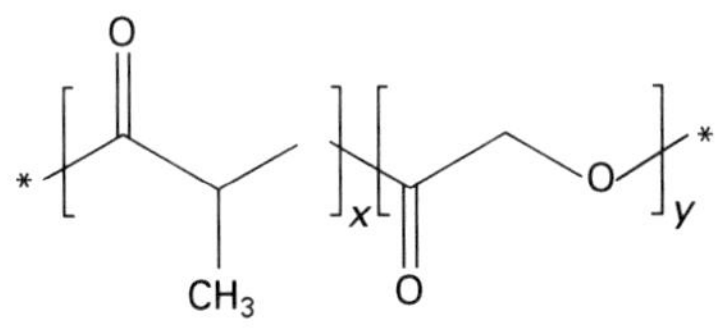

O
*
x
O
*
y
CH_3
O

1.5 Poly(lactic-co-glycolic acid).

which is responsible for degradation phenomenon. This blend allowed the introduction of new suture threads with the commercial name of Vicryl.

Lactic acid contains a carbon atom with four different substituting groups, and thus has two enantiomeric forms: L- and D-lactic acid (Fig. 1.6). This implies that four morphologically different poly(lactic acid) (PLA) polymers can be obtained: poly-L-lactic acid (PLLA), poly-D-lactic acid (PDLA) and the racemic form poly-D,L-lactic acid (PDLLA). The fourth form, meso PLA, synthesized from D- and L-lactide, is rarely used (Ratner, 2004). PLLA and PDLA are stereoregular and have a high crystalline ratio, thus making them suitable for applications where high mechanical strength is required. However, PLLA is employed more frequently because L-lactic acid is the monomer recognized by human body, being involved in the Krebs's cycle. PDLLA is an amorphous polymer, suitable for drug delivery where a homogeneous drug dispersion into a monophasic matrix is needed.

A crucial aspect of the synthesis of these polymers is water removal; the polycondensation reaction produces water which causes polymer hydrolysis during the process, since the reaction is reversible, reducing the molecular weight of the final product. Moreover, in order to obtain high molecular weights, these reactions are carried out with a catalyst, such as $SnCl_2$ or $Ti(BuO)_4$ (Harshe *et al.*, 2007). Another example of aliphatic polyesters is a material called 'Bionolle' (Ishioka *et al.*, 2005), a bioresorbable polymer obtained from a polycondensation of glycols (such as ethylene glycol and 1,4-butanediol) with dicarboxylic acids (such as oxalic acid and succinic acid) (Fig. 1.7). By varying the initial monomer composition it is possible to obtain materials with different properties. Two examples of Bionolle are poly(butylene succinate) (PBS) and poly(butylene succinate-adipate) (PBSA).

The fourth category involves polymers which are synthesized following the ROP mechanism, a particular step-growth polymerization, where cyclic monomers are involved. The most representative material belonging to this

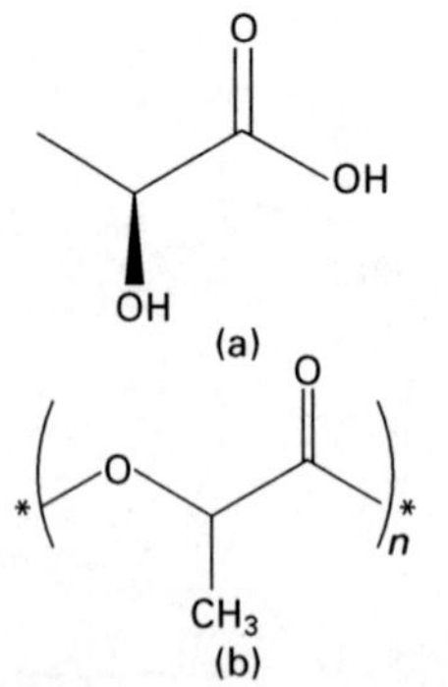

O
OH
OH
(a)
O
O
*
*
n
CH_3
(b)

1.6 (a) L-Lactic acid and (b) poly(lactic acid).

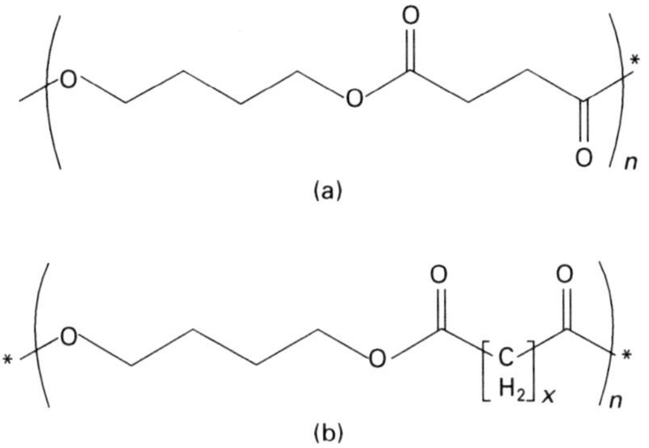

1.7 Bionolle structures: (a) poly(butylene succinate) and (b) poly(butylene succinate adipate).

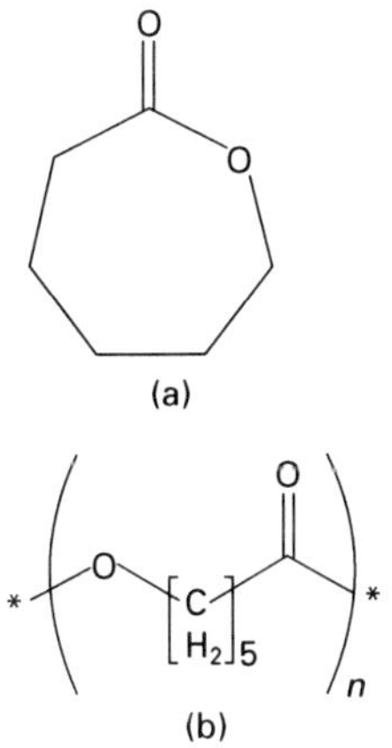

1.8 (a) ε-Caprolactone and (b) poly-ε-caprolactone.

category is poly-ε-caprolactone (PCL); the monomer, ε-caprolactone, is a cyclic ester with a ring of seven carbon atoms (Fig. 1.8).

Polymerization is carried out using stannous octoate as catalyst and alcoholic compounds as initiators. PCL is a crystalline polymer with a low melting point (about 60 °C) and it degrades because of hydrolysis; nevertheless, its characteristic degradation time is very large compared with that of other commonly used aliphatic polyesters, such as PLA. This feature allows its use in medical devices and drug delivery systems that remain active for over a year (Ratner, 2004). Moreover, this material is compatible with a good range of other polymers, and thus PCL blends can be easily obtained (Gunatillake and Adhikari, 2003). ROP can be also used to realize polymerization of PLA and PGA with high molecular weights. L-Lactic acid is condensed in small oligomers with low molecular weight as described; these short chains are depolymerized with a catalyst and subjected to a back-biting reaction which produces L-lactide, a cyclic compound (Tsuji, 2005) (Fig. 1.9). L-Lactide

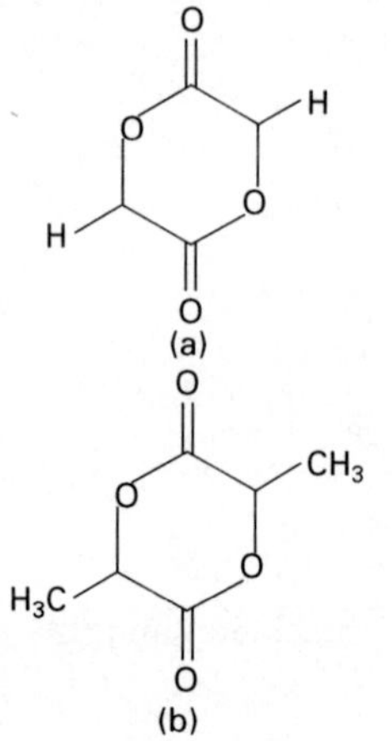

1.9 (a) Glycolide and (b) lactide.

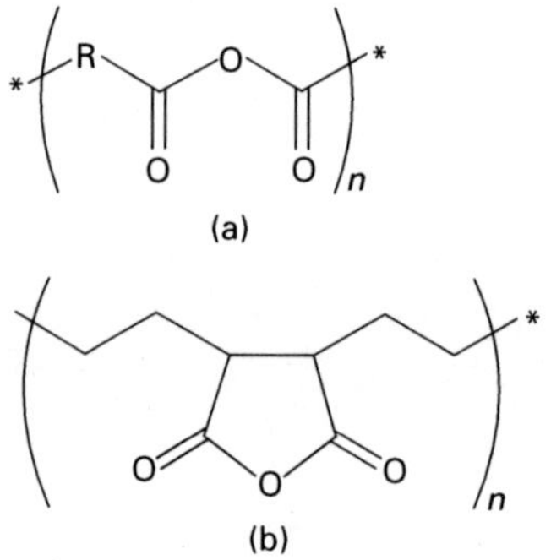

1.10 Anhydride groups (a) in backbone and (b) as side chain.

is polymerized to PLA using a catalyst and an initiator, obtaining a high molecular weight polymer because this process does not produce water, avoiding the main difficulty of this kind of polycondensation synthesis (Yu *et al.*, 2009). For what concerns molecular weight distribution, a similar result can be achieved during the production of high MW-PGA, obtained starting from glycolide and a catalyst (Gunatillake and Adhikari, 2003).

Other examples of monomers involved in ROP are β-propiolactone (β-PL), β-butyrolactone, γ-butyrolactone, δ-valerolactone (δ-VL).

1.3 Polyanhydrides

Polyanhydrides are characterized by anhydride bonds connecting monomers along the chain, or by anhydride groups located on the side of the chain and not along the backbone. Indeed, poly(malic anhydride) is a polyethylene chain with anhydride groups as side chains (Fig. 1.10).

In general terms, polyanhydrides have a hydrophobic backbone where anhydride bonds are subjected to hydrolysis because they are very water-labile; these polymers degrade with a surface erosion. The depolymerization reaction is too fast to allow water penetration into the matrix, which is eroded gradually on the surface. Polyanhydrides have a number of advantages. They are produced from available and cheap resources, obtaining a well-defined polymeric structure whose degradation rate can be computed. In particular, hydrolitic degradation can be modulated by realizing a copolymer with hydrophobic groups along the chain; fatty acids are suitable for this purpose, because they are hydrophobic natural body components. Moreover, they can be easily processed at low temperatures and sterilized with γ-irradiation without serious effects for the material; degradation products are dicarboxylic acids, which are metabolized by human body itself. Polyanhydrides also have disadvantages; they must be stored in moisture-free frozen conditions because of their hydrolytic instability and, because at room temperature or above, they may spontaneously depolymerize. Polyanhydrides can be synthesized with various techniques, including melt condensation, ROP, interfacial condensation, and dehydrochlorination; solution polymerization does not allow to obtain high molecular weights.

Polyanhydrides have been classified into several categories (Kumar *et al.*, 2002, Kumar *et al.*, 2005):

- Aliphatic polyanhydrides presenting saturated bonds along the chain and a crystalline structure.
- Unsaturated polyanhydrides exhibiting unsaturated bonds along the chain and thus being suitable for the synthesis of a crosslinked matrix. Unsaturated bonds remain intact during polymerization.
- Aromatic polyanhydrides containing aromatic groups; since homopolymers belonging to this category melt at temperatures above 200 °C and cannot be properly processed, copolymers obtained from different aromatic diacids are commonly employed.
- Aliphatic–aromatic polyanhydrides, which are synthesized starting from diacids, having aliphatic and aromatic moieties.
- Poly(ester anhydrides) and poly(ether anhydrides) presenting ether and/or ester linkages along the chain (in addition to anhydride bonds). Aliphatic and aromatic moieties are also present in the backbone.
- Fatty acid-based polyanhydrides derived from dimers or trimers of unsaturated fatty acid, which have two carboxylic groups available for the reaction. Natural fatty acids possess only one reactive group and can be employed as chain terminators. Chemical and physical properties can be modulated by choosing adequate monomers and their relative amount.
- Amino acid-based polymers synthesized from naturally occurring amino acids, for example by amidation of the amino group of an amino acid

with a cyclic anhydride or by the amide coupling of two amino acids with a diacid chloride.

- Branched polyanhydrides.
- Crosslinked polyanhydrides with three dimensional networks, showing high mechanical strength and a slow degradation rate.

The properties of polyanhydrides can be modified by changing polymer composition and structure. This is obtained by realizing copolymers, polymer blends, crosslinking between chains, partial hydrogenation and reaction with epoxides. Low molecular weight PLA, PHB and PCL are miscible with polyanhydrides whereas high molecular weight polyesters are not.

Polyanhydrides have been investigated as potential materials suitable for controlled-release devices of drugs, chemotherapeutic agents, local anesthetics, anticoagulants, neuroactive drugs, and anticancer agents, since the *in vivo* compatibility is very good (Lanza *et al.*, 2007). Representative polyanhydrides are poly(1,3-bis-*p*-carboxyphenoxypropane anhydride) (PCPP) and its copolymers with sebacic acids (PCPP-SA) (Fig. 1.11).

Indeed, PCPP-SA systems were clinically tested in order to deliver an anticancer agent into the brain for the treatment of brain neoplasm in rats, rabbits and monkeys, showing a satisfactory biocompatibility without adverse effects (Domb *et al.*, 1997). Nowadays, this material is FDA approved and is currently in clinical use for the treatment of brain cancer (Lanza *et al.*, 2007).

1.4 Poly(ortho esters)

Poly(ortho esters) (POE) contain ortho ester groups along the chain; an ortho ester is a functional group containing three alkoxy groups attached to one carbon atom. Degradation results from a hydrolysis mechanism. These polymers can be formulated in order to obtain a surface erosion degradation.

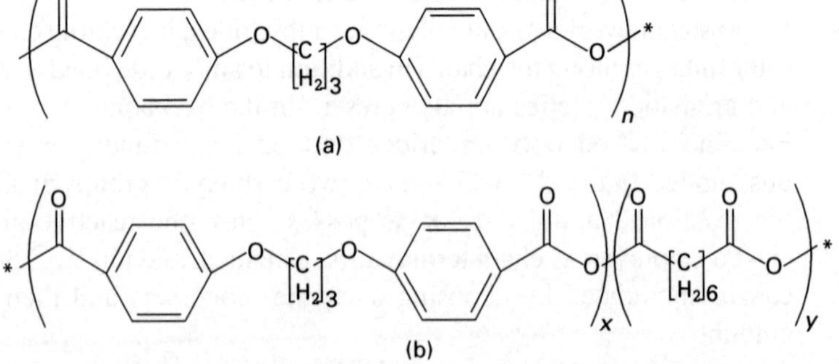

1.11 (a) PCPP and (b) PCPP-SA.

This means that with slab-like devices, if the drug is uniformly dispersed, its release is carried out at constant rate, whereas in PLA devices, for example, the drug release is a combination of erosion and diffusion because bulk degradation takes place. Poly(ortho esters) are divided in four families (Heller *et al.*, 2002):

- POE I,
- POE II,
- POE III, and
- POE IV.

The following paragraphs review each of these families.

POE I polymers are synthesized from 2,2′-dimethoxyfuran and a diol. Hydrolysis of POE I materials produces γ-butyrolactone which becomes γ-hydroxybutyric acid (Fig. 1.12). This compound enhances degradation since ortho ester linkages are acid sensitive; it is necessary to stabilize the polymer with a basic compound such as Na_2CO_3 in order to avoid autocatalytic and uncontrollable hydrolysis degradation. POE I polymers have been investigated for clinical devices, but the autocatalytic nature of the degradation and the low glass-transition temperature limited applications for these materials, that nowadays are not under development.

POE II polymers are synthesized starting from 3,9-diethylidene-2,4,8,10-tetraoxaspiro[5.5]undecane (a diketene acetal) and a diol; another example is the addition of a diol with 1,1,4,4-tetramethoxy-1,3-butadiene. Their synthesis is simpler because it is only necessary to dissolve the monomers in a polar solvent and to add traces of an acidic catalyst (Fig. 1.13). Molecular weights

H_3CH_2CO OCH_2CH_3 + HO–R–OH → * O O–R * n + OH

(a)

* O O–R * n $\xrightarrow{H_2O}$ O + OH → HO OH O

(b)

1.12 POE I: (a) synthesis and (b) hydrolysis.

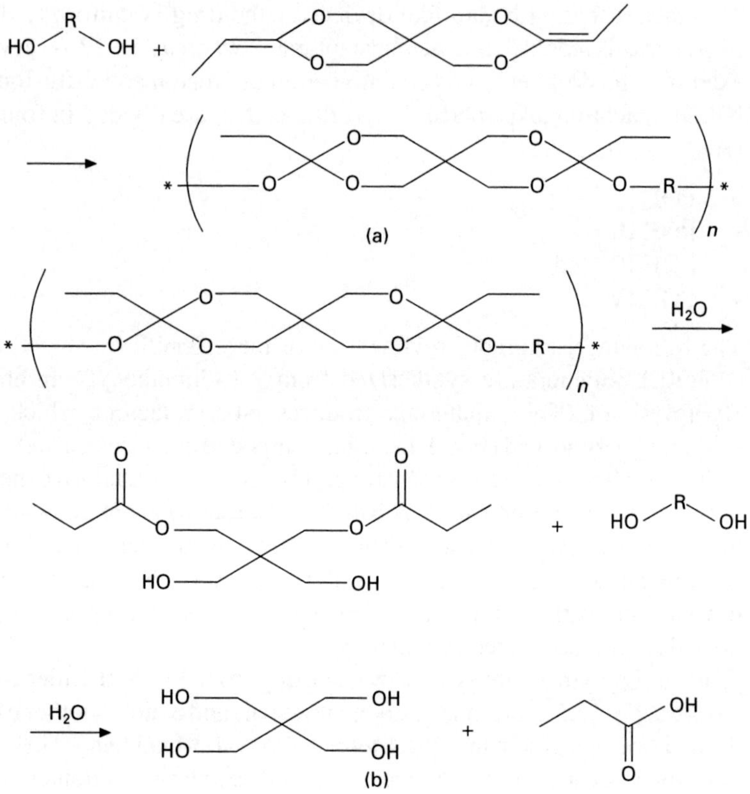

1.13 POE II: (a) synthesis and (b) hydrolysis.

can be controlled by use of stoichiometry. Hydrolysis initially produces neutral fragments that do not affect degradation, so there are no autocatalytic effects. By using alcohols with more than two functional groups (triols, and so on) it is possible to obtain crosslinked matrices which completely degrade in small water soluble fragments. POE II polymers are hydrophobic, water uptake is limited and thus in physiological conditions they are very stable. Since ortho ester linkages are affected by acids but are stable in base, by adding a basic compound such as $Mg(OH)_2$ hydrolysis can be controlled even if the matrix is in an aqueous environment; $Mg(OH)_2$ stabilizes the bulk of the matrix and erosion occurs only on the surface where the base has been eluted or neutralized. Moreover, mechanical and thermal properties can be adjusted by using diols with different chain flexibility.

POE III polymers are synthesized with a triol (whose functional groups are placed on the first, the second, and the last carbon atom) and a 1,1,1-triethoxy compound (Fig. 1.14). When 1,2,6-hexanetriol is employed, the polymer is semisolid at room temperature. Drugs can be incorporated by simply mixing and the material can be injected. Degradation also occurs

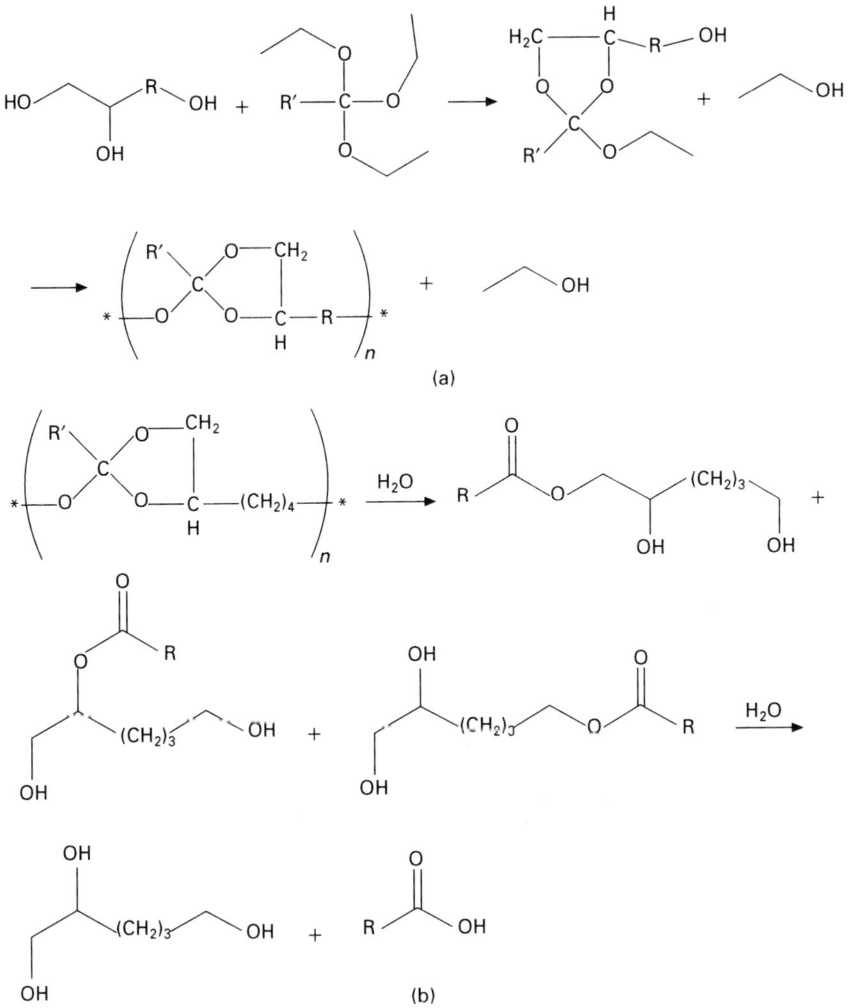

(a)

(b)

1.14 POE III: (a) synthesis and (b) hydrolysis.

because of hydrolysis for POE III polymers. However, the synthesis presents some problems such as long reflux times and ethanol removal in order to obtain high molecular weight. It is difficult to obtain reproducible results and a control on molecular weight, and thus POE III were discarded, even if they had shown a very good ocular compatibility.

Synthesis of POE IV materials is similar to POE II reaction, but mono/dilactide or mono/diglycolide are included in the backbone (Fig. 1.15). These fragments can be considered as 'latent acids' because hydrolysis of POE IV polymers produces lactic acid or glycolic acid which act as catalysts for the hydrolysis of ortho ester linkages. The advantage of these polymers is the

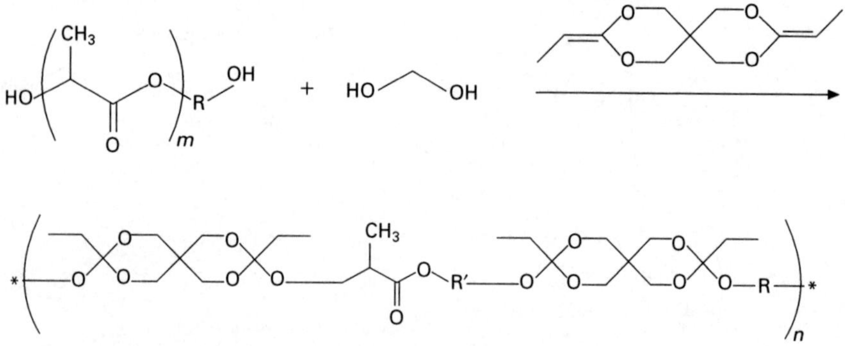

1.15 POE IV synthesis.

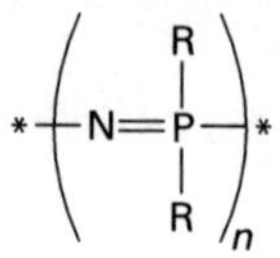

1.16 Structure of polyphosphazene.

control on properties and degradation rate by varying the diol, the latent acid diol, and the proportion between these two. For low latent acid concentration there is an induction period, which is the result of the hydrophobic nature of the material, because an adequate amount of water must diffuse into the matrix in order to start hydrolysis. The induction period can be decreased by increasing matrix hydrophilicity, the amount of latent acid diol and by using lower molecular weight materials. This induction period can be very useful if the aim is a delayed drug release.

Nowadays, POE IV are the most promising poly(ortho esters); they were tested for treatment of postsurgical pain (with short-term delivery of analgesic agents), release of peptides and proteins, and postoperative treatment of cancer (with drug delivery systems containing antineoplastic agents in order to destroy tumor cells that were not removed during surgery) (Heller *et al.*, 2000, Heller and Barr, 2004).

1.5 Polyphosphazenes

Polyphosphazenes are a particular class of inorganic polymers, which do not have carbon atoms in their backbone. Their structure exhibits alternate sequences of nitrogen and phosphorus atoms, with two side groups of various nature (organic, inorganic, organometallic …) (Mark *et al.*, 1992). The bonding structure along the chain shows an alternate sequence of single and double bonds (Fig. 1.16).

Synthesis of polyphosphazenes dates back to 1895 when H. N. Stokes obtained this type of polymer via ROP of hexachlorotriphosphazene $[(NPCl_2)_3]$ (Lakshmi *et al.*, 2003). The first polyphosphazene was a colorless crosslinked material with high molecular weight, that is, an inorganic rubber which was insoluble in all solvents and unstable with respect to hydrolysis; the degradation products were ammonia, phosphates and hydrochloric acid. Because of its poor stability, this material did not find proper applications. The first stable linear polydichlorophosphazene was obtained by Allcock *et al.* in 1996 (Deng *et al.*, 2010), controlling the time and the temperature of the ROP (Fig. 1.17). Hydrolytic instability results from the polar and highly reactive chlorine-phosphorus bond; stability was achieved by exploiting the reactivity of this bond and substituting chlorine with organic or organometallic nucleophiles. Thus, as said before, several different polyphosphazenes can be obtained by varying the groups which will substitute the chlorine atoms.

Four main ways to synthesize polyphosphazenes have been identified (Zhu and Qiu, 2005):

- replacement of halogen atoms in polydichlorophosphazene;
- ROP of cyclic phosphazene trimers containing organic groups;
- condensation polymerization of organophosphoranimines, $CF_3CH_2OR_2P{=}NSiMe_3$, by thermal or anionic catalyzed techniques;
- denitrogenation of phosphine azides, R_2PN_3.

It is also known that the nitrogen–phosphorus backbone can become instable to hydrolysis by inserting adequate side groups, a feature that makes polyphosphazenes suitable for biomedical application. Moreover, degradation products are usually non-toxic compounds such as phosphates, ammonia, and the side groups. Thus, a variety of bioresorbable polyphosphazenes can be prepared with the proper choice of substituent groups and their ratio (Fig. 1.18). Bioresorbable polyphosphazenes are usually prepared using the first aforementioned synthesis method, and can be roughly divided in two groups, according to the side groups (Lakshmi *et al.*, 2003):

- Aminated polyphosphazenes present amines with a low value of pKa as side groups, and constitute the most studied class of bioresorbable polyphosphazenes. Amino acid ester and imidazole-substituted polyphosphazenes appear to be two good candidates for drug delivery applications, because of their good hydrolysis degradation and low

250 °C

1.17 Synthesis of polydichlorophosphazene.

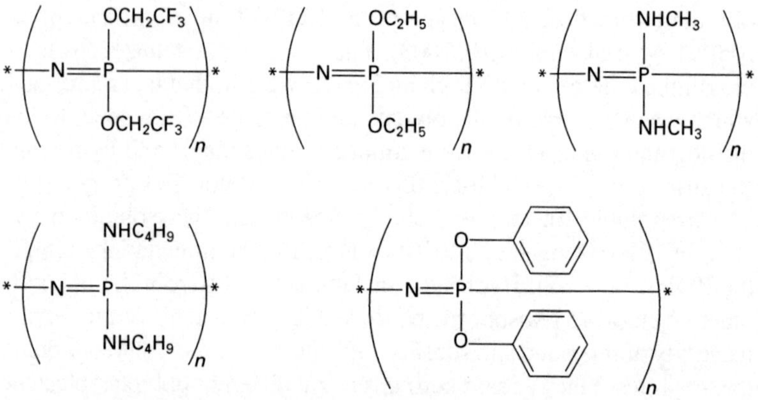

1.18 Examples of linear polyphosphazenes.

toxicity of degradation products. Two kinetic pathways have been proposed to explain hydrolytic degradation, which involve protonation of atoms in the backbone and in the side groups. Protonation of skeletal nitrogen leads directly to ring cleavage and to conversion to ammonium ion, phosphoric acid, and free amine salt. Protonation of a side group nitrogen, followed by a nucleophilic water attack at phosphorus, leads to a monohydroxycyclophosphazene, which would be subject to ring cleavage and eventual degradation by further hydrolysis (Allcock *et al.*, 1982).

- Alkoxy-substituted polyphosphazenes present activated alcohols as substituting groups. The first example of this kind of polymers is a glyceryl-substituted phosphazene, obtained by Allcock and Kwon (1988). Since glycerol is a three-functional molecule, two of the hydroxyl groups were protected in order to avoid crosslinking reactions. Starting from this polymer, it is thus possible to obtain polyphosphazene-based hydrogels using crosslinking agents without protecting hydroxyl groups. Ambrosio *et al.* (2002) also synthesized alkoxy-substituted polyphosphazenes bearing esters of glycolic or lactic acid as side groups.

Bioresorbable polyphosphazenes can be classified also according to their function (Zhu and Qiu, 2005):

- Hydrophobic polyphosphazenes.
- Water-soluble polyphosphazenes.
- Polyphosphazene–drug conjugates.

Polyphosphazenes have already been investigated for biomedical applications, especially in controlling the release of chemotherapeutic agents (Cho and Allcock, 2007) (and thus in the drug delivery field) and in the temporary replacement of body parts (Deng *et al.*, 2010). For example, following the 'tissue guided regeneration', Passi *et al.* (2000) promoted healing of rabbit tibia by using membranes of polyphosphazene with amino acid ester side groups (POP). Moreover, as previously stated, polyphosphazenes are suitable for synthesizing hydrogels: Allcock and Ambrosio (1996) obtained pH-sensitive hydrogels starting from poly(organophosphazenes).

1.6 Poly(amino acids) and 'pseudo' poly(amino acids)

From 1970, amino acids-based homo- and copolymers were studied for biomedical applications; the idea was quite intuitive, because proteins are made of amino acids. However, initial studies showed that most poly(amino acids) could not be employed for biomedical applications because of immunogenicity problems and poor mechanical properties. Only a small number of poly(γ-substituted glutamates) possess adequate characteristics to be interesting. In order to improve mechanical and physiological features of these materials, amino acids can be used as monomeric building blocks in polymers that do not have a backbone with the conventional structure which can be found in peptides. These materials are the so called 'non-peptide amino acids-based polymers' or 'amino-acid-derived polymers with modified backbone', and can be divided into four main categories (Bourke and Kohn, 2003):

- Synthetic polymers with amino acid side chains: these have a synthetic backbone where amino acids and peptides are present as side chains. These materials show a polyelectrolytic and metal complexation behavior. Polymethacrylamides with glycylglycine and phenylalanine are a good example of such systems.
- Copolymers of α-L-amino acids and non-amino acid monomers: this class comprises a wide range of copolymers synthesized starting from α-L-amino acid (an α-amino acid has the amino group attached to the carbon atom adjacent to the carboxylate group) and acid monomers, obtaining various features and mechanical properties. For example, ring-opening copolymerization of 2,5-morpholinedione derivatives and D,L-lactide gave copolymers of poly(α-aminoacid-co-D,L-lactic acid), which belong to the family of poly(amino esters), whose interesting feature is that they degrade primarily through the ester bonds. Another example is the family of poly(anhydride-co-imides) obtained with naturally occurring α-amino acids and ω-amino acids linked through anhydride bonds. Allcock *et al.* (1993) synthesized poly[(amino acid ester) phosphazenes] films and studied release of small molecules from these scaffolds.
- Pseudo poly(amino acids): in order to improve the properties of poly(amino acids), Kohn and Langer (1986) synthesized polymers where amino acids were not linked through amide bonds but through their side chains,

obtaining, for example, ester, iminocarbonate, and carbonate bonds. Thus, the final polymers, called 'pseudo' poly(amino acids), contain amino acids as monomers similar to conventional poly(amino acids) but do not have a peptide-like backbone.

- Block-copolymers containing peptide or poly(amino acid) blocks: these polymers usually have a A–B or A–B–A copolymer block structure, where A is poly(ethylene glycol) and B is a conventional poly(amino acid) or a peptide.

Nowadays, the most promising materials of this field are tyrosine-based polymers. Tyrosine is a non-essential (i.e., it is produced by human body itself) amino acid with a polar side group (Fig. 1.19).

Industrially, diphenols such as bisphenol A are frequently used in order to increase the stiffness of polymers thanks to their aromatic backbone (Fig. 1.20). However, for biomedical applications diphenols cannot be used as monomers because they are cytotoxic. Tyrosine (2-amino-3-(4-hydroxyphenyl) propanoic acid) is the only major natural nutrient containing an aromatic hydroxyl group. Thus, tyrosine dipeptide (where the terminal amino group and terminal carboxylic group are protected) can be seen as replacing diphenols for biomedical devices.

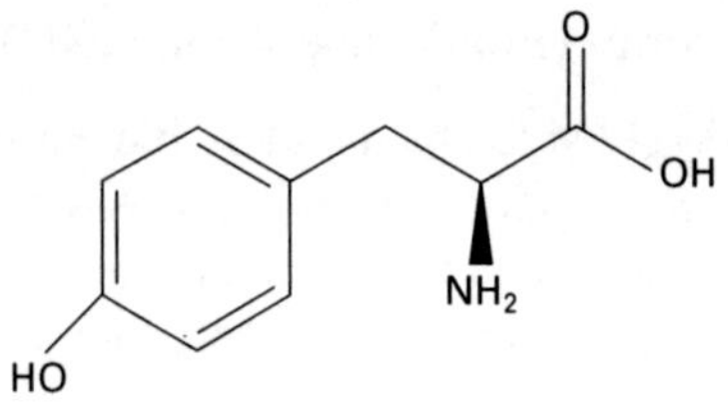

1.19 Tyrosine.

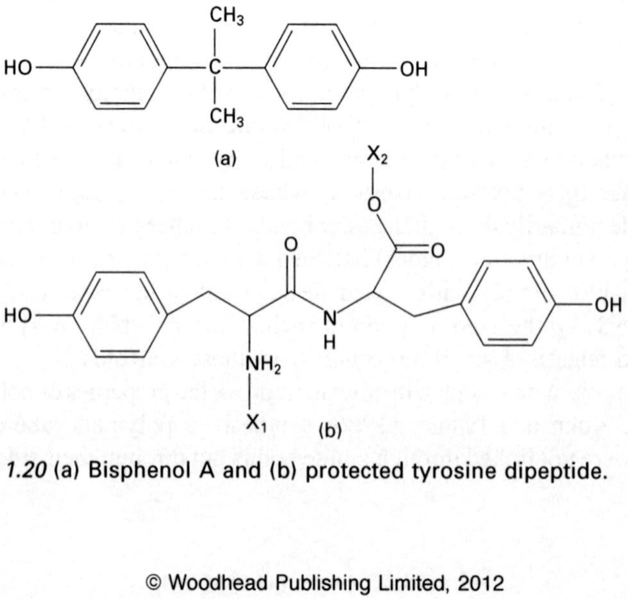

1.20 (a) Bisphenol A and (b) protected tyrosine dipeptide.

This approach makes it possible to obtain tyrosine-based materials. The protecting groups have a role in determining the properties of the final product; the challenge is identifying suitable groups that will lead to a non-toxic and bioresorbable material. However, this was not achieved, and tyrosine dipeptide was substituted with a dimer of tyrosine and L-tyrosine, or desaminotyrosine [3-(4'-hydroxyphenyl)propionic acid], finally obtaining a fully biocompatible substitute for diphenols (Fig. 1.21). However, diphenolic monomers used in this field are obtained from desaminotyrosine and alkyl esters of tyrosine (Sen Gupta and Lopina, 2002). The resulting pendent chain protects carboxylic group.

There are four main categories of tyrosine-based polymers (Bourke and Kohn, 2003):

- Tyrosine-derived polycarbonates (Fig. 1.22): they are a group of carbonate–amide copolymers which differ in the length of their alkyl ester pendent chains. Monomers are subjected to polymerization using phosgene or bis(chloromethyl) carbonate triphosgene. Weight-average molecular weight in the range of 100 000–400 000 can be reached. Chemical and physical properties can be easily modulated by changing the length of the alkyl ester pendent chain, even if this does not influence degradation rate. Properties of such polymers have already been investigated (Bourke and Kohn, 2003).
- Tyrosine-derived polyarylates (Fig. 1.23): these materials are obtained starting from the tyrosine-derived monomers described above and alkyl

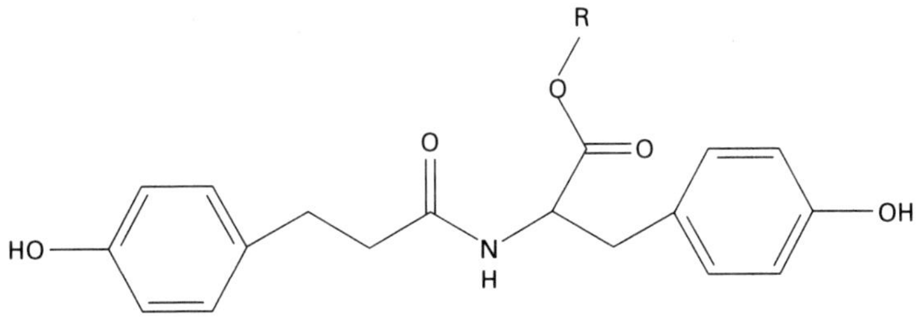

1.21 Tyrosine-derived monomer.

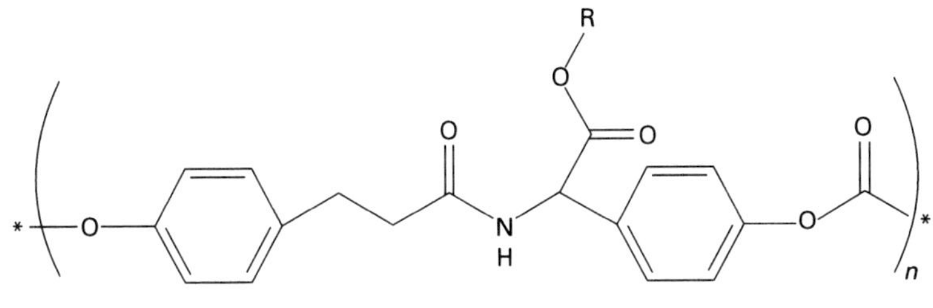

1.22 Tyrosine-derived polycarbonates.

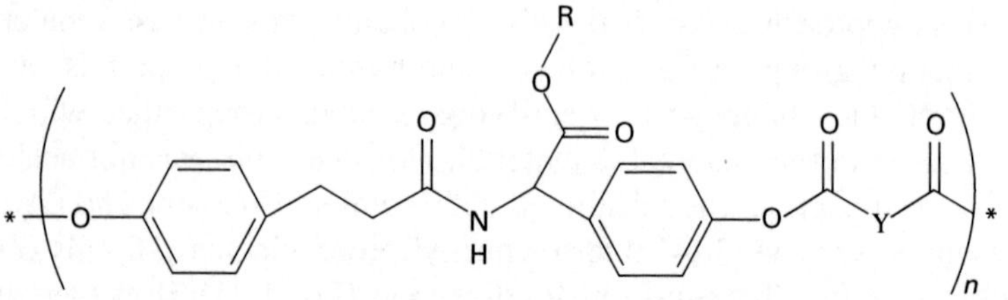

1.23 Tyrosine-derived arylates.

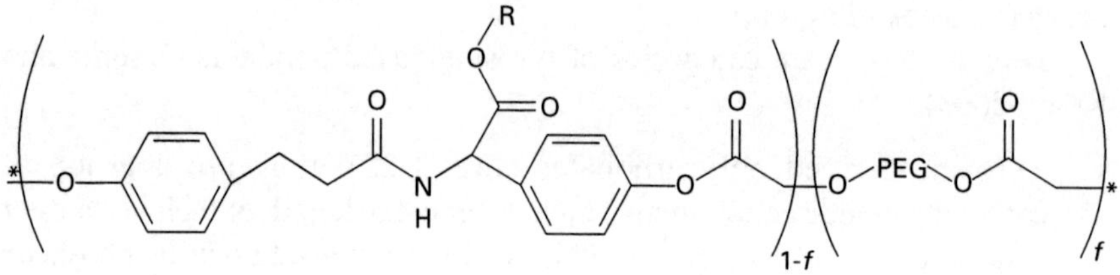

1.24 Tyrosine-containing poly(DTR-PEG carbonates).

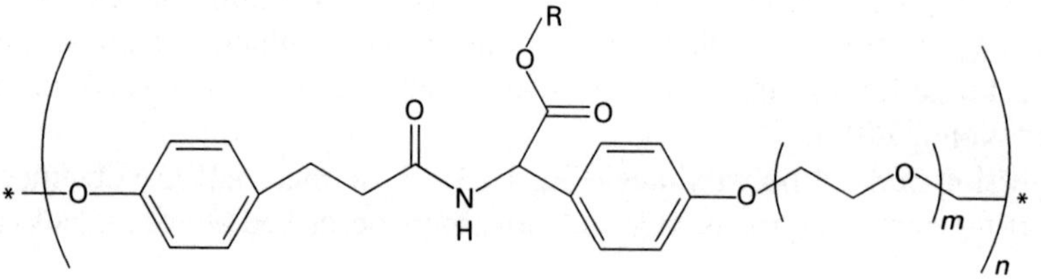

1.25 Tyrosine-containing poly(DTR-PEG ethers).

diacids (such as succinic, adipic, suberic and sebacic acids) in order to modify backbone structure and thus polymer properties.

- Tyrosine-containing poly(DTR-PEG carbonates) (Fig. 1.24): these polymers are obtained with a copolymerization of tyrosine-derived diphenolic monomers with blocks of poly(ethylene glycol) (PEG). There are three main degrees of freedom that allow to modulate material properties: mole fraction of PEG, molecular weight of PEG, and the pendent alkyl group. PEG increases material hydrophilicity and thus water uptake; when the amount of PEG is 15% (mol) the material has a hydrogel-like behavior, whilst with a PEG content of about 70% (mol) the material becomes water soluble. Moreover, as PEG fraction increases, polymer becomes less stiff and more flexible, and degradation is more rapid.
- Tyrosine-containing poly(DTR-PEG ethers) (Fig. 1.25): these polymers are synthesized by copolymerization of tyrosine-derived monomers and methylsulfone-activated PEG.

Tyrosine-derived polycarbonates have been tested for orthopedic implants, because of their high mechanical strength. Polyacrylates, instead, are used where a more flexible material is needed, for example for 'thrombo-resistant' coating for blood-contacting devices.

1.7 Polyalkylcyanoacrylates

Polyalkylcyanoacrylates (PACA) are considered interesting polymers because of the high reactivity of the corresponding monomer, which can polymerize in various media, and also in water. In particular, monomers are cyanoacrylate esters where alkyl chain length varies from methyl to decyl (Fig. 1.26).

Cyanoacrylate monomers, in pure form, are quite unstable; they must be treated with acid stabilizers or radical scavengers in order to avoid spontaneous polymerization. However, polymerization follows both a free radical mechanism or an anionic/zwitterionic mechanism. Free radical mechanism is characterized by a high value of activation energy (125 kJ mol^{-1}) (Domb *et al.*, 1997); the process is slow and strongly dependent on temperature and radical amount. Anionic/zwitterionic polymerization is more interesting because it is more rapid and easier to perform; it also takes place in weak bases. Classical initiators are ionic (I^-, Br^-, OH^-, etc.) and nucleophilic compounds, such as tertiary bases (phosphine, pyridine). The propagation reaction occurs because of the formation of carbanions that react with other monomers; termination is realized with a cation, adding a strong mineral acid. However, in the case of zwitterionic polymerization, termination occurs with the formation of intra- or intermolecular bonds (Fig. 1.27). In the former, polymer cyclization takes place, whereas in the latter, chain length doubling is obtained (Domb and Jain, 2011).

Polymerization of polyalkylcyanoacrylates can be carried out in various ways:

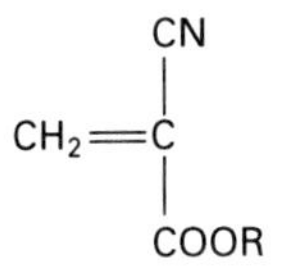

CN
CH_2=C
COOR

1.26 Cyanoacrylate monomer.

CN CN CN CN
COOR COOR COOR COOR n

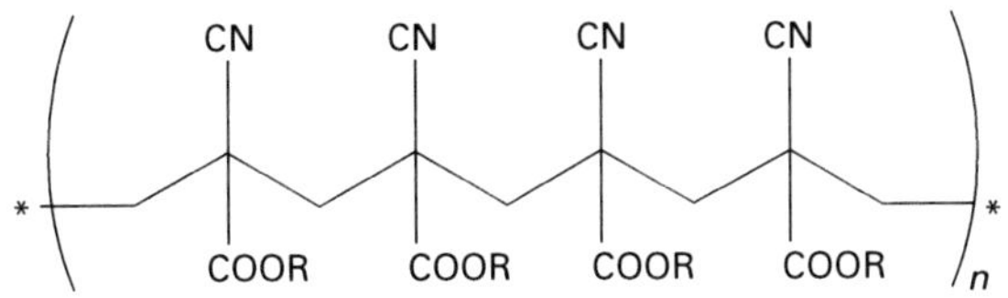

1.27 Polyalkylcyanoacrylate structure.

- bulk polymerization;
- polymerization in organic solvents;
- emulsion polymerization (suitable for nanoparticles); and
- interfacial polymerization (suitable for nanocapsules).

In particular, PACA nanoparticles have been widely investigated (Dossi *et al.*, 2010); they have been used as delivery systems for anticancer drugs, proteins and peptides, and oligonucleotides (Lanza *et al.*, 2007). PACA nanospheres have also been used for ocular therapies, in order to bypass the issue of the short half-life time of eye drops (Vauthier and Couvreur, 2005). Polycyanoacrylates are also employed as tissue adhesives for the closure of skin wounds, and as embolytic material in endovascular surgery. As regards degradation, two mechanisms have been proposed. In the first, the hydrolysis products formaldehyde and alkylcyanoacetic esters are formed, an inverse Knoevenagel reaction; the reaction is subjected to equilibrium which depends on pH, temperature, and alkylcyanoacrylate ester involved. This mechanism is slow and competes with other more rapid processes; moreover, degradation rate depends on the physical form of the polymer. The second kinetic path comprises hydrolysis of the alkyl side chains at basic pH, with alcohol and poly(cyanoacrylic acid) as degradation products (Vauthier and Couvreur, 2005). This mechanism is catalyzed by various esterases, and thus it is believed to be the main degradation process for *in vivo* applications. Even if formaldehyde has been found to be a possible hydrolysis product, PACA shows low toxicity, both in form of nanoparticles or implantation.

1.8 Poly(propylene fumarate) (PPF), poloxamers, poly(*p*-dioxanone) (PPDO), polyvinyl alcohol (PVA)

Poly(propylene fumarate) (PPF) is an unsaturated linear polyester and degrades into fumaric acid and propylene glycol, which are both biocompatible compounds (Fig. 1.28). PPF can be subjected to crosslinking with a vinyl monomer, because of the presence of a double bond of the fumarate. This material has been tested for bone repair surgery (Domb *et al.*, 1997).

Poloxamers are copolymers composed of two polyoxyethylene blocks separated by a polyoxypropylene block (Fig. 1.29). Polyoxyethylene content can vary from 10 to 90% in weight terms. Poloxamers are soluble in water and in polar solvents; they can be solid, liquid, or paste depending on POE/POP ratio and molecular weight. This material has been investigated for drug delivery applications. However, since poloxamers contain ether linkages, they are not readily metabolized and thus are not truly bioresorbable (Domb *et al.*, 1997).

Poly(*p*-dioxanone) (PPDO) is an aliphatic poly(ether ester) (Domb *et al.*,

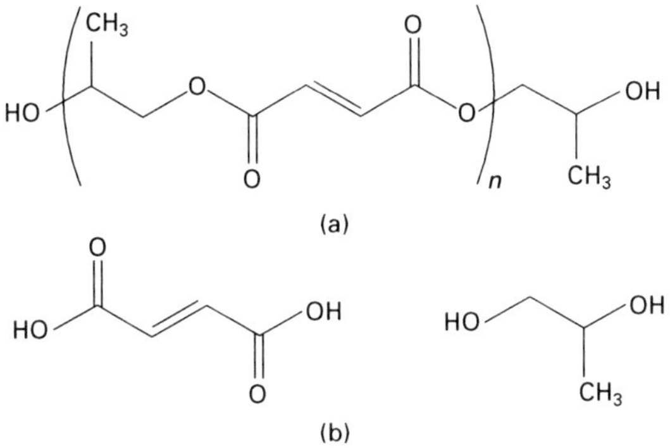

1.28 (a) Structure and (b) degradation products (fumaric acid and propylene glycol) of poly(propylene fumarate).

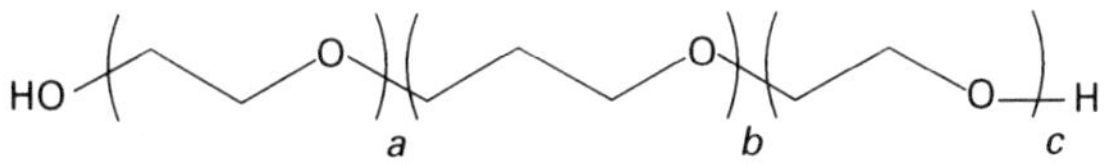

1.29 Poloxamers structure.

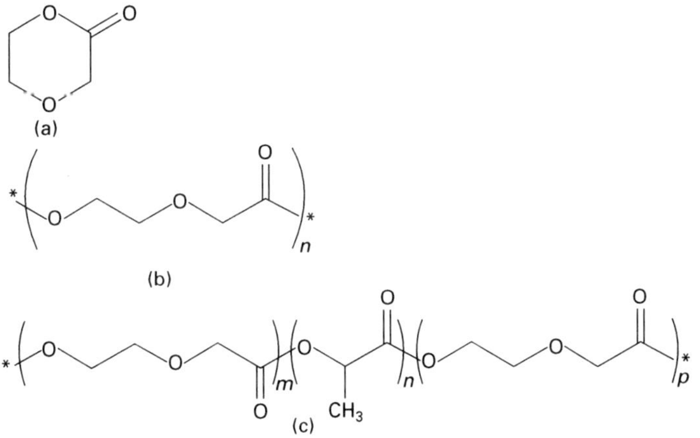

1.30 (a) *p*-Dioxanone, (b) PPDO and (c) poly(*p*-dioxanone-co-L-lactide).

1997); the ether bond provides both hydrophilicity and flexibility (Fig. 1.30). It is prepared with ROP of *p*-dioxanone. The main unit contains one ether bond, one ester bond and no side chains. PPDO degradation results from hydrolysis which follows a mechanism similar to that of aliphatic polyesters, even if in these materials hydrophilicity is more marked because of the presence of ether bonds. PPDO is mainly used for bioresorbable suture threads because of its good tensile strength (Nishida, 2005, Lanza *et al.*, 2007). Moreover, copolymers such as poly(*p*-dioxanone-co-L-lactide) have been synthesized.

Polyvinyl alcohol (PVA) is a polyhydroxy polymer, produced by the

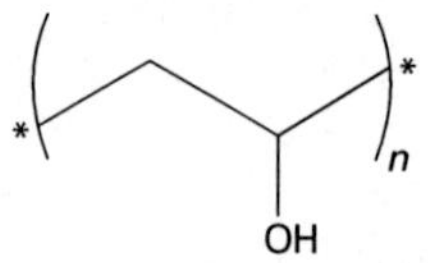

1.31 Polyvinyl alcohol.

hydrolysis of polyvinyl acetate. Vinyl alcohol does not exist in nature, since it becomes acetaldehyde because of keto–enol tautomerism. PVA is composed mainly of 1,3-diol units, with a very small amount of head-to-head 1,2-diol units (Fig. 1.31). This material has a great number of applications in the industrial field, and it is also bioresorbable and non-toxic. These features make PVA suitable for biomedical applications; indeed, it has been tested for the synthesis of PVA-based hydrogels or films for drug delivery (Matsumura, 2005).

1.9 References

Abe, H. & Doi, Y. 2005. Molecular and material design of polyhydroxyalkanoates (PHAs). *Biopolymers Online*, Part 3b. Polyesters.

Albertsson, A. C. & Varma, I. K. 2005. Aliphatic polyesters. *Biopolymers Online*, Part 4. Polyesters.

Allcock, H. R. & Ambrosio, A. M. A. 1996. Synthesis and characterization of pH-sensitive poly(organophosphazene) hydrogels. *Biomaterials*, **17**, 2295–2302.

Allcock, H. R., Fuller, T. J. & Matsumura, K. 1982. Hydrolysis pathways for aminophosphazenes. *Inorganic Chemistry*, **21**, 515–521.

Allcock, H. R. & Kwon, S. 1988. Glyceryl polyphosphazenes: synthesis, properties, and hydrolysis. *Macromolecules*, **21**, 1980–1985.

Allcock, H. R., Pucher, S. R. & Scopelianos, A. G. 1993. Poly[(amino acid ester) phosphazenes] as substrates for the controlled release of small molecules. *Biomaterials*, **15**, 563–569.

Ambrosio, A. M. A., Allcock, H. R., Katti, D. S. & Laurencin, C. T. 2002. Degradable polyphosphazene/poly(alpha-hydroxyester) blends: degradation studies. *Biomaterials*, **23**, 1667–1672.

Batycky, R. P., Hanes, J., Langer, R. & Edwards, D. A. 1997. A theoretical model of erosion and macromolecular drug release from biodegrading microspheres. *Journal of Pharmaceutical Sciences*, **86**, 1464–1477.

Bourke, S. L. & Kohn, J. 2003. Polymers derived from the amino acid L-tyrosine: polycarbonates, polyarylates and copolymers with poly(ethylene glycol). *Advanced Drug Delivery Reviews*, **55**, 447–466.

Cho, S. Y. & Allcock, H. R. 2007. Dendrimers derived from polyphosphazene–poly(propyleneimine) systems: Encapsulation and triggered release of hydrophobic guest molecules. *Macromolecules*, **40**, 3115–3121.

Deng, M., Kumbar, S. G., Wan, Y. Q., Toti, U. S., Allcock, H. R. & Laurencin, C. T. 2010. Polyphosphazene polymers for tissue engineering: an analysis of material synthesis, characterization and applications. *Soft Matter*, **6**, 3119–3132.

Domb, A. J. & Jain, J. P. 2011. *Biodegradable polymers in clinical use and clinical development*, Hoboken, NJ, Wiley.

Domb, A. J., Kost, J. & Wiseman, D. M. 1997. *Handbook of biodegradable polymers*, Amsterdam, Harwood Academic Publishers.

Dossi, M., Storti, G. & Moscatelli, D. 2010. Synthesis of poly(alkyl cyanoacrylates) as biodegradable polymers for drug delivery applications. *Macromolecular Symposia*, **289**, 124–128.

Freiberg, S. & Zhu, X. 2004. Polymer microspheres for controlled drug release. *International Journal of Pharmaceutics*, **282**, 1–18.

Gunatillake, P. A. & Adhikari, R. 2003. Biodegradable synthetic polymers for tissue engineering. *European Cells and Materials*, **5**, 1–16.

Harshe, Y. M., Storti, G., Morbidelli, M., Gelosa, S. & Moscatelli, D. 2007. Polycondensation kinetics of lactic acid. *Macromolecular Reaction Engineering*, **1**, 611–621.

Heller, J. & Barr, J. 2004. Poly(ortho esters) – from concept to reality. *Biomacromolecules*, **5**, 1625–1632.

Heller, J., Barr, J., Ng, S. Y., Abdellauoi, K. S. & Gurny, R. 2002. Poly(ortho esters): synthesis, characterization, properties and uses. *Advanced Drug Delivery Reviews*, **54**, 1015–1039.

Heller, J., Barr, J., Ng, S. Y., Shen, H. R., Schwach-Abdellaoui, K., Emmahl, S., Rothen-Weinhold, A. & Gurny, R. 2000. Poly(ortho esters) – their development and some recent applications. *European Journal of Pharmaceutics and Biopharmaceutics*, **50**, 121–128.

Ishioka, R., Kitakuni, E. & Ichikawa, Y. 2005. Aliphatic polyesters: 'Bionolle'. *Biopolymers Online*, Part 4. Polyesters.

Kim, J. M., Seo, K. S., Jeong, Y. K., Lee, H. B., Kim, Y. S. & Khang, G. 2005. Co-effect of aqueous solubility of drugs and glycolide monomer on *in vitro* release rates from poly(D,L-lactide-co-glycolide) discs and polymer degradation. *Journal of Biomaterials Science-Polymer Edition*, **16**, 991–1007.

Kohn, J. & Langer, R. 1986. Polymerization reactions involving the side chains of alpha-L-amino acids. *Journal of the American Chemical Society*, **109**, 817–820.

Kumar, N., Albertsson, A. C., Edlund, U., Teomim, D., Rasiel, A. & Domb, A. J. 2005. Polyanhydrides. *Biopolymers Online*, Part 4. Polyesters.

Kumar, N., Langer, R. S. & Domb, A. J. 2002. Polyanhydrides: an overview. *Advanced Drug Delivery Reviews*, **54**, 889–910.

Lakshmi, S., Katti, D. S. & Laurencin, C. T. 2003. Biodegradable polyphosphazenes for drug delivery applications. *Advanced Drug Delivery Reviews*, **55**, 467–482.

Lanza, R. P., Langer, R. S. & Vacanti, J. 2007. *Principles of tissue engineering*, Amsterdam; Boston, Elsevier/Academic Press.

Lee, S. Y. & Park, S. J. 2005. Biosynthesis and fermentative production of SCL and MCL polyhydroxyalkanoates (SCL-MCL-PHAs). *Biopolymers Online*, Part 3a. Polyesters.

Liggins, R. T. & Burt, H. M. 2001. Paclitaxel loaded poly(L-lactic acid) microspheres: properties of microspheres made with low molecular weight polymers. *International Journal of Pharmaceutics*, **222**, 19–33.

Loo, S. C. J., Tan, Z. Y. S., Chow, Y. J. C. & Lin, S. L. I. 2009. Drug release from irradiated PLGA and PLLA multi-layered films. *Journal of Pharmaceutical Sciences*, **99**, 3060–3071.

Marchessault, R. H. & Yu, G. 2005. Crystallization and material properties of polyhydroxyalkanoates (PHAs). *Biopolymers Online*, Part 3b. Polyesters.

Mark, J. E., Allcock, H. R. & West, R. 1992. *Inorganic polymers*, Englewood Cliffs, N.J., Prentice Hall.

Matsumura, S. 2005. Biodegradation of poly(vinyl alcohol) and its copolymers. *Biopolymers Online*, Part 9. Miscellaneous Biopolymers and Biodegradation of Polymers.

Mochizuki, M. 2005. Properties and application of aliphatic polyester products. *Biopolymers Online*, Part 4. Polyesters.

Nishida, H. 2005. Biodegradation of polydioxanone. *Biopolymers Online*, Part 9. Miscellaneous biopolymers and biodegradation of polymers.

Nishimura, Y., Takasu, A., Inai, Y. & Hirabayashi, T. 2005. Melt spinning of poly(L-lactic acid) and its biodegradability. *Journal of Applied Polymer Science*, **97**, 2118–2124.

Osswald, T. A. & Hernández-Ortiz, J. P. 2006. *Polymer processing: modeling and simulation*, Munich; Cincinnati, Hanser Publishers.

Ottenbright, R. M. & Scott, G. 1992. *Biodegradable polymers and plastic*, London, Royal Society for Chemistry.

Park, T. G. 1995. Degradation of poly(lactic-co-glycolic acid) microspheres – effect of copolymer composition. *Biomaterials*, **16**, 1123–1130.

Passi, P., Zadro, A., Marsilio, F., Lora, S., Caliceti, P. & Veronese, F. M. 2000. Plain and drug loaded polyphosphazene membranes and microspheres in the treatment of rabbit bone defects. *Journal of Materials Science-Materials in Medicine*, **11**, 643–654.

Peppas, N. A. 1986. *Hydrogels in medicine and pharmacy*, Boca Raton, Fla., CRC Press.

Perale, G., Casalini, T., Barri, V., Muller, M., Maccagnan, S. & Masi, M. 2010. Lidocaine release from polycaprolactone threads. *Journal of Applied Polymer Science*, **117**, 3610–3614.

Ratner, B. D. 2004. *Biomaterials science: an introduction to materials in medicine*, Amsterdam; Boston, Elsevier Academic Press.

Rehm, B. H. A. & Steinbuchel, A. 2005. Polyhydroxyalkanoate (PHA) syntheses: the key enzymes of PHA synthesis. *Biopolymers Online*, Part 3a. Polyesters.

Satkowski, M. M., Melik, D. H., Autran, J.-P., Green, P. R., Noda, I. & Schechtman, L. A. 2005. Physical and processing properties of polyhydroxyalkanoate (PHA) copolymers. *Biopolymers Online*, Part 3b. Polyesters.

Sen Gupta, A. & Lopina, S. T. 2002. L-Tyrosine-based backbone-modified poly(amino acids). *Journal of Biomaterials Science-Polymer Edition*, **13**, 1093–1104.

Siepmann, J., Streubel, A. & Peppas, N. A. 2002. Understanding and predicting drug delivery from hydrophilic matrix tablets using the 'sequential layer' model. *Pharmaceutical Research*, **19**, 306–314.

Tsuji, H. 2005. Polylactides. *Biopolymers Online*, Part 4. Polyesters.

Vauthier, C. & Couvreur, P. 2005. Biodegradation of poly(alkylcyanoacrylates). *Biopolymers Online*, Part 9. Miscellaneous biopolymers and biodegradation of polymers.

Wang, L., Yasuyuki, I., Hajime, O. & Tsuge, S. 1999. Characterization of natural resin shellac by reactive pyrolysis – gas chromatography in the presence of organic alkali. *Analytical Chemistry*, **71**, 1316–1322.

Wang, Q., Du, Y. M. & Fan, L. H. 2005. Properties of chitosan/poly(vinyl alcohol) films for drug controlled release. *Journal of Applied Polymer Science*, **96**, 808–813.

Williams, S. F. & Martin, D. P. 2005. Applications of polyhydroxyalkanoates (PHA) in medicine and pharmacy. *Biopolymers Online*, Part 4. Polyesters.

Yu, Y. C., Storti, G. & Morbidelli, M. 2009. Ring-opening polymerization of L,L-lactide: kinetic and modeling study. *Macromolecules*, **42**, 8187–8197.

Zhu, K. & Qiu, L. 2005. Biodegradation of polyphosphazenes. *Biopolymers Online*, Part 9. Miscellaneous Biopolymers and Biodegradation of Polymers.

Zurita, R., Puiggali, J. & Rodriguez-Galan, A. 2006a. Loading and release of ibuprofen in multi- and monofilament surgical sutures. *Macromolecular Bioscience*, **6**, 767–775.

Zurita, R., Puiggali, J. & Rodriguez-Galan, A. 2006b. Triclosan release from coated polyglycolide threads. *Macromolecular Bioscience*, **6**, 58–69.

2

The effect of molecular structure on the properties of biomedical polymers

G. PERTICI, Industrie Biomediche Insubri SA, Switzerland

Abstract: A review is presented on the effects of the molecular structure of polymers on their properties. The influence of such variables as molecular weight, macromolecular conformation and crystallisation, amorphous states and the glass transition temperature are discussed. Biphasic systems are explored and the properties of thermoplastic and thermosetting polymers are investigated.

Key words: amorphous state, crystallinity, average molecular weight, polydispersity, glass-transition temperature.

2.1 Introduction: the molecular structure of polymers

Natural and synthetic polymers are comprised of macromolecules. These are formed from many concatenated structural units and limited terminal moieties (Fig. 2.1) (Cowie, 1991). The structural units are usually carbon atoms linked to hydrogen, oxygen or nitrogen, but often it is possible to find other chemical elements such as: Si, Cl, B, P, F and S. This involves considerable modification of properties (Figs 2.2–2.4) [Mark and SpringerLink (Online Service), 2007].

ABBBBBBBBBBBBBBBBBBBBBBBBBBBA

2.1 Polymer representation (A = terminal moiety, B = structural unit).

$\cdots\!-\!CH_2\!-\!CH_2\!-\!CH_2\!-\!CH_2\!-\!CH_2\!-\!CH_2\!-\!\cdots$

2.2 Polyethylene (PE).

$\cdots\!-\!CH_2\!-\!CH_2\!-\!O\!-\!CH_2\!-\!CH_2\!-\!\cdots$

2.3 Polyethylene glycol (PEG) or polyethylene oxide (PEO) or polyoxyethylene (POE).

$\cdots\!-\!CH_2\!-\!CH(Cl)\!-\!\cdots$

2.4 Polyvinyl chloride (PVC).

Polymer preparation is based on chemical reactions (polymerisation) of gas (e.g. ethylene) or liquid (e.g. styrene) substances with low molecular weight. These molecules (monomers) are bi- or poly-functional because they show two or more reactive moieties [Nicholson and Royal Society of Chemistry (Great Britain), 2006]. As an example, the reaction between ethylene glycol and terephthalic acid promotes the formation of polyethylene terephthalate (PET, a polyester), (Fig. 2.5) (Liangbin *et al.*, 2001).

Bifunctional monomers produce linear macromolecules, whereas polyfunctional monomers create a ramified (crosslinked) structure. Linear polymers are represented only by the repeating structural units, because the terminal moieties are not relevant. As an example, polyethylene is represented as shown in Fig. 2.6. In this formula 'n' represents the degree of polymerisation. It is calculated by the ratio between the molecular weight of polymer and molecular weight of the monomer.

Representing crosslinked polymers is more complicated. There is the same difficulty in nomenclature for crosslinked polymers. As a result, standard denominations were introduced for this class of polymers. After the prefix 'poly', there is the name of the functional group that bonds the repetition units (polyaldehyde, polyamide, polycarbonate, polyester, polysulfide, polyphosphonitrile, etc.) (Rudin, 1999).

2.1.1 Isomers

After identifying the main structure of a polymer, it is useful to consider the structure in more detail. As an example, if two polymers are formed by the same monomer but use two different polymerisation procedures, they are still given the same name. In this case the concept of isomer could help to provide a more precise identification. There are three basic classes of isomerism (Kricheldorf *et al.*, 2005):

- position,
- structural, and
- steric.

As an example, a vinyl monomer (CH_2=CHR) usually proceeds with a 'head

$$n\,\underset{\text{OH}}{\underset{|}{CH_2}}-\underset{\text{OH}}{\underset{|}{CH_2}} + n\,HOOC-C_6H_4-COOH \xrightarrow[-H_2O]{} \left(-O-\overset{O}{\overset{\|}{C}}-C_6H_4-\overset{O}{\overset{\|}{C}}-O-CH_2-CH_2-\right)_n$$

2.5 PET formation.

$$(-CH_2-CH_2-)_n$$

2.6 Polyethylene (PE).

to tail' polymerisation. Sometimes it is possible to find 'head to head' and 'tail to tail' (Figs 2.7 and 2.8). These structures are isomers for the position of *R*-groups (side chains). In the next example a structural isomerism is shown (Figs 2.9 and 2.10). These examples include steric isomerism; in polybutadiene 1–4 the *cis–trans* configuration is applicable (Okada and Furuya, 2002).

2.1.2 Copolymers

This class of polymers (heteropolymers) is obtained by the simultaneously polymerisation of two or more monomers to achieve useful properties. Well known commercial copolymers for biomedical applications are produced by Boehringer Ingelheim GmbH, Germany (i.e. Resomer LC 703 S) and Purac, Netherlands (i.e. Purasorb PDLG). A possible configuration for a random polymerisation of two monomers (unit A and unit B) is shown in Fig. 2.11. The fundamental parameters for the characterisation become composition and disposition. Composition is not too difficult to determine because it relates to the percentage of a unit inside the structure.

Block copolymers are an interesting class where the disposition is as shown in Fig. 2.12. By synthesis it is also possible to obtain graft copolymers;

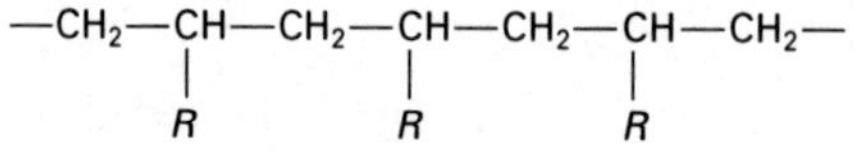

$$-CH_2-\underset{R}{\underset{|}{CH}}-CH_2-\underset{R}{\underset{|}{CH}}-CH_2-\underset{R}{\underset{|}{CH}}-CH_2-$$

2.7 Head to tail.

$$-CH_2-\underset{R}{\underset{|}{CH}}-\underset{R}{\underset{|}{CH}}-CH_2-CH_2-\underset{R}{\underset{|}{CH}}-CH_2-$$

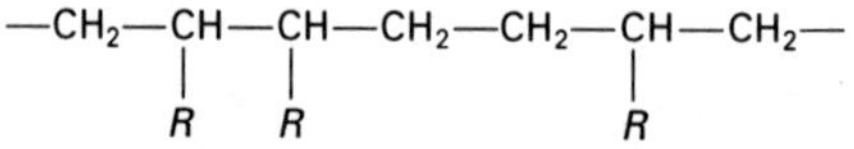

2.8 Head to head, tail to tail.

$$-CH_2-CH=CH-CH_2-CH=CH-CH_2-$$

2.9 1, 4-Polybutadiene.

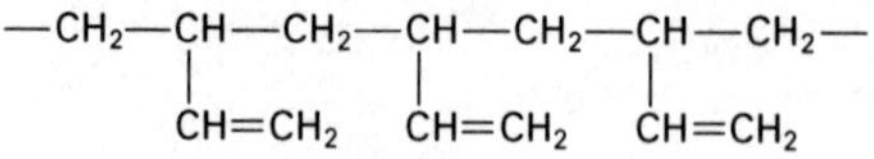

$$-CH_2-\underset{CH=CH_2}{\underset{|}{CH}}-CH_2-\underset{CH=CH_2}{\underset{|}{CH}}-CH_2-\underset{CH=CH_2}{\underset{|}{CH}}-CH_2-$$

2.10 1, 2-Polybutadiene.

-ABABBBAABAAABABAAB-

2.11 Random copolymer.

-AAAAABBBBBAAAAAABBBBBBAAAAAAAA-

2.12 Block copolymers.

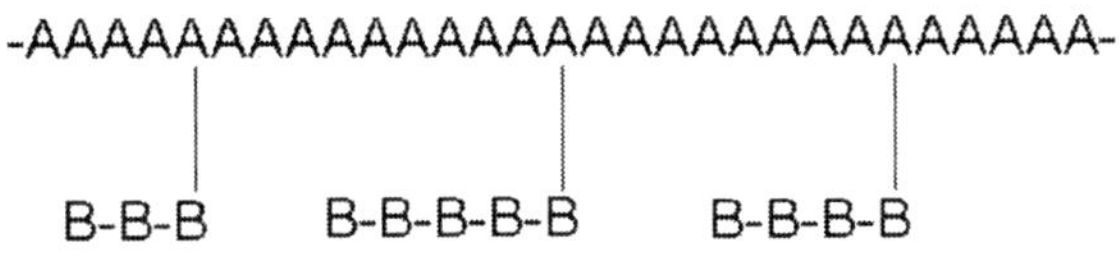

2.13 Graft copolymers.

this is a special kind of branched copolymer in which the side chains are structurally distinct from the main chain (Fig. 2.13) (Hadjichristidis *et al.*, 2003).

2.2 Molecular weight and polymer properties

In general, polymers are defined as 'polydisperse' because they show a non-uniform molecular size. This parameter is important in determining many physical properties such as transition temperature, strength, viscosity, toughness and stiffness. For this reason it is necessary to identify an average value of molecular weight (Misra, 1993). In polymer science the most practical way to identify polymer molecular weights is the average molecular weight ($\bar{M}_n$) and the weight average molecular weight ($\bar{M}_w$). Let n_i be the number of molecules with molecular weight M_i, then the number average molecular weight is:

$$\bar{M}_n = \frac{\Sigma n_i M_i}{\Sigma n_i} \quad [2.1]$$

If the polymer property is dependent on the weight of each polymer molecule, the weight average molecular weight is:

$$\bar{M}_w = \frac{\sum_{i=1}^{\infty} n_i M_i^2}{\sum_{i=1}^{\infty} n_i M_i} = \sum_{i=1}^{\infty} w_i M_i \quad [2.2]$$

where w_i represents the weight fraction of polymer with molecular weight *i*.

These parameters are very important for the mechanical properties of the polymer. A high value of average molecular weight corresponds to high mechanical resistance (Gowariker *et al.*, 1986). The polydispersity index (PDI) is a measure of the distribution of molecular mass in a given sample:

$$\text{PDI} = M_w/M_n \quad [2.3]$$

For a theoretical monodisperse polymer, PDI = 1, whereas PDI > 1 for polydisperse polymers (Chanda and Roy, 2007).

2.2.1 Average molecular weight and the properties of polymers

All mechanical characteristics of polymers are strictly correlated with average molecular weight. The degree of polymerisation has a dramatic effect on the mechanical properties of a polymer. As chain length increases, mechanical properties such as ductility, tensile strength, and hardness rise sharply and eventually level off. This is schematically illustrated by the dashed line in Fig. 2.14 (Gowariker *et al.*, 1986). As a result, in the production of medical polymers it is usually desirable to have a high molecular weight.

However, in polymer melts, for example, the flow viscosity at a given temperature rises rapidly with the increasing degree of polymerisation, as shown by the continuous line in Fig. 2.14. As a result, using high molecular weight polymers can cause problems of viscosity during common polymer processes (extrusion, spinning, moulding) owing to a low melt flow index (MFI). MFI is a measure of the ease of the melt flow of a thermoplastic polymer. It is defined as the mass of a polymer (g), flowing in 10 min through a capillary of specific dimensions by a pressure applied via prescribed gravimetric weights at prescribed temperatures (the method described in ASTM D1238 and ISO 1133). MFI is an indirect measure of molecular weight and at the same time, it is a measure of the ability of the material to flow under pressure at specific temperature (Scheirs, 2000).

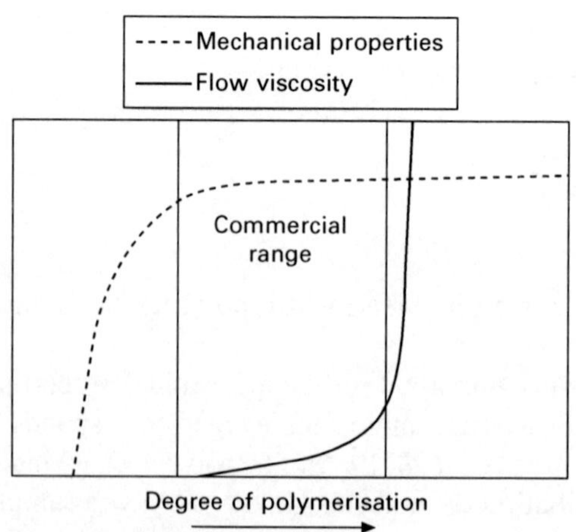

2.14 Degree of polymerisation.

2.3 Macromolecular conformation, crystallisation and polymer properties

The conformation of a polymer is defined as a *statistical chain* owing to the possibility of rotation around the simple carbon–carbon bond (–C–C–). The enormous number of possible conformations is reduced by steric impediments. However, the structure of a polymer is similar to a filament hank known as *random coil* (Figs 2.15 and 2.16) (Gedde, 1995). In the melted and solid amorphous (or glass-like) state, the macromolecular conformation of

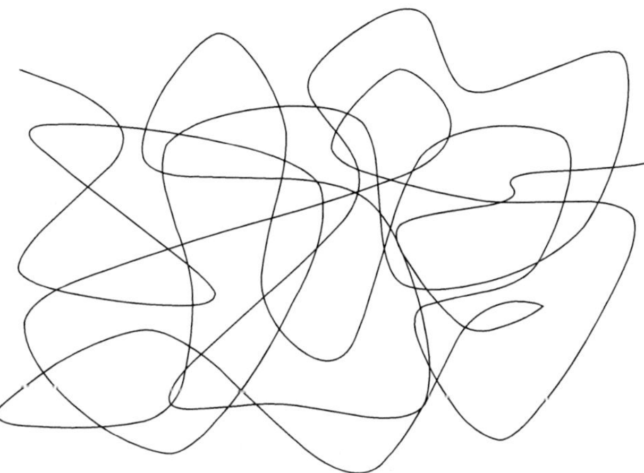

2.15 Random coil conformation for linear amorphous polymers (single molecule).

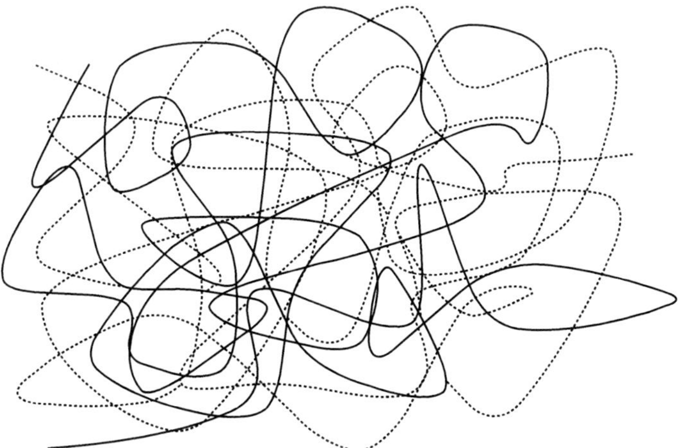

2.16 Random coil conformation for linear amorphous polymers (double molecules).

polymers is totally irregular; an amorphous crosslinked polymer is shown in Fig. 2.17. In the solid crystalline state, the polymer chains find stretched and regular positions that allow organisation in a crystal lattice (Fig. 2.18) (Perez, 1998). A stack of polymer chains folded back on themselves (as shown in Fig. 2.18) are called *lamellae* (Bassett, 1981).

Polymers that show a high regular structure at room temperature (T_{amb}) are usually solid crystalline materials with good mechanical properties until the melting point. Conversely, an amorphous status characterises polymers with insufficient regularity. These polymers display adequate mechanical properties if they are in glass-like state. They are used when the glass transition temperature (T_g) is above T_{amb}. In particular, T_g is the temperature at which the amorphous phase of the polymer is converted between the rubbery and glassy states (section 2.4).

The mechanical properties of amorphous polymers are determined by two fundamental parameters:

- the intrinsic rigidity of the polymeric chain, and
- the intensity of intermolecular forces.

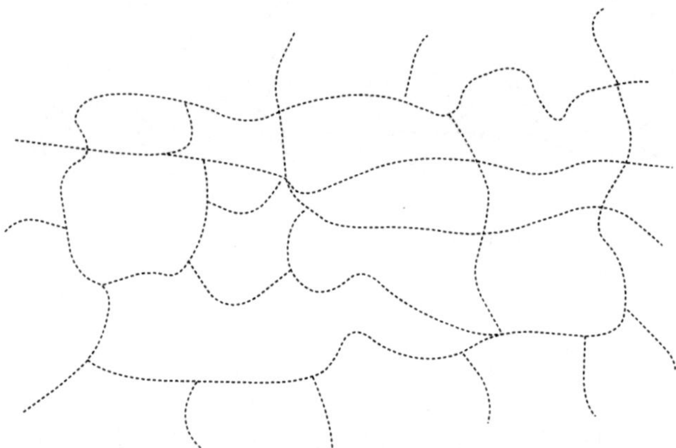

2.17 Crosslinked polymer (amorphous).

2.18 Crystalline polymer.

Analysis by X-ray scattering shows that there are no complete ordered structures for crystalline polymers; fusion usually occurs inside an interval of temperature (Ward and Sweeney, 2004).

The mechanism of polymer crystallisation comprises two simultaneous processes:

- macromolecules stiffening in axial conformation, and
- macromolecular aggregation through parallel axes ('bundles' linked by intermolecular forces).

The primary morphological element is therefore the lamella, which can propagate in two directions. In conditions of high viscosity, one direction is preferred to the other and a *fibril* is formed. The fibrils grow like the spokes of a bicycle wheel from a central nucleus, forming a spherulite (Figs 2.19 and 2.20). The development of spherulites is arrested by the contact with other growing spherulites (Kausch and SpringerLink (Online Service), 2005). The number of nuclei that are formed is in direct proportion to the difference between crystallisation temperature (T_C) and melting point. This is very important because changing the T_C makes it possible to obtain different mechanical properties.

Crystallisation kinetics are described by the Avrami equation:

$$\frac{V - V_\infty}{V_0 - V_\infty} = e^{-\mathrm{K}t^n} \qquad [2.4]$$

where V is the specific volume at the starting point (V_0), at a specific moment (V) and at the end of crystallisation (V_∞). The constants (K and n) are dependent on the kind of nucleation, and t represents the time (Sperling, 2006). The traditional model adopted to describe crystalline polymers is the '*fringed micelle model*' of Hermann *et al.* (1930). This is shown in Fig. 2.21. The model gives this definition of degree of crystallinity:

$$w_c = \frac{\varphi_c \rho_c}{\rho} \qquad [2.5]$$

where w_c represents the mass fraction, φ_c is the volume fraction, while ρ and ρ_c are the densities of entire sample and crystalline fraction, respectively.

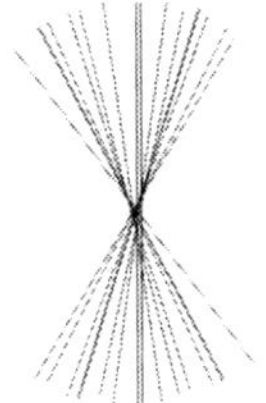
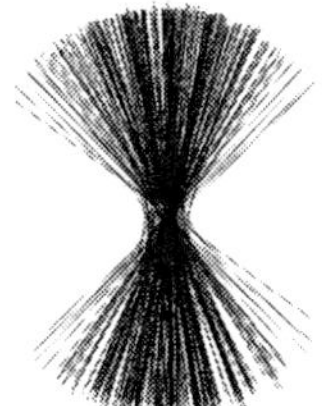
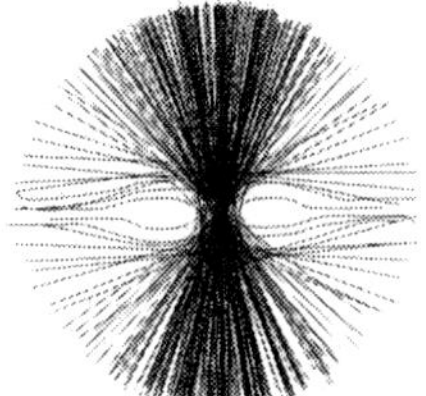

2.19 Spherulite formation.

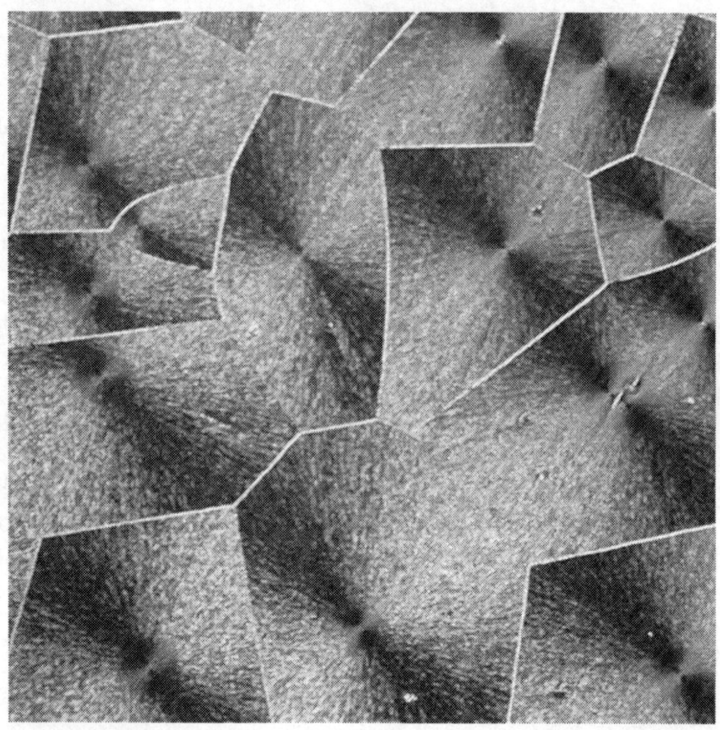

2.20 Spherulites in a PEO film viewed by optical microscope between crossed polarisers.

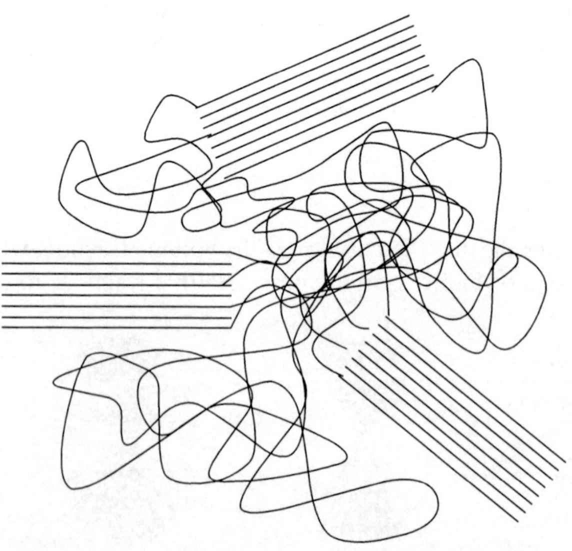

2.21 Two-phase model (fringed micelle).

This model is a very useful way to describe the physical and mechanical behaviour of polymers with low crystallinity. It is important to note that the model disregards some important parameters:

- the ordered zones sometimes show reticular defects;
- the presence of low ordered structures close to interfaces;
- the fact that the density and the structure of unordered zones are influenced by the presence of ordered areas.

The degree of crystallinity can be determined by several experimental procedures: X-ray diffraction, calorimetry, infrared (IR) spectroscopy and density measurements. Some disagreement among the results of quantitative measurements of crystallinity by different methods is frequently encountered because imperfections in crystals are not easily distinguished from the amorphous phase. Moreover, these techniques may be affected to different extents by imperfections and interfacial effects (Bower, 2002).

As the temperature of a crystalline polymer increases, the phase transition is achieved when the crystallinity is dissolved. This process is known as 'fusion' and is investigated by X-ray diffraction, specific volume, double refraction or calorimetry measurements. Using this last test, it is quite easy to identify the melting point, because this process is accompanied by an increase in enthalpy (heat absorption at constant pressure) (Fig. 2.22).

In general, the presence of impurities and defects brings a decrease in the degree of crystallinity and an increase of melt temperature range. Sometimes the degradation temperature is very close to the melting point. For this reason it can be useful to decrease the melting point by introducing some impurities through copolymerisation. This technique can improve some material properties such as resilience, flexibility and elongation at break (Riga and Judovits,

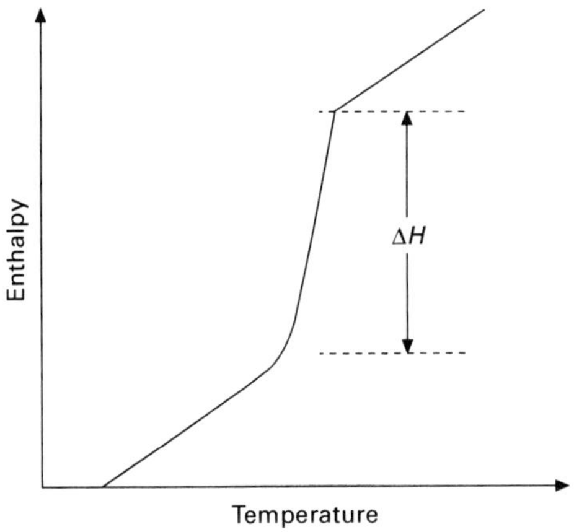

2.22 Enthalpy versus temperature graph for a crystalline polymer.

2001). A crystalline polymer in an amorphous state is usually stiffer, but also more resistant to gas permeability and solvent. These characteristics are not adequate for practical applications because a high crystalline state produces fragile materials with low flexibility and fatigue resistance.

Polymer properties can be improved by thermal and mechanical treatments. For example a fast cooling from the melt state produces polymers with low crystallinity and density. Polymers with high crystallinity can be cold-stretched in order to obtain fibres with high tensile strength (e.g. surgical sutures based on nylon 6,6). Performing X-ray analysis after the treatment of these fibres, it can be observed that the degree of crystallinity is maintained but the amorphous and crystalline regions are oriented in the axial direction (Fig. 2.23) (Ward, 1997).

2.4 The effect of the amorphous state and glass transition temperature on polymer properties

In the amorphous state the macromolecular conformation of polymers is totally irregular, whereas in the crystalline state, the polymer chains find stretched and regular positions that allow organisation into a crystal lattice. Polymers with high regular structure at room temperature usually are solid crystalline materials with good mechanical properties up to the melting point. Conversely, the amorphous state of polymers, with low regularity, displays materials with appropriate mechanical properties if they are in glass-like state i.e. when the glass transition temperature (T_g) is above T_{amb}. T_g is the temperature where the amorphous phase is converted between the rubbery and glassy states.

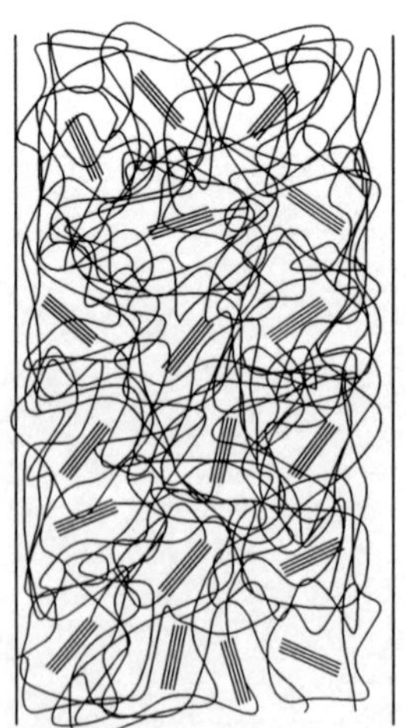
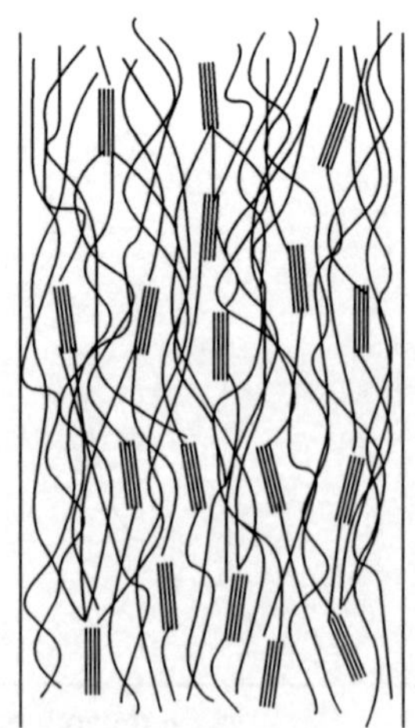

2.23 Crystalline polymer non-oriented and oriented.

In this class of amorphous polymers, there are many biomedical polymers such as phenolic resins (adopted for production of surgical instruments), unsaturated polyester resins (used in bone repair) (Kharas *et al.*, 1997), polystyrene (e.g. Petri dishes for cell culture) and polymethyl methacrylate (PMMA, used in bone cements, intraocular lens, and dental fillings) (Stuart, 2002). These are highly crosslinked polymers (resins in particular) or linear thermoplastic polymers that do not show structural macromolecular regularity.

Crosslinked amorphous polymers at T_{amb} are very stiff and devoid of plasticity. They have a high Young's modulus, high tensile strength, and low elongation at break. Linear amorphous polymers show properties with large variability depending on the temperature, caused by variations in molecular structure and chemical composition. At high temperatures decomposition phenomenon starts in crosslinked polymers. Under the same conditions, thermoplastics become viscous liquids (ASM International, 2003).

Decreasing the temperature in linear amorphous polymers increases viscosity owing to the reduction of macromolecular mobility. Cooling this type of polymer creates a supercooled liquid with properties similar to the glassy state. Below the glass transition temperature, a molecule is confined with very limited group or branch movement, and its free volume is relatively small. For whole molecules, there is no possibility of moving away from each other. For this reason T_g is a direct measurement of molecular mobility. It is well known that T_g is not a material constant, but depends on many parameters such as heating rate, cooling rate and physical ageing (Fig. 2.24). The values of T_g may vary in the range of 10 to 20% depending on differences in cooling and heating rates (Seyler, 1994). A typical (though now obsolete) test for T_g evaluation is to measure the specific volume of a polymeric sample by changing the temperature. As it is shown in Fig. 2.24, for the amorphous state there is a sudden variation in grade line around the –70 °C, representing the T_g point for this sample (Dissado and Fothergill, 1992). In the other case shown in Fig. 2.24, there is first a decrease of specific volume owing to crystallisation inside the sample; then there is a secondary transition caused by the non-crystallisable regions that move to the glassy state.

Considering the linear coefficient of thermal expansion, there is a discontinuity around the T_g value:

$$\alpha = \left(\frac{1}{V}\right)\left(\frac{\partial V}{\partial T}\right)_{P} \qquad [2.6]$$

The glass transition is a typical kinetic phenomenon and its position depends on cooling rate. A lower T_g is achieved by an increase in cooling speed (Askadskii, 2003). There is no enthalpy leap in this transition, but a heat capacity C_P leap (Hatakeyama and Hatakeyama, 1995):

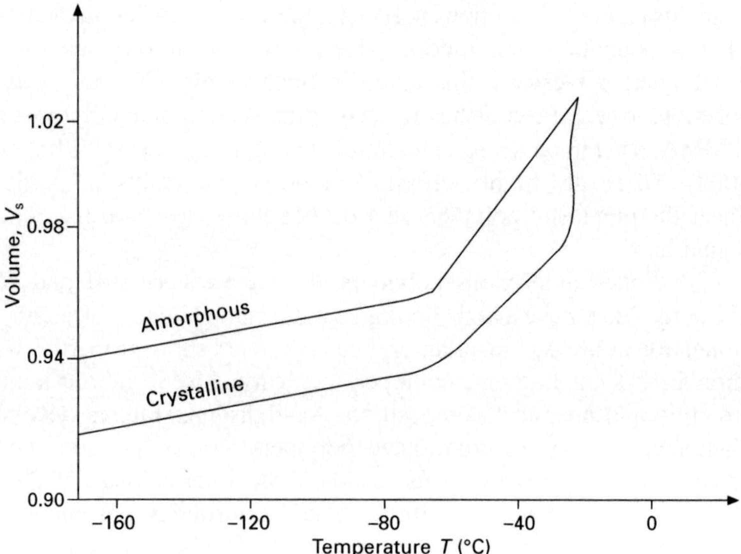

2.24 Dilatometric diagram of a hypothetic polymer, obtainable in crystalline and amorphous state.

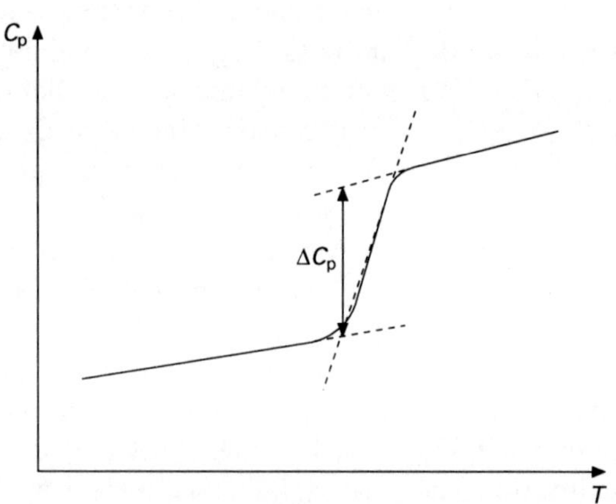

2.25 Schematic differential scanning calorimetry (DSC) graph showing ΔC_p for amorphous polymers.

$$C_P = \left(\frac{\partial H}{\partial T}\right)_P \qquad [2.7]$$

Polymers containing polar groups (–Cl, –F, –CN, $-OCH_3$, $-COOCH_3$), either in the main structure or in lateral chains, show higher transition points than similar non-polar structures (Fig. 2.25).

This is because the polarity allows the augmentation of intermolecular forces by electrostatic effects or hydrogen bonds. Thus, comparing the transition points of poly(vinyl chloride) and polypropylene (low polarity), a difference of 85 °C is found.

Plasticised PVC is the most widely utilised material for the production of blood and blood-component contacting devices, including blood storage bags, catheters and tubing for extracorporeal circuits (Fig. 2.26) (Manfredini *et al.*, 2003), whereas polypropylene has a wide use in medical disposables and as surgical implantable meshes (Alariqi *et al.*, 2009). Poly(vinyl chloride) and polypropylene have the same main chemical structure and also a similar steric burden given by the methyl group (–CH_3) and chlorine atom (–Cl), but, in this case, the polarity plays an important role (Fig. 2.27). The presence of large molecular groups limiting chain movements can promote a transition point rise. An example is the presence of aromatic rings.

The glass transition temperature is therefore a fundamental material parameter for manufacturing and future applications. Polymers such as PVC are usually processed by compression/injection moulding or extrusion and an adequate manufacturing temperature is required (normally 50–100 °C over the T_g point). The application temperature must be significantly higher than T_g (typically 50–60 °C) in order to avoid mechanical problems such as creep.

Table 2.1 records glass transition temperatures for some common biomedical polymers. It allows comparisons between polymers such as polypropylene, poly(vinyl chloride) and polystyrene.

Linear amorphous polymers in the solid state usually show a behaviour very close to inorganic glasses: very stiff, devoid of plasticity, with high Young's modulus, high tensile strength and low elongation at break. There are a number of exceptions. Some linear amorphous polymers in a glass-like state display certain flexibility and a moderate plasticity. The reason is the presence inside the macromolecule of very flexible chain segments (methylene sequence) or short lateral chains. This allows some local molecular movement below T_g. In these cases, as temperature decreases, there is a secondary transition temperature which results in freezing the macromolecule structure (Stuart, 2002; Dattelbaum and Rae, 2004).

Besides the Young's modulus, *mechanical damping* is a good criterion

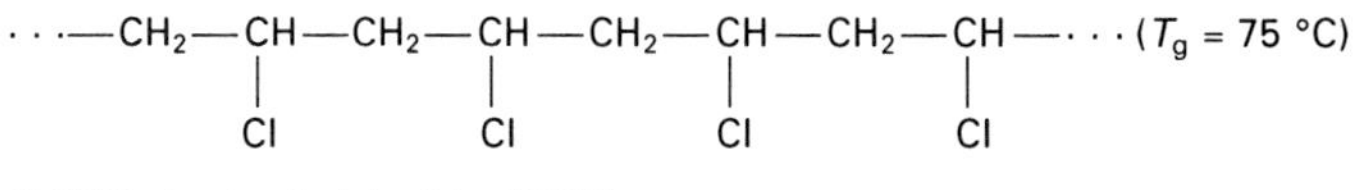

2.26 Polyvinyl chloride (PVC).

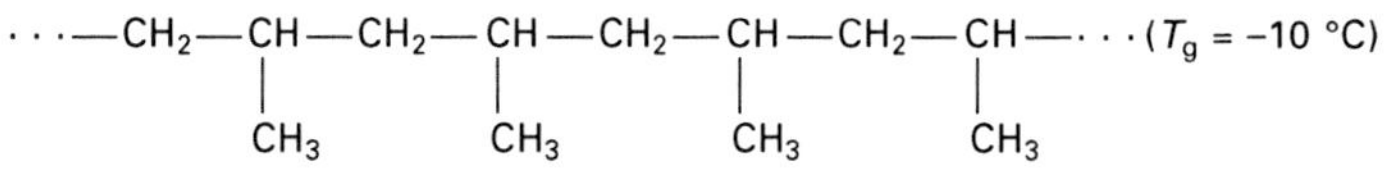

2.27 Polypropylene (PP).

Table 2.1 Glass transition temperature for some common biomedical polymers

Polymer	Formula of repeating unit	T_g(°C)
Polytetrafluoroethylene (PTFE) (crystalline)	$-CF_2-CF_2-$	−100
Polyethylene (PE) (crystalline)	$-(CH_2-CH_2)-$	−80
Polycaprolactone (PCL) (crystalline)	$-(C(=O)-(CH_2)_5-O)-$	−61
Polypropylene (PP) (crystalline)	$-(CH_2-CH(CH_2))-$	−10
Polyvinyl acetate (PVA) (amorphous)	$-(CH_2-CH(O-C(=O)-CH_3))-$	30
Nylon 6,6 (crystalline)	$-(C(=O)-(CH_2)_4-C(=O)-NH-(CH_2)_6-NH)-$	45
Polylactide (PLA) (amorphous)	$-(C(=O)-CH(CH_3)-O)-$	58
Poly(vinyl chloride) (PVC) (amorphous)	$-(CH_2-CH(Cl))-$	75
Polystyrene (PS) (amorphous)	$-(CH_2-CH(C_6H_5))-$	100
Polymethyl methacrylate (PMMA) (amorphous)	$-(CH_2-C(CH_3)(COOCH_3))-$	120

for evaluating transitions in polymer properties. Damping is defined as the rate of damping in a free vibration, or as the tangent of the loss angle in vibration experiments. The damping ($\tan \delta$) displays a maximum at T_g, and less pronounced maxima at the secondary glass transitions T_{sec} (Fig. 2.28). A

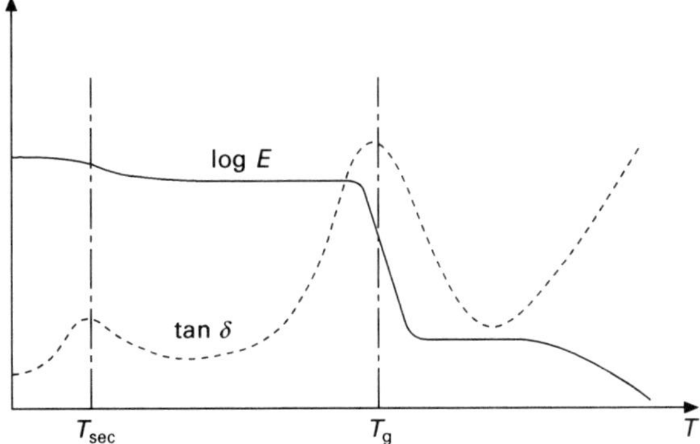

2.28 Secondary glass transition temperature for an amorphous polymer.

secondary glass transition is important for the *impact strength* of a polymer. It makes it possible to dissipate energy in situations of shock loading, making the polymer less fragile. This can be seen for polystyrene and polymethyl methacrylate (PMMA), which show many similar properties. However, comparing mechanical characteristics, in particular ductility and shock resistance, PMMA displays better properties. The reason is the presence in PMMA of flexible lateral groups. This is underlined by high values of dielectric constant in the glassy state (van der Vegt, 2006).

2.5 Biphasic systems: linear crystalline polymers and their properties

Linear crystalline polymers always contain a fraction of amorphous material. For this reason they are usually considered biphasic systems. They show the typical transitions of amorphous polymers (glass and secondary) but also the common transitions of crystalline polymers (polymorphic, order–disorder, melting). Mechanical and physical properties of this category of polymers depend on morphology and amorphous/crystalline ratio, but also on the molecular mobility of the amorphous phase.

In Fig. 2.29, a typical Young's Modulus temperature graph for a generic crystalline polymer is shown. At very low temperatures, E (Young's Modulus) is very high owing to the rigidity of crystalline and amorphous molecules. With temperature rise, E slightly decreases until T_g. At this point, there is a sudden drop in E with activation of molecular movement of the amorphous chain segments. As seen in Fig. 2.29, this drop depends on the amorphous/crystalline ratio, between T_g and T_m (melting temperature). From a mechanical point of view, the material is considered semirigid. At this point, the mechanical behaviour of the material is controlled by the crystalline zone.

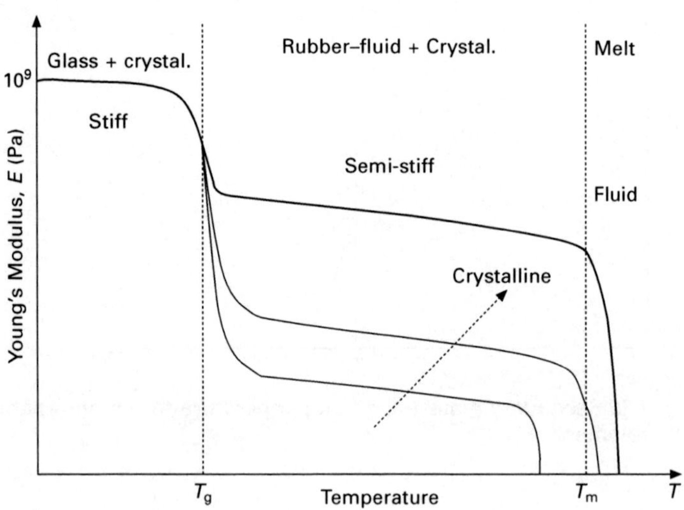

2.29 Schematic representation of *E*–*T* curve for a generic crystalline polymer.

In the proximity of T_m, there is a mechanical collapse owing to gradual crystallite fusion (Braun, 2005).

2.5.1 Thermoplastic and thermosetting polymers

The behaviour described in the previous section occurs in thermoplastic polymers, where the single molecules are bonded together by thermosensitive intermolecular attractive forces (van der Waals, dipole–dipole, hydrogen bonding). Crosslinked polymers (thermosetting polymers) show a different behaviour owing to primary bonds between main chains. These types of bonds are not thermosensitive and they limit viscous flows. The segments of chain, included between transversal bonds, are obstructed in their movement.

In general, thermosetting polymers are in amorphous state (Fig. 2.30). The presence of a high density of transversal bonds can produce the disappearance of the glass transition. Thermosetting polymers thus maintain shape stability until high temperature and then thermal decomposition occurs. Typical examples of thermosetting polymers are unsaturated polyesters, epoxy resins, phenolic and urea–formaldehyde resins (Pascault, 2002). Urea–formaldehyde resins are not widely used in biomedical applications owing to their potentially toxic, allergenic and carcinogenic characteristics. Unsaturated polyesters have been considered as potential bone cement and scaffolds in bioresorbable composite materials for tissue engineering (Kharas *et al.*, 1997). Epoxy resins have been used in combination with other biomaterials for plates in bone fixation devices (Ramakrishna *et al.*, 2001). Phenolic resins have been used to develop activated carbon for many biomedical applications (Cai *et al.*, 2004).

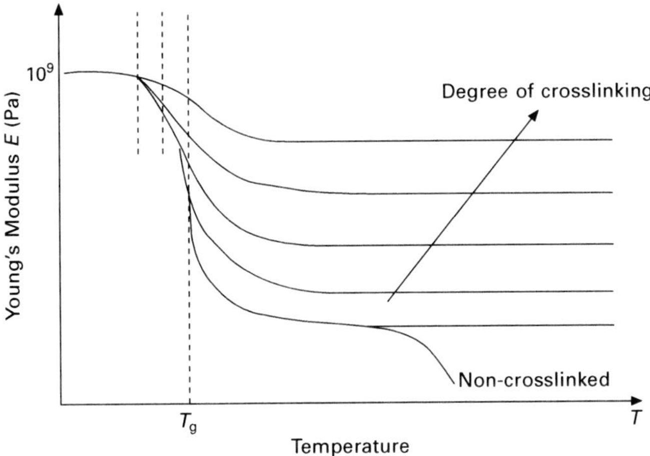

2.30 Schematic representation of *E–T* curve for thermosetting polymers.

2.6 References

Alariqi, S. A. S., Kumar, A. P., Rao, B. S. M. & Singh, R. P. 2009. Effect of γ-dose rate on crystallinity and morphological changes of γ-sterilized biomedical polypropylene. *Polymer degradation and stability*, **94**, 6.

Askadskii, A. A. 2003. *Computational materials science of polymers*, Cambridge, UK, Cambridge International Science Pub.

ASM International. 2003. *Characterization and failure analysis of plastics*, Materials Park, OH, ASM International.

Bassett, D. C. 1981. *Principles of polymer morphology*, Cambridge, England; New York, Cambridge University Press.

Bower, D. I. 2002. *An introduction to polymer physics*, Cambridge; New York, Cambridge University Press.

Braun, D. 2005. *Polymer synthesis: theory and practice: fundamentals, methods, experiments*, Berlin; New York, Springer.

Cai, Q., Huang, Z.-H., Kang, F. & Yang, J.-B. 2004. Preparation of activated carbon microspheres from phenolic-resin by supercritical water activation. *Carbon*, **42**, 9.

Chanda, M. & Roy, S. K. 2007. *Plastics technology handbook*, Boca Raton, FL, CRC Press/Taylor & Francis Group.

Cowie, J. M. G. 1991. *Polymers: chemistry and physics of modern materials*, Glasgow, New York, Blackie; Chapman and Hall.

Dattelbaum, D. M. & Rae, P. J. 2004. The properties of poly(tetrafluoroethylene) (PTFE) in compression. *Polymer*, **45**, 11.

Dissado, L. A. & Fothergill, J. C. 1992. *Electrical degradation and breakdown in polymers*, London, P. Peregrinus.

Gedde, U. W. 1995. *Polymer physics*, London; New York, Chapman & Hall.

Gowariker, V. R., Viswanathan, N. V. & Sreedhar, J. 1986. *Polymer science*, New York, Wiley.

Hadjichristidis, N., Pispas, S. & Floudas, G. 2003. *Block copolymers: synthetic strategies, physical properties, and applications*, Hoboken, NJ, Wiley-Interscience.

Hatakeyama, T. & Hatakeyama, H. 1995. Effect of chemical structure of amorphous polymers on heat capacity difference at glass transition temperature. *Thermochimica Acta*, **267**, 9.

Kausch, H. H. & Springerlink (Online Service) 2005. *Intrinsic molecular mobility and toughness of polymers II. Advances in polymer science No. 188*. Berlin; New York: Springer.

Kharas, G. B., Kamenetsky, M., Simantirakis, J., Beinlich, K., C., Rizzo, A.-M., T., Caywood, G., A. & Watson, K. 1997. Synthesis and characterization of fumarate-based polyesters for use in bioresorbable bone cement composites. *Journal of Applied Polymer Science*, **66**, 15.

Kricheldorf, H. R., Nuyken, O. & Swift, G. 2005. *Handbook of polymer synthesis*, New York, Marcel Dekker.

Liangbin, L., Rui, H., Ling, Z. & Shiming, H. 2001. A new mechanism in the formation of PET extended-chain crystal. *Polymer*, **42**, 5.

Manfredini, M., Marchetti, A., Atzei, D., Elsener, B., Malagoli, M., Galavotti, F. & Rossi, A. 2003. Radiation-induced migration of additives in PVC-based biomedical disposable device. Part. 1 Surface morphology by AFM and SEM/XEDS. *Surface and interface analysis*, **35**, 8.

Mark, J. E. & Springerlink (Online Service) 2007. *Physical properties of polymers handbook*. 2nd ed. New York: Springer.

Misra, G. S. 1993. *Introductory polymer chemistry*, New York, J. Wiley & Sons.

Nicholson, J. W. & Royal Society of Chemistry (Great Britain) 2006. *The chemistry of polymers*, Cambridge, UK, Royal Society of Chemistry.

Okada, O. & Furuya, H. 2002. Molecular dynamics simulation of *cis*-1,4-polybutadiene. 1. Comparison with experimental data for static and dynamic properties. *Polymer*, **43**, 6.

Pascault, J.-P. 2002. *Thermosetting polymers*, New York, Marcel Dekker.

Perez, J. 1998. *Physics and mechanics of amorphous polymers*, Rotterdam; Brookfield, VT, A. A. Balkema.

Ramakrishna, S., Mayer, J., Wintermantel, E. & Leong, K., W. 2001. Biomedical applications of polymer-composite materials: a review. *Composites Science and Technology*, **61**, 36.

Riga, A. T. & Judovits, L. 2001. *Materials characterization by dynamic and modulated thermal analytical techniques*, West Conshohocken, PA, ASTM.

Rudin, A. 1999. *The elements of polymer science and engineering: an introductory text and reference for engineers and chemists*, San Diego, Academic Press.

Scheirs, J. 2000. *Compositional and failure analysis of polymers: a practical approach*, Chichester; New York, Wiley.

Seyler, R. J. 1994. *Assignment of the glass transition*, Philadelphia, PA, ASTM.

Sperling, L. H. 2006. *Introduction to physical polymer science*, Hoboken, N.J., Wiley.

Stuart, B. 2002. *Polymer analysis*, Chichester; New York, J. Wiley.

Van Der Vegt, A. K. 2006. *From polymers to plastics*, VSSD.

Ward, I. M. 1997. *Structure and properties of oriented polymers*, London; New York, Chapman & Hall.

Ward, I. M. & Sweeney, J. 2004. *An introduction to the mechanical properties of solid polymers*, Chichester; Hoboken, NJ, Wiley.

3
Processing of bioresorbable and other polymers for medical applications

T. CASALINI and G. PERALE, Politecnico di Milano, Italy

Abstract: Established polymer processing techniques are reviewed and the particular challenges in applying them successfully to biopolymers are examined. Mixing, molding, shaping, calendering, coating, foaming and solvent casting processes are examined. Problem areas, such as electrospinning, are investigated.

Key words: biopolymers, extrusion, molding, calendering, solvent casting.

3.1 Introduction

Polymer processing is an established industrial reality able to produce a huge variety of objects of different shapes, dimensions, structures and properties. However, not all of the steps in conventional polymer processing are suitable for biopolymers. The properties that make them useful in the biomedical field create significant challenges when it comes to processing. In this chapter, the key steps in conventional polymer processing are reviewed and how these steps need to be modified to maximize the functionality of bioresorbable medical polymers, is investigated.

The main steps in polymer manufacturing can be summarized broadly as follows (Osswald and Hernández-Ortiz, 2006):

- Shaping operations: polymer pellets, powders or resin are transformed into a preform or into the final product, using extrusion or molding processes.
- Secondary shaping operations: preforms are transformed into the final product using techniques such as thermoforming or blow molding.
- Joining operations: two or more parts are assembled physically or through bonding or welding operations.

One or more of these steps can be involved in polymer processing. However, most parts require shaping operations such as extrusion, which is discussed in more detail below.

3.2 Extrusion

In the extrusion process, a polymer melt is pumped through a shaping die and formed into a profile which can be, for example, a plate, a film, or a tube (Osswald and Hernández-Ortiz, 2006). For this purpose, ram and screw extruders are used. The ram extruder uses a positive displacement pump based on pressure. In this process, the volume is reduced, the fluid is moved from one point to another and the pressure rises. A screw extruder is a viscosity pump based on the pressure gradient and fluid deformation. Currently, single-screw extruders are the most common equipment used in the polymer industries. Twin-screw extruders are widely used as mixing and compounding devices.

Single-screw plasticating extruders are different because they are not directly fed with a melted polymer but with solid pellets or powders (Fig. 3.1). Plasticating extruders can be divided into three zones:

- the solid conveying zone,
- the transition (or melting) zone, and
- the pumping (or metering) zone.

The solid feed descends via gravity into the hopper and into the screw channel, where it is conveyed and compressed, and then melted (or 'plasticated') directly into the screw channel. Melted polymer is mixed in order to obtain a homogeneous melt. It is then removed and finally pumped through the die.

The overall extrusion process can be divided in four elementary steps:

- the handling of solid particulate,
- melting,

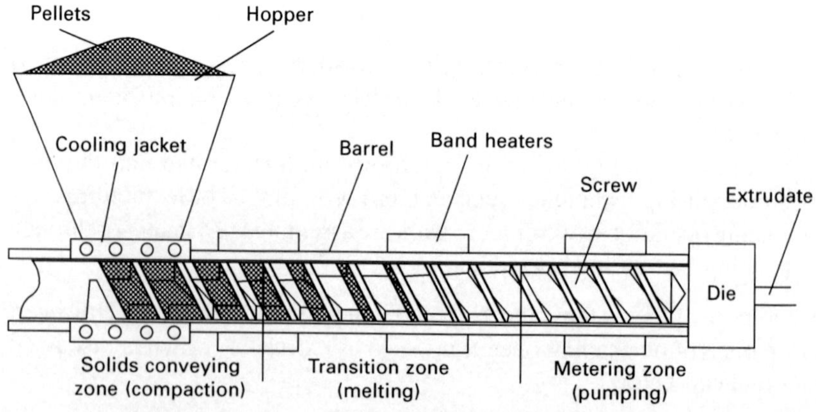

3.1 Plasticating single-screw extruder (from Osswald and Hernández-Ortiz, 2006).

- mixing, and
- pumping.

The solid conveying zone moves the solid from the hopper to the screw channel, where the material is compacted and transported along the channel. This process (compacting and moving pellets) can take place only if friction at the barrel surface exceeds the friction at the screw surface; otherwise there would not be any movement in axial direction. In order to maintain a high friction coefficient between the barrel and the polymer, the feed section is cooled with cold-water cooling lines. These frictional forces cause a pressure rise in the feed zone that compresses the solid bed which moves along the channel until it reaches the transition zone. The simplest mechanism that ensures an adequate friction along the channel between the polymer and the barrel is grooving the barrel surface in an axial direction.

The transition zone is where polymer melting occurs; the length of this zone is a function of material properties, screw geometry and process conditions. During melting, the size of the solid bed shrinks as the melt pool forms at its side. The solid bed profile is an important aspect of screw design, as well as knowing where the melt pool begins and ends. However, there are large variations in experimental bed profile. In order to have a defined profile, Maillefer screws and barrier screws are used. The former maintains a constant solid bed width, whereas the latter ensures a gradually decreasing solid bed width. In the metering zone the generated pressures are monitored to ensure they are sufficient for pumping. The screw diameter determines the pumping capacity of the extruder.

The extrusion die, at the end of the extruder, gives the final shape to the polymer melt. It can be used to obtain, for example, films, sheets, pipes and tubular films, filaments, open and hollow profiles. There are some aspects to consider when designing an extruded plastic profile. Thick sections must be avoided because they are expensive, and hollow sections must be minimized because they make the die more difficult to clean. It is important to generate profiles with a constant wall thickness because this allows easier thickness control and a better crystallinity distribution of semicrystalline materials.

The coat-hanger sheeting die is one of the most widely used extrusion dies (Fig. 3.2; Osswald and Hernández-Ortiz, 2006). It is formed by a manifold which distributes the melt to the approach or land region, where the fluid is carried to the die lips. Here the final shaping is performed. The flow through the manifold and the land region is strongly dependent on the non-Newtonian properties of the melt. A die designed for one material may therefore not work for another polymer. Tubular dies are used to extrude tubular films and plastic tubes; polymer melt exits through an annulus. Spiral dies are commonly used to obtain tubular blown films.

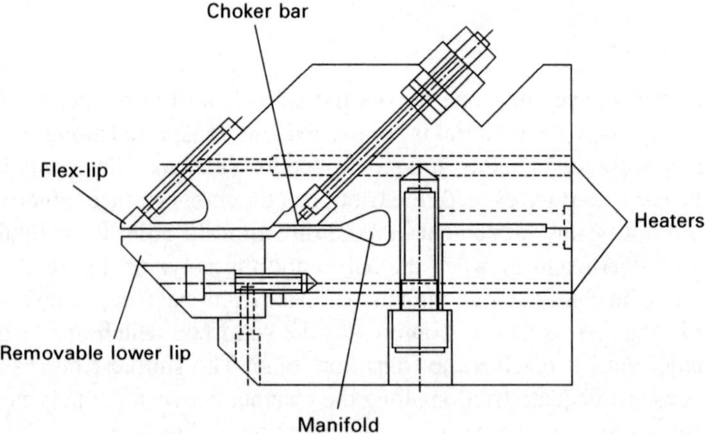

3.2 Coat hanger die section (from Osswald and Hernández-Ortiz, 2006).

3.3 Mixing processes

The quality of finished products also depends on how well the material was mixed. Material properties are also influenced by mixing quality (Tadmor and Gogos, 2006). Single screw extruders have a mixing zone, but mostly twin screw extruders are used as mixing devices. Polymer blending or mixing is performed by distributing or dispersing a secondary component in a primary component which acts as a matrix. The major component is intended as a continuous phase in which a second phase is dispersed. A polymer blend will probably be melted again for a shaping process and this must be taken into account in mixing. Indeed, a rapidly cooled mixture, frozen as a homogeneous blend, can exhibit phase separation when melted again, giving a blend which is not processable.

There are three general types of motion involved in mixing:

- molecular diffusion,
- eddy motion, and
- bulk flow or convection.

Molecular diffusion results from concentration gradients and takes place spontaneously. Eddy motion is caused by turbulent flow, and bulk flow is caused by large-scale matter flows. In polymer processing, the viscosity of polymer melts is very high. Flow is laminar and eddy motion owing to turbulence is absent. Molecular diffusion is too slow. Convection is thus the dominant mixing process.

There are three general categories of mixtures that can be created:

- homogeneous mixtures of compatible polymers,

- single-phase mixtures of partly incompatible polymers, and
- multiphase mixture of incompatible polymers.

The morphological development of these polymer mixtures is determined by two possible mechanisms:

- dispersive or intensive mixing and
- distributive or extensive mixing.

Dispersive or intensive mixing involves the reduction of the size of a component having a cohesive character within a continuous liquid phase. This component can be a solid phase or non-compatible liquid phase. Agglomerates are broken and dispersed in the liquid phase. The cohesive character of the added component is the result of Van der Waals forces and surface tension. The most common example of dispersive mixing is the dispersion of carbon black in a rubber compound. Incompatible droplets tend to assume a spherical shape in order to minimize interphasic surface. It is necessary to impose a stress high enough to achieve surface tension. Distributive or extensive mixing involves the distribution of droplets of a compatible liquid in the primary phase. By imposing a strain, the interfacial area increases and the local dimension of the secondary phase decreases. Large strains are insufficient to ensure a homogeneous mixing, because the type of mixing device, the initial orientation and the position of the two fluids have a significant role.

The final properties of a polymeric material strongly depend on the mixing process. Mixing efficiency must also be evaluated, because the amount of power necessary to obtain the highest mixing quality can be unrealistic or unachievable. Static mixers are pressure-driven continuous-mixing devices, through which the melt is pumped, rotated and divided with no use of moving parts. The twisted tape static mixer is the most common static mixer. In this device, the polymer melt is shorn and rotated 90° by a dividing wall, thus increasing the interfaces between fluids. This sequence is repeated until a homogeneous mixture is obtained.

Internal batch mixers are high-intensity mixers that generate complex shearing and elongational flows. They work well with dispersions of solid particles in polymeric matrices, because intensive mixing is able to break up solid agglomerates. Solid dispersion is a function of rotor speed, mixing time, temperature, and rotor blade geometry. Mixing is also achieved in the extruder screw channel, as said before. Mixing can be enhanced by adding pins (Osswald and Hernández-Ortiz, 2006) in the flow channel on the screw or barrel surface (Fig. 3.3). Pins reorient surfaces between fluids and split the flow, creating new surfaces. An extruder with adjustable pins on the barrel surface is called a QSM-extruder (QSM stands for *Quer Strom Mischer*, the German for crossflow mixing). Pin-type extruders are necessary when operating with high-viscosity mixtures such as rubber compounds.

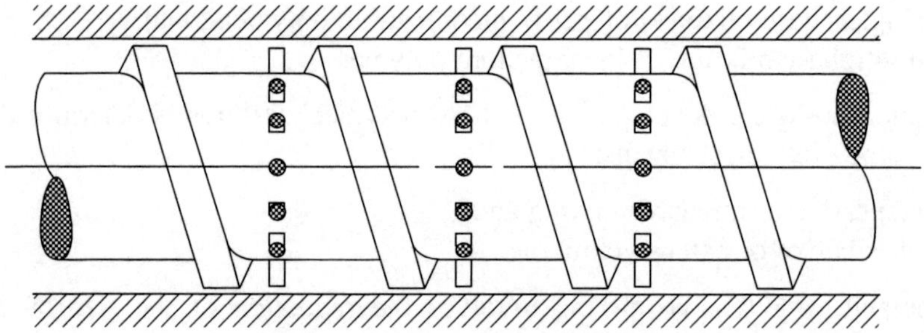

3.3 Pin screw (from Osswald and Hernández-Ortiz, 2006).

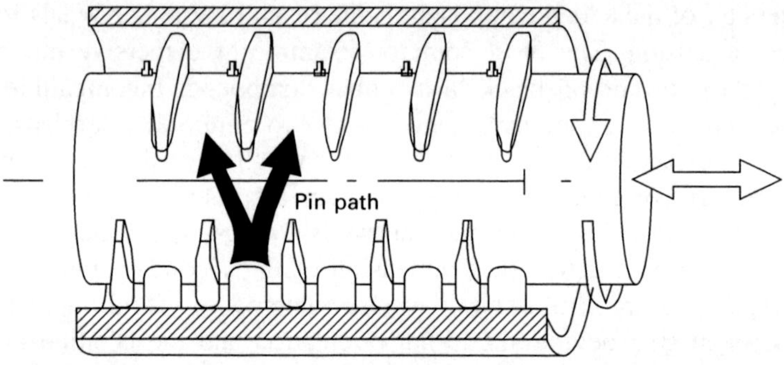

3.4 Self-cleaning single-screw extruder design (from Osswald and Hernández-Ortiz, 2006).

As already noted, when dispersive mixing is required, the mixture must be subjected to large stresses in order to break up agglomerates. In this instance, barrier-type screws can be used, because the mixture is forced through narrow gaps, inducing high stresses. It must also be noted that any disruption to flow causes a pressure drop and viscous heating during extrusion. Another example of a mixing extruder is a single-screw extruder with pins on the barrel surface and a screw that oscillates in an axial direction (Fig. 3.4). Pins on the barrel wipe the entire surface of the screw, making this design the only self-cleaning single-screw extruder (Osswald and Hernández-Ortiz, 2006). The reduced residence time is advantageous when operating with thermally sensitive materials. The pins disrupt the solid bed, creating dispersed melting which improves the overall melting rate.

Twin-screw extruders are continuous-mixing devices and can be classified as follows (Fig. 3.5; Tadmor and Gogos, 2006):

- intermeshing or not intermeshing
- co-rotating or counter-rotating.

The intermeshing twin-screw extruder has a self-cleaning effect that reduces

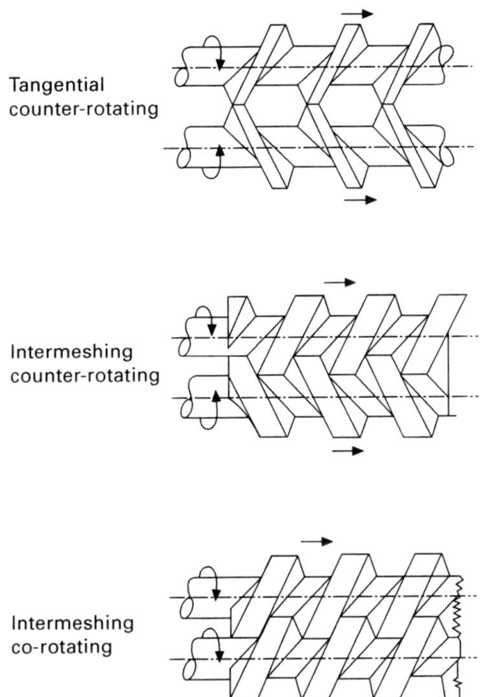

3.5 Screws configurations (from Tadmor and Gogos, 2006).

residence time. In co-rotating systems, screws move in the same direction; they have a high pumping efficiency caused by the double transport action of the two screws. Counter-rotating systems apply high stresses because of the calendering action of the screws which allows dispersal of pigments and lubricants.

3.4 Molding processes

The following molding processes are discussed here:

- injection molding,
- reactive injection molding,
- compression molding, and
- rotational molding.

3.4.1 Injection molding

Injection molding is now the most important molding process in manufacturing polymeric products (Osswald and Hernández-Ortiz, 2006, Han, 2007).

Indeed, more than one third of all thermoplastic materials are processed with injection molding (Fig. 3.6; Han, 2007). This is because of the suitability of injection molding to mass production of parts with complex shapes and precise dimensions. Injection molding machines are classified using an international convention, based on the T/P ratio, where T is the clamping force (tonne), and P is defined as:

$$P = \frac{V_{max}\, p_{max}}{1000}$$

where V_{max} is the maximum shot size (cm^3) and p_{max} is the maximum injection pressure (bar). Injection molding can be considered to be the sum of two distinct processes. The first process involves solid transport, melt generation, mixing, pressurization and flow, which are phenomena that take place in the injection unit. The second process is the product shaping occurring into the mold cavity.

In injection molding, the polymer melt is forced into a cavity in order to reproduce its shape (Fig. 3.6). The injection molding cycle begins when the mold closes, followed by the injection of the polymer melt into the mold cavity. To perform this, the melt must be pressurized with a piston or a screw. Once the cavity is filled, a holding pressure is required in order to compensate for material shrinkage. When the part has reached a sufficiently low temperature, it is ejected. The design is similar to a single-screw plasticating extruder. The screw can, however, slide back and forth in order to accumulate and inject the melt. The presence of vents allows extraction of moisture and residual gaseous monomer from the melt. At the end of the screw there is a non-return valve which enables the screw to work like a plunger during injection and to prevent the back flow of the melt which is injected in the mold through a nozzle. The clamping unit has the task of opening and closing the mold, avoiding the risk of flash during filling and holding.

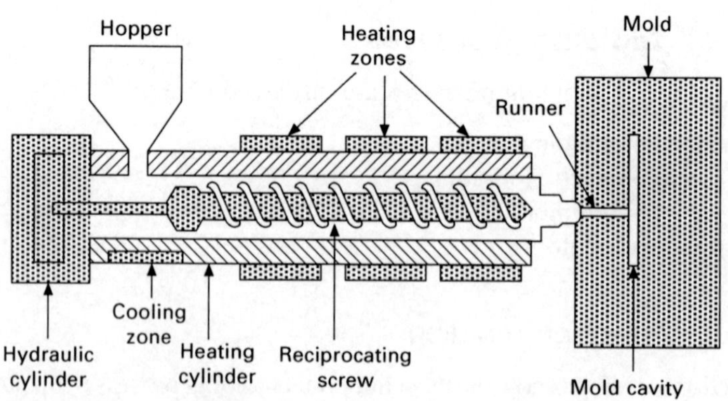

3.6 Screw-injection molding machine (from Han, 2007).

The mold cavity is the central point of every injection molding machine. It distributes the melt into and throughout the cavities, shapes the part, cools the melt, and ejects the final product. During mold filling, the melt flows from a nozzle through a sprue (the overall entrance into the mold). It is distributed by a runner system which brings the hot melt into the mold cavity. Runners are designed in order to produce small drops at low pressure, while ensuring a low amount of material waste generation and slow cooling. There are two types of runners:

- cold runners and
- hot runners.

Cold runners are ejected with the part and trimmed after removal. Hot runners keep the polymer at melting temperature. Finally, the melt is distributed in mold cavities through gates which control polymer flow and isolate mold cavities from the rest of the system.

Total cycle time can be expressed as a sum of three terms: closing time, cooling time and ejection time. Closing and ejection can take a fraction of a second or a few seconds according to the size of the mold and the machine. Cooling time depends on the maximum thickness of the part. The process can be divided into five steps which can be represented, for example, by plotting specific volume against temperature in a *v–T* diagram (Fig. 3.7; Osswald and Hernández-Ortiz, 2006):

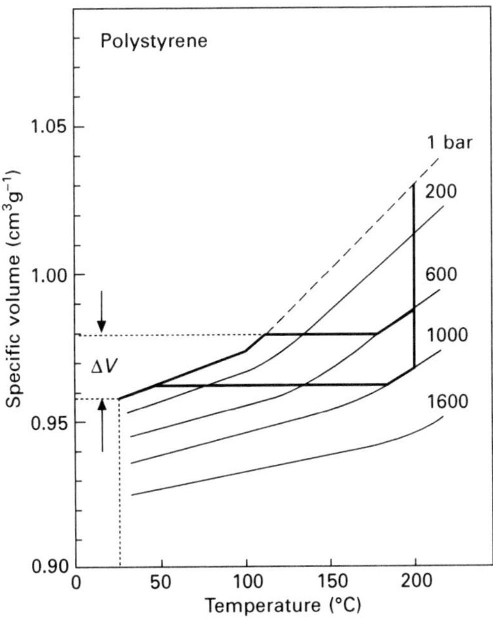

3.7 A *v–T* diagram (from Osswald and Hernández-Ortiz, 2006).

- isothermal injection,
- pressure rising to the holding pressure,
- isobaric cooling process,
- isochoric cooling process, and
- a second isobaric cooling process to room temperature.

The point where the final cooling begins determines the total shrinkage of the part. This point is influenced by melt temperature and holding pressure (Tadmor and Gogos, 2006). There are many combinations of operating temperatures and pressures, bounded by minimum and maximum values. Incorrect temperatures and pressures reduce product quality. As an example, too low a melt temperature can result in an unfilled cavity, whereas thermal degradation of the material occurs at very high temperatures. A low holding pressure can cause excessive shrinkage, whereas high pressure can cause the flash phenomenon that occurs when pressure is higher than the machine clamping force and the melt flows across the mold parting lines. Another critical aspect is the presence of defects and residual stresses (that can lead to breaking stresses) in the final product (Fig. 3.8; Tadmor and Gogos, 2006). Sink marks are caused by material shrinkage during cooling. Deformations are caused by process conditions that lead to asymmetric residual stresses through the part thickness. Residual stresses are mainly owing to rapid cooling.

There are several important variations in molding processes, such as:

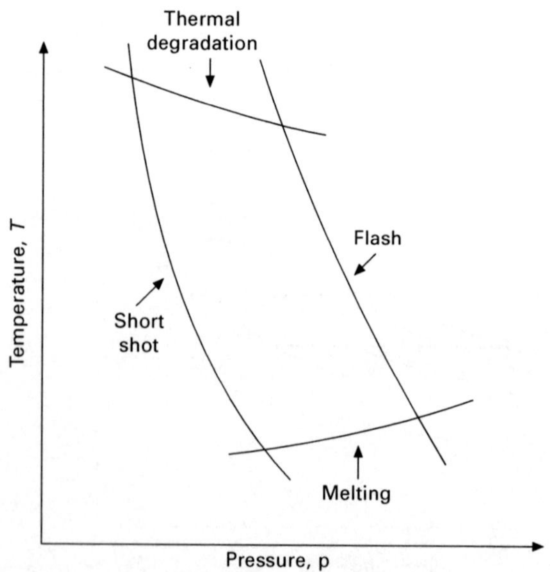

3.8 Molding diagram (from Tadmor and Gogos, 2006).

- Multicolor and multicomponent molding: these injection molding processes occur when two or more polymers, or equal polymers of different colors, are injected through different runners at different stages during the molding process. Every component has its own plasticating unit.
- Co-injection molding: this process, unlike multicomponent and multicolor molding, uses the same runner system. The component which forms the outer skin of the part is injected first, followed by the core component.
- Gas-assisted injection molding: this process is similar to co-injection molding, but the second component is nitrogen, which is injected through a needle into the polymer melt and blown against mold walls.

3.4.2 Reactive injection molding

When the size of the product to be molded increases, two aspects in injection molding become critical:

- ensuring sufficient homogeneous melt in the injection molding machine; and
- generating an adequate clamping pressure in order to keep the mold closed during the filling and packing stages.

Reactive injection molding was developed to avoid these issues. Two or more low-viscosity (0.1–1 Pa s) liquid flows are mixed and injected into large cavities. Even if part of the polymerization reaction occurs during the filling phase, it mostly takes place after the filling step, and even after the removal from the hot mold. Thus, injection pressures needed for filling molds are usually small. The heat generated by the reaction increases the volume of the mix. The viscosity also increases because of the increase in molecular weight and/or crosslinking. A small amount of foaming agent is introduced to ensure that the final component conforms to the shape of the cavity. This means that complex-shaped cavities can be used with a small injection pressure and small clamping presses. Reaction molding processes must guarantee high polymerization rate in order to be competitive with other molding processes. Not all polymeric systems are suitable for this process. The most commonly used materials are linear or crosslinked polyurethans, where di- or trialcohols and di- or tri-isocyanates are the main reactant species. It is important to ensure good temperature control of the reactant system, stoichiometric metering of reactants and an adequate reactant mixing (Han, 2007, Tadmor and Gogos, 2006).

3.4.3 Compression molding

In the compression molding process, a thermoplastic or a partially polymerized thermosetting polymer is placed in a heated cavity. The material is usually preheated and preshaped with a form roughly similar to that of the cavity. The mold is closed and pressure is applied in order to force the material to fill the mold cavity. In the process, the polymer undergoes complete polymerization or crosslinking. At the end, the mold is opened, the part is ejected and the cycle can start again. This process wastes very little material. However, it is difficult to produce parts with close tolerances because the final size of compression molded products depends on the exact amount of the preform. Moreover, it is not possible to obtain parts with a complex shape, for example with deep undercuts (Osswald and Hernández-Ortiz, 2006, Tadmor and Gogos, 2006).

3.4.4 Rotational molding

Rotational molding is used to produce hollow objects. Rotational molding can produce large parts with uniform thickness at low costs compared with injection molding. It can be seen as a sequence of six different steps:

- induction or initial temperature rise,
- melting and sintering,
- bubble removal and densification,
- precooling,
- crystallization of the polymer melt, and
- final cooling.

To begin with, a certain amount of a powdered polymer is loaded in the mold. The mold is closed and placed in an oven where it turns around two axes while the polymeric powder melts. During the heating and melting phases, the polymer is deposited uniformly on the mold walls. At the end of the process, the mold is cooled and the final product is removed. The cooling rate is particularly important because it affects residual stresses in the molded object. If cooling is too fast, objects can be warped. The mold undergoes a slow initial cooling using air, followed by a faster quenching using a water spray. The main disadvantage of rotational molding is the long time required to heat the powder and the mold, and then to cool the mold. Induction time can be reduced by preheating the polymeric powder, whereas bubble removal and cooling stage times can be decreased by pressurizing the material in the mold. Melting and sintering depend on the rheology and geometry of the particles (Osswald and Hernández-Ortiz, 2006).

3.5 Secondary shaping

Secondary shaping operations take place when the extruded pellet exits from the equipment. These operations include:

- fiber spinning,
- cast film extrusion,
- film blowing,
- blow molding, and
- thermoforming.

3.5.1 Fiber spinning

In this process, the melt is first extruded through a filter in order to eliminate small contaminants, and then it goes into a die with multiple holes called a spinneret. Formed fibers are drawn to their final diameter, solidified and wound into a spool (Fig. 3.9; Han, 2007). In addition to melt spinning, there are two other spinning methods. Using wet spinning, the polymer is dissolved in a solvent and extruded through a spinneret immersed in a chemical solution. In dry spinning, a polymer solution is extruded and the solvent is removed

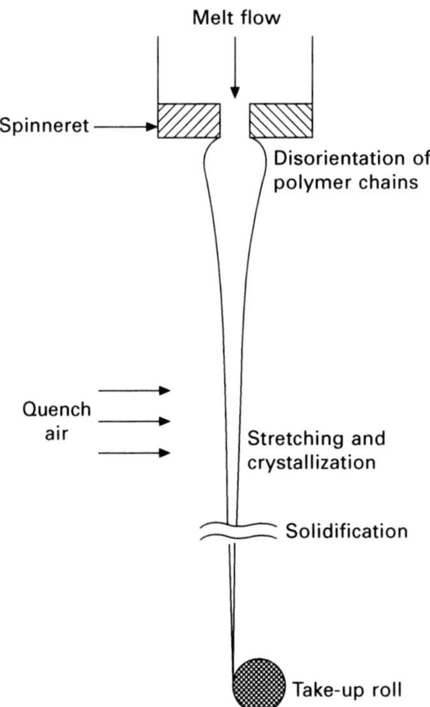

3.9 Schematic of fiber-spinning process (from Han, 2007).

via evaporation. Melt spinning is, however, the most common commercial process. Fibers solidification occurs either in a water bath or for forced convection. Final properties of the filament, such as breaking strength, Young Modulus and flex loss, are determined by the spinning process. When the molten filament exits from the spinneret to a take-up roll, it is simultaneously stretched and cooled, and these phenomena orient polymer chains and induce crystallization in the polymer. The spinning process is thus not only a shaping process but also a structuring process (Tadmor and Gogos, 2006, Osswald and Hernández-Ortiz, 2006).

3.5.2 Cast film extrusion

In cast film extrusion a thin film is extruded through a slit. It passes through a chilled turning roller where it is quenched from one side. The film is sent to a second roller in order to cool the other side. Finally, the film is wound in a roll by passing through a final system of rollers (Fig. 3.10; Osswald and Hernández-Ortiz, 2006). Film thickness depends on roller speed.

3.5.3 Film blowing

In film blowing, a tubular film is extruded upwards. It is blown upwards, with air introduced below the die, into a larger tubular film which is then picked up by a pair of nip rolls that seals the bubble (Fig. 3.11; Han, 2007). An external stream of chilled air cools and solidifies the film at a certain point called the freeze line, where the temperature of the film is equal to the melting temperature. A feature of this process is that the film is stretched biaxially, improving mechanical properties. Tangential circumferential stretching depends on blow-up ratio, i.e. the ratio between the tubular film diameter after air introduction and the initial tubular film diameter. This parameter is determined by the pressure level within the bubble. Axial stretching depends

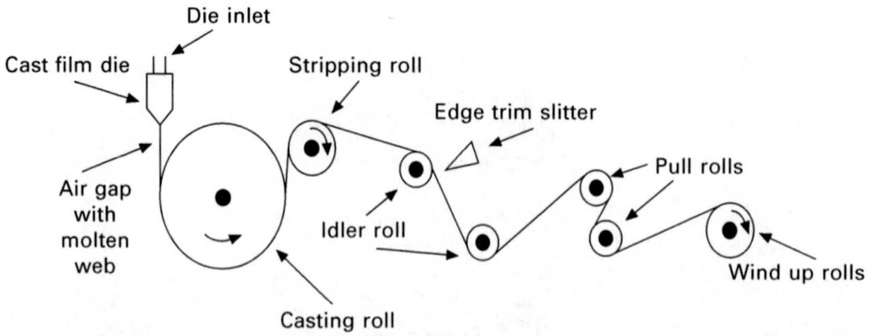

3.10 Schematic of film-casting (from Osswald and Hernández-Ortiz, 2006).

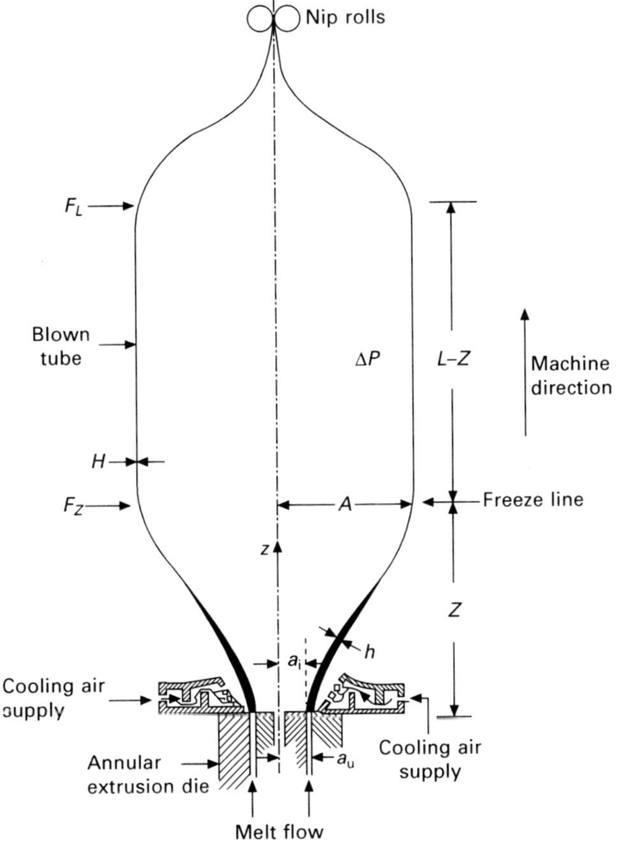

3.11 Schematic of film-blowing process (from Han, 2007).

on the take-up speed of nip rolls. Using film blowing, film thickness varies between 10 and 100 μm, with high production rates.

3.5.4 Blow molding

Blow molding is a process 'borrowed' from the glass industry and is used to produce hollow shapes. There are three types of blow molding process:

- extrusion blow molding,
- injection blow molding, and
- stretch blow molding.

The first step in extrusion blow molding is the formation of a molten tube called a parison. The parison is engaged between two mold halves and, after closing the mold, is inflated by using compressed air, ensuring the polymer adheres to the mold shape. The material solidifies in contact with the cold walls of the mold. It is also possible to obtain products with several layers of material by coextrusion blow molding.

In the injection blow molding process, the parison is obtained by injection molding of a preshaped parison onto a steel rod. The rod with the molten thread is moved to the blowing station where inflation takes place. Injection stretch blow molding is a variation of the process, which introduces a biaxial orientation in crystalline polymers, improving product properties (Fig. 3.12, Osswald and Hernández-Ortiz, 2006). The perform is molded, cooled and transported to the stretch blow molding station, where it is reheated in order to reach a temperature which is above glass transition temperature, but well below melting point. Material is stretched with an axially moving rod and simultaneously blown in a mold. This process is used, for example, to produce PET bottles. The aim of thermal conditioning is to allow crystallization during biaxial stretching, thus inducing a structural improvement (Han, 2007, Tadmor and Gogos, 2006, Osswald and Hernández-Ortiz, 2006).

3.5.5 Thermoforming

In a thermoforming process, a plastic sheet is warmed and formed into a cavity (or over a tool) using vacuum, air pressure or mechanical means. The plastic

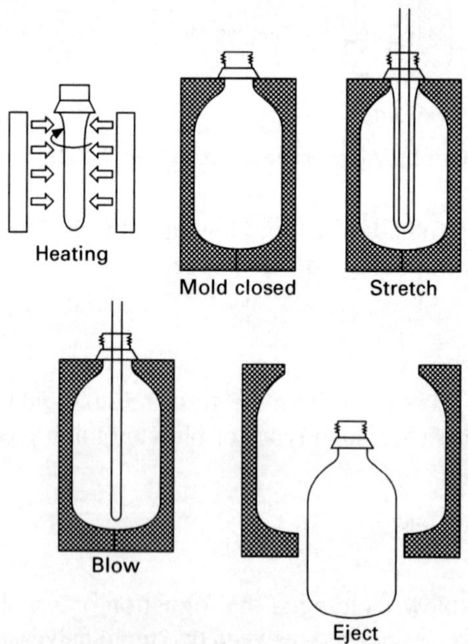

3.12 Schematic of stretch blow-molding process (from Osswald and Hernández-Ortiz, 2006).

sheet is heated in order to reach a temperature that is slightly above the glass transition temperature for amorphous polymers and slightly below the melting temperature for semicrystalline polymers. The process is most suitable for amorphous materials because they have a wide rubber temperature range. At these temperatures, the polymer can be easily shaped and it conserves enough rigidity to avoid sheet sagging. The risk with semicrystalline polymers is that the material rapidly loses its strength when the crystalline structure is broken. Heating is achieved through radiative heaters. The temperature must be high enough to allow sheet shaping and the forming temperature profile must be uniform to obtain an optimal process.

One of the main problems in thermoforming is minimizing thickness differences throughout the product. This can be achieved with a plug-assisted system (Fig. 3.13). The plug pushes the sheet into the cavity. Because of this, only the part of the sheet not touching the plug is subjected to stretching. This is followed by use of a vacuum for the final shaping. Once cooled, the product is removed. The sheet can also be prestretched at the beginning of the process (Osswald and Hernández-Ortiz, 2006).

3.6 Calendering

In the calendering process, a polymer melt is transformed into film and sheet shapes by squeezing it between co-rotating pairs of rollers. The number of rollers depends on the material processed and the final product. Rubber can be calendered with a two-roller system. Other thermoplastic polymers require a four-roller system to ensure good surface quality. A typical calendering system is composed of:

- a plasticating unit,

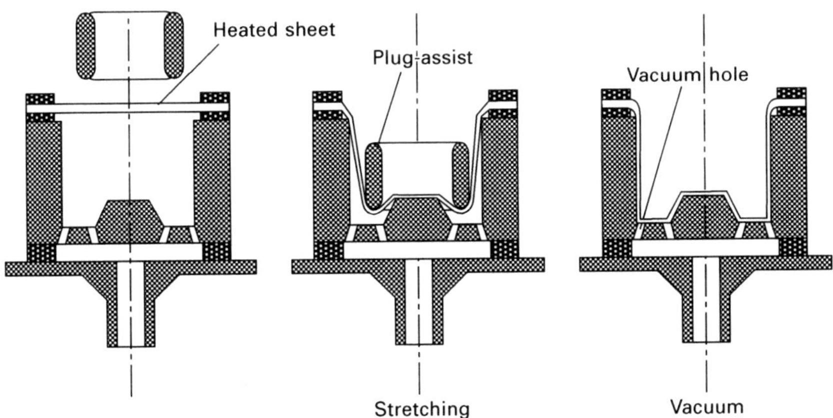

3.13 Plug-assisted system (from Osswald and Hernández-Ortiz, 2006).

- a calender,
- a cooling unit,
- an accumulator, and
- a wind-up station.

In the plasticating unit, the material is melted, mixed, and continuously fed through the nip of the first two rollers. This step controls the feeding rate with the remaining rollers controlling product thickness. In a four-roller system the polymer passes through three nip regions:

- The first pass is the feed pass.
- The second pass is the metering pass.
- The third pass is the sheet formation pass.

Rollers come in different types such as I-type, F-type, L-type, inverted L-type, and Z-type configurations (Fig. 3.14).

After passing the main calender, the sheet passes through a system of chilling rollers where it is cooled from both sides. At the end of the process, the sheet is wound. The calendering process is suitable for shaping high melt viscosity thermoplastic sheets and for polymers which undergo thermal degradation or which contain solid additives. A calender system is able to convey large rates of melt using a smaller amount of energy than an extruder. The thickness of the product should be uniform in both the machine and the cross-machine directions.

A variation in the gap size between the rollers (which can be caused by poor roller dimensions, setting, thermal effects or roller distortion because of high pressure in the gap region) causes a non-uniformity in the cross-machine

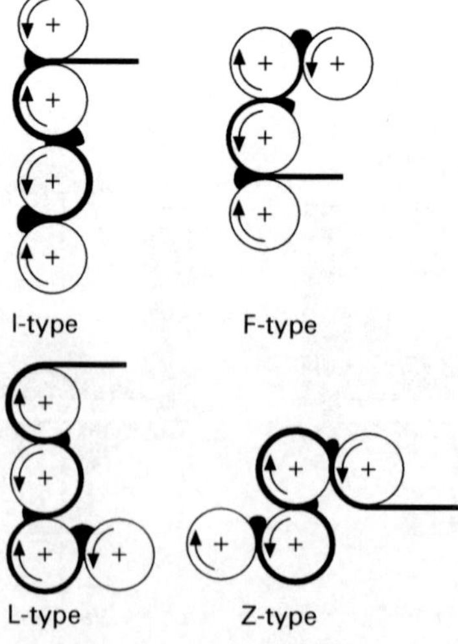

3.14 Calender configurations.

direction. Non-uniformity in the machine direction is caused by eccentricity of the roller with respect to its axis, roller vibration or a non-uniform feed. The gap size can also change during operation because of hydrodynamic forces that take place in the nip which deflect the rollers. In this situation, the final product is thick in the middle and thin at the borders. In order to avoid this problem, three methods have been developed:

- roll-crown,
- roll-crossing, and
- roll-bending.

In the roll-crown method, the roll diameter in the center is slightly greater than at the edges. This allows for compensation of roller deviation. Roll-crossing and roll-bending involve a continuous adjustment of gap size distribution. In the roll-bending method, a bending moment is applied on roll ends by additional bearings in order to increase or decrease bending caused by hydrodynamic forces. Roll bowing is another problem caused by pressure that occurs in the nip region. This problem can be overcome by placing rolls in a slightly crossed pattern rather than completely parallel. The knowledge of pressure distribution in the nip is necessary to evaluate gap thickness distribution and the load on the bearings. A calender line requires a long time to reach the steady state, or, in other words, to stabilize. As a result calender lines are used for long runs (Han, 2007, Tadmor and Gogos, 2006, Osswald and Hernández-Ortiz, 2006).

3.7 Coating

In the coating process, a liquid film is deposited on a substrate. Wire coating is a good example of this type of process. It is used for primary insulation of conducting wires, as well as increasing wire mechanical strength and providing protection. The unwound bare wire is preheated to a temperature above the glass transition temperature or the melting temperature of the polymer that is to become the coating layer. This promotes adherence of the layer to the bare wire and removes moisture or oils from the conductor surface. The wire is fed into a 'guider tube' of a die. At the exit it meets the molten plastic that covers it circumferentially. The coated wire is then exposed to an air or gas flame for surface annealing and melt relaxation which improves coating gloss. The coated wire then enters a cooling trough with water usually employed as cooling fluid. Trough length depends on wire speed, wire diameter and insulation thickness. It increases as these parameters increase. It is longer for crystalline polymers, because crystallization is an exothermic phenomenon.

After cooling, the wire passes over a capstan where its tension is controlled and further cooling takes place. It then passes through a capacitance-measuring device which detects flaws and thickness variations. The device is used to adjust the speed of the pulling device. The process is closely monitored because it is difficult to reprocess a defective wire. Two types of dies are used in wire coating. The first die type is an annular flow or tubing die. A thin-walled tube is extruded and the molten tube drawn onto the conductor by vacuum after it leaves the die. The vacuum is applied through the clearance between the conductor and the guide, which is about 0.2 mm. Tube dies are usually employed for coating very thin wires with a viscous polymer melt. The second die type is the 'pressure' type, where the melt contacts the conductor inside the die. The clearance between the guide and the conductor is quite small, around 0.05 mm, because at the guide tip, the melt is under pressure.

There are other coating techniques such as dip coating, knife coating, roll coating, slide coating and curtain coating. Dip coating is the simplest coating operation. A substrate is immersed in a fluid and withdrawn with one side or both sides covered by a polymeric layer. Coating thickness is determined by fluid viscosity and density, and by speed and angle of the surface. Knife coating is achieved by spreading the coating material on a surface using a flexible or rigid knife. The knife can be parallel to the substrate or at an angle, and the bottom edge can be flat or tapered. Layer thickness is roughly equal to half the gap between the knife edge and the surface. In the roll-coating process the substrate and the coating polymer pass simultaneously through the nip region between two rolls. The physics of this process is similar to calendering but, in this case, the fluid adheres both to the substrate and the opposing roll. The coating material is usually a low viscosity mixture, taken from a bath by the lower roll and applied to one side of the surface. Layer thickness is controlled by the gap between the rolls and polymer viscosity. This process can use co-rotating rolls (forward roll coating) or counter-rotating rolls (reverse roll coating). This configuration leads to a more accurate thickness control. Slide coating and curtain coating are commonly used to apply multilayered coatings (Osswald and Hernández-Ortiz, 2006).

3.8 Foaming

A foamed polymer is characterized by a porous structure which is generated with physical or chemical blowing agents. The foaming process can be divided in three steps:

- cell nucleation,
- cell growth, and
- cell stabilization.

Nucleation occurs when, at a certain pressure and temperature, the solubility of a gas is reduced and saturation is reached, thus leading to gas bubble formation. Nucleating agents, such as powders of metal oxides, are used for the initial formation of bubbles. In physical foaming, a gas such as nitrogen or carbon dioxide is introduced into the polymer melt. Physical foaming can also be achieved by heating a melt which contains a low boiling point liquid (such as pentane) that vaporizes. Physical blowing agents are introduced into the plasticating zone. Nitrogen is widely used for this purpose. Chemical foaming occurs when the chemical blowing agent thermally decomposes, releasing large amounts of gases. The most widely used agent is azodicarbonamide. In mechanical foaming, a gas is dissolved in a polymer and it undergoes expansion after reducing the pressure of the process (Han, 2007, Osswald and Hernández-Ortiz, 2006).

3.9 Solvent casting

Solvent casting is a technique used to create polymeric films. The polymer is first dissolved in a solvent to create a viscous solution. Viscosity typically increases from 1500 to 80 000 mPa s. In order to obtain a more stable solution, with a reasonable viscosity and solid concentration, additives are used. Dissolution can be carried out increasing the pressure and/or the temperature, thus improving the process. Other additives can be added in order to provide specific properties to the final film, such as chelating agents, pigments, and electrically conductive substances. The impact of the addition of these components on solution viscosity must be taken into account. The stirring process, mechanical shear rate and temperature have to be carefully monitored to control viscosity. The dissolution process usually takes several hours. The final solution is degassed (with heat exchangers or vacuum equipment), in order to prevent air bubbles during film forming, and clarified with two or three filtration steps. The solution is then pumped to the belt machine. The belt (which is moved by a drum) acts as a support for the film that is formed. Belt tension is adjusted in order to ensure a constant flatness, avoid vibrations and to offset the effect of thermal expansion of belt length caused by temperature differences. The commonest support material is stainless steel. The polymeric mixture is uniformly distributed by a spreader, in order to ensure a constant thickness profile. The temperature of the liquid must be constant because temperature changes cause viscosity variations and thus an inhomogeneous thickness distribution. Liquid film is then dried using a stream of hot air (Siemann, 2005).

3.10 Challenges in biopolymer processing

Biopolymers introduce new challenges in processing related to the chemical/physical properties of the processed material and to final product attributes and applications. The most important challenge is to avoid biopolymer degradation resulting from such factors as high temperature and the presence of moisture. It is also critical to ensure that any chemicals used in processing are not harmful. As an example, solvent casting and melt spinning are suitable processes for biomaterials, but there are very strict requirements governing the presence of residual solvent in devices that are used for tissue engineering or drug eluting systems.

High temperatures (that are often required in processes such as injection molding and extrusion, for example) increase the risk of polymer degrading. This implies a great reduction in mean molecular weight and a wider distribution, thus worsening mechanical features of the final device. This sharp variation in molecular weight and distribution modifies degradation and drug release rates. This means that final device behavior is very different from predicted performance. If drug delivery devices are being manufactured, drug thermal degradation must also be taken into account. Biopolymer processing also requires the absence of moisture and residual water because hydrolysis results in biopolymer degradation, particularly at higher temperatures. Biopolymer pellets are often dried in a vacuum environment in order to remove residual moisture.

The following examples review process issues relating to biopolymers. They deal mainly with poly-L-lactic acid (PLLA) processing, because it is the most widely studied biomaterial.

3.10.1 Injection molding and melt extrusion

Harris and Lee (2008) studied the increase of crystallinity of injection molded poly(lactic acid) (PLA). The PLA was first dried and dry mixed with fillers. It was then melt extruded with a twin screw extruder in a temperature range of 160–190 °C with a screw speed of 230 rpm. Extruded pellets were dried and injection molded at various mold temperatures. They found that material crystallinity was enhanced by addition of nucleating agents (about 2%), by annealing injection molded samples or by directly molding the material in a preheated mold.

Taubner and Shishoo (2001) studied the effect of process parameters during the extrusion of PLLA pellets. Extrusion was performed at 210 and 240 °C with a rotational screw speed of 20 and 120 rpm. At 210 °C and 20 rpm, the loss in molecular weight increased. They found that molecular weight drop, at high temperature, does not depend on residual moisture because thermal degradation becomes more important than hydrolysis. Using dry pellets, they showed a dramatic loss in molecular weight at 240 °C and 20 rpm, where it varied from 44 000 to 13 600 g mol^{-1}. Mechanical properties decreased with the decrease in molecular weight.

Jiang *et al.* (2008) prepared a composite material of poly(3-hydroxybutyrate-co-3-hydroxyvalerate) (PHBV) and cellulose by extrusion blending, using a co-rotating twin screw extruder with a temperature profile ranging from 160 to 145 °C. PHBV pellets were dried, dry mixed with a cellulose nanowhisker powder and extruded. The extrudate was cooled in a water bath and the final pellets were dried. This material did not have the same mechanical properties and the same cellulose dispersion as the analogous composite prepared with solvent casting process. It was necessary to add a compatibilizer to improve the dispersion.

Rothen-Weinhold *et al.* (1999) compared extrusion and injection molding processes in the preparation of biodegradable implants, analyzing the behavior of matrices made of PLLA loaded with a somatostatin analogue, *i.e.* vapreotide pamoate. They extruded a powder of PLLA and the drug in a ram extruder at 80 °C. Injection molding was carried out at 100 °C with a cooling temperature of 14 °C and a pressure of 130 bar. Extrusion is a simple technique for manufacturing drug delivery devices because it needs low temperatures, thus avoiding the risk of degradation both of material and the active compound. Injection molding is more appropriate for large scale production, but this process presents some disadvantages such as high temperatures, high amounts of material needed for initial trials and high loss of material during the process. However, both extrusion and injection molding appeared to be suitable methods for device manufacturing. The effect of processing on drug release was also investigated. The vapreotide release rate *in vitro* is higher for extruded implants because injection molding leads to products with a higher crystalline ratio which implies a slower release. Injection molding is a feasible technique for drug loaded devices, but processing conditions have to be modified according to the chemical/physical properties of the drug, *i.e.* in order to avoid degradation of the active compound.

Wang *et al.* (2008) monitored PLLA thermal degradation during melt extrusion, using UV–vis (ultraviolet–visible) spectroscopy. There is a correlation between UV–vis absorption of the melt and the decrease of the molar mass of the extrudate, related to the thermal degradation that occurs during the process. When processing dry PLLA, loss in molecular weight mainly results from thermal degradation, which is linked to heat input (direct heating and conversion of mechanical energy, that depends on screw speed) and to residence time in the barrel. The presence of moisture does not affect UV–vis spectra but it causes further degradation. The degradation rate *in vitro* of extruded samples increases as molecular weight decreases because of processing.

Weir *et al.* (2004) studied the effect of compression molding and extrusion on PLLA. They confirmed that the thermal history of the material has a strong influence on a device's final properties (*i.e.*, molecular weight and mechanical behavior). Perale *et al.* (2008) studied microextrusion of PLLA and poly(glycolic acid) (PGA). They found that this process did not show losses of mean molecular weights. Limited degradation observed during this process makes microextrusion promising for production of biomedical devices.

3.10.2 Melt spinning

Nishimura *et al.* (2005) produced PLLA fibers using a melt spinning process. PLLA was first dried in vacuum at 70 °C, melted and extruded at a melt temperature of 220 °C in order to avoid thermal degradation. Pellets were extruded with a single-screw extruder, at the end of which a spinning nozzle with 12 holes was placed. Extrusion took place in a water bath kept at 45 °C, and spun fibers were drawn at 98 °C in order to have enough energy to achieve solvent evaporation. The mechanical and other properties of the PLLA fibers were preserved.

3.10.3 Solvent casting

Rhim *et al.* (2006) compared two different methods for obtaining PLLA films, *i.e.* solvent casting and thermocompression. In the first case, dried PLLA pellets were dissolved in chloroform at room temperature. The solution was spread on a casting surface (made of Teflon) and allowed to dry for 24 h at room temperature. In the thermocompression process, PLLA was placed in a press formed by two plates of stainless steel lined with aluminum foil, heated to 190 °C. Then, a pressure of about 69 MPa was applied for 3 min. Using the solvent-casting method, PLLA films retained up to 10% of the solvent, which acted as a plasticizer and affected film properties. Thermocompressed film showed a greater thermal stability and better mechanical properties; moreover, they did not contain residual solvent.

Jiang *et al.* (2008) prepared a composite material from PHBV and cellulose using solvent casting. They dissolved PHBV, cellulose nanowhiskers and polyethylene glycol (as a compatibilizer) in *N,N*-dimethylformamide (DMF), and cast the solution on a glass plate at 50 °C in order to realize DMF evaporation. The final material showed a homogeneous dispersion of cellulose nanowhiskers, which improved mechanical properties.

3.10.4 Electrospinning

Electrospinning is a method which uses a high voltage electric field (10–20 kV) to produce fibers from a suspended droplet of polymer melt or solution through a nozzle. The electrostatic field is applied to the end of a capillary tube where the polymer is suspended. A polymer jet is formed when the surface tension of the droplet is overcome by the electrostatic charge. The solvent evaporates from the jet, which elongates and becomes thinner. An electrically charged polymer is left behind, which is solidified and collected on a surface. Electrospinning is useful in the biomedical field because it allows production of fibers with diameters in the nanometer range. Chung *et al.* (2010) produced fibers made of a copolymer [poly(L-lactide-co-ε-caprolactone)] using an electrospinning technique with two different solvents, acetone and 1,1,1,3,3,3-hexafluoro-2-propanol (HFIP). Fiber diameters ranged from 200 to 800 nm with acetone, and from 400 to 1200 with HFIP. The effect of residual solvent was investigated by observing cell behavior on electrospun fibers. They found that solvent traces did not significantly affect cell proliferation.

3.10.5 Preparation of porous structures

The synthesis of porous structures is important in the biomedical field, because these devices are suitable for cell proliferation and tissue regeneration. Zhang and Ma (2000) prepared nanoscale fibrous matrices of PLLA, poly(L-galactic acid) (PLGA) and poly(D, L-lactic acid) (PDLLA) with a five-step procedure: polymer dissolution, phase separation and gelation, solvent extraction from gel with water, freezing and freeze-drying under vacuum. Salerno *et al.* (2008) obtained biodegradable foams using a gas foaming process, with CO_2 as physical foaming agent, and NaCl nanoparticles in order to increase pore-wall opening during foaming and to create additional interconnectivity after leaching. This technique, where particles are used to control porosity and then removed, is named particle leaching. Wei and Ma (2006) used particle leaching to obtain porous PLLA scaffolds, mixing a polymer solution with sugar spheres, and removing them with distilled water. Kramschuster and Turng (2010) combined injection molding and foaming processes. A polymer melt was mixed with supercritical CO_2 at high pressure. In order to ensure a single-phase solution, a pressure of about 200 bar was maintained in the barrel. A pressure drop during injection induces a thermodynamic instability of the solution and the gas emerges from the melt, forming microscale cells.

3.10.6 Preparation of microparticles

Biopolymer microparticles (Freiberg and Zhu, 2004) are gaining a great importance in the drug delivery field, because they allow release of the active compound in a controlled and targeted manner. Microparticles can be obtained starting with monomer polymerization. This process requires a colloidal solution with the monomer dispersed in a liquid with the presence of a surfactant. Polymerization can be achieved with various techniques such as:

- emulsion,
- suspension, and
- dispersion.

The emulsion process allows the production of particles with a diameter in the nanometer range (10–10^4 nm). The monomer is dispersed in water with a water-soluble initiator and a surfactant which forms uniform micelles. Polymerization occurs inside micelles, in which the monomer is able to diffuse, because the initiator is not miscible in the dispersed monomer phase.

The dispersion process produces particles in the range of 0.5–10 μm. Monomer, initiator and stabilizer are dissolved in an organic medium. The initiator is soluble in monomer droplets stabilized by the surfactant. Polymerization takes place at this point. Polymer droplets are not soluble in the organic medium and therefore form a precipitate. Aggregation is avoided by the stabilizer. Suspension polymerization produces micrometer-sized particles (50–500 μm). The monomer is dispersed in water with a stabilizer. The initiator is soluble in the monomer phase where polymerization occurs.

Microspheres can also be prepared using linear polymers with techniques such as spray drying or the solvent evaporation method. Microspheres can be obtained by the evaporation of an organic solvent from dispersed oil droplets containing both polymer and drug, thus also achieving drug loading. The drug is first dissolved in water. This aqueous phase is then dispersed in an organic solvent (such as dichloromethane) which contains the polymer, forming a water/oil emulsion. This is dispersed in a stabilized aqueous medium to obtain the final oil/water emulsion. Organic solvent evaporation is realized, forming the polymer microspheres, which encapsulate the drug.

3.11 Conclusions

It can be seen that injection molding and melt extrusion are suitable methods for biomaterial processing. Injection molding increases the crystallinity of the material. This improves device performance because degradation is reduced and mechanical strength increases. Solvent casting and melt spinning are also suitable methods for the production of biomedical devices, provided that the residual solvent amount is below the minimum value. Electrospinning allows the production of fibers with diameters in the range of nanometers as long as the solvent is removed. Porous structures can be obtained both using foaming process or particle leaching technique. This last technique allows control of pore diameter in tissue scaffold materials. Polymeric microparticles, which are of growing importance in drug delivery, can also be synthesized in ways that avoid thermal degradation or residual solvent traces.

3.12 References

Chung, S. W., Ingle, N. P., Montero, G. A., Kim, S. H. & King, M. W. 2010. Bioresorbable elastomeric vascular tissue engineering scaffolds via melt spinning and electrospinning. *Acta Biomaterialia*, **6**, 1958–1967.

Freiberg, S. & Zhu, X. 2004. Polymer microspheres for controlled drug release. *International Journal of Pharmaceutics*, **282**, 1–18.

Han, C. D. 2007. *Rheology and processing of polymeric materials*, Oxford; New York, Oxford University Press.

Harris, A. M. & Lee, E. C. 2008. Improving mechanical performance of injection molded PLA by controlling crystallinity. *Journal of Applied Polymer Science*, **107**, 2246–2255.

Jiang, L., Morelius, E., Zhang, J. W., Wolcott, M. & Holbery, J. 2008. Study of the Poly(3-hydroxybutyrate-co-3-hydroxyvalerate)/cellulose nanowhisker composites prepared by solution casting and melt processing. *Journal of Composite Materials*, **42**, 2629–2645.

Kramschuster, A. & Turng, L. S. 2010. An injection molding process for manufacturing highly porous and interconnected biodegradable polymer matrices for use as tissue engineering scaffolds. *Journal of Biomedical Materials Research Part B–Applied Biomaterials*, **92B**, 366–376.

Nishimura, Y., Takasu, A., Inai, Y. & Hirabayashi, T. 2005. Melt spinning of poly(L-lactic acid) and its biodegradability. *Journal of Applied Polymer Science*, **97**, 2118–2124.

Osswald, T. A. & Hernández-Ortiz, J. P. 2006. *Polymer processing: modeling and simulation*, Munich; Cincinnati, Hanser Publishers.

Perale, G., Pertici, G., Giordano, C., Daniele, F., Masi, M. & Maccagnan, S. 2008. Non-degradative microextrusion of resorbable polyesters for pharmaceutical and biomedical applications: The cases of poly-lactic-acid and poly-caprolactone. *Journal of Applied Polymer Science*, **108**, 1591–1595.

Rhim, J. W., Mohanty, A. K., Singh, S. P. & Ng, P. K. W. 2006. Effect of the processing methods on the performance of polylactide films: Thermocompression versus solvent casting. *Journal of Applied Polymer Science*, **101**, 3736–3742.

Rothen-Weinhold, A., Besseghir, K., Vuaridel, E., Sublet, E., Oudry, N., Kubel, F. & Gurny, R. 1999. Injection-molding versus extrusion as manufacturing technique for the preparation of biodegradable implants. *European Journal of Pharmaceutics and Biopharmaceutics*, **48**, 113–121.

Salerno, A., Iannace, S. & Netti, P. A. 2008. Open-pore biodegradable foams prepared via gas foaming and microparticulate templating. *Macromolecular Bioscience*, **8**, 655–664.

Siemann, U. 2005. Solvent casting technology – the most suitable tool for LCD polarizer film production. *Proceedings of the Twenty-Fifth International Display Research Conference – Eurodisplay 2005*, 240–242.

Tadmor, Z. & Gogos, C. G. 2006. *Principles of polymer processing*, Hoboken, N.J., Wiley-Interscience.

Taubner, V. & Shishoo, R. 2001. Influence of processing parameters on the degradation of poly(L-lactide) during extrusion. *Journal of Applied Polymer Science*, **79**, 2128–2135.

Wang, Y. M., Steinhoff, B., Brinkmann, C. & Alig, I. 2008. In-line monitoring of the thermal degradation of poly(L-lactic acid) during melt extrusion by UV-vis spectroscopy. *Polymer*, **49**, 1257–1265.

Wei, G. B. & Ma, P. X. 2006. Macroporous and nanofibrous polymer scaffolds and polymer/bone-like apatite composite scaffolds generated by sugar spheres. *Journal of Biomedical Materials Research Part A*, **78A**, 306–315.

Weir, N. A., Buchanan, F. J., Orr, J. F., Farrar, D. F. & Boyd, A. 2004. Processing, annealing and sterilisation of poly-L-lactide. *Biomaterials*, **25**, 3939–3949.

Zhang, R. Y. & Ma, P. X. 2000. Synthetic nano-fibrillar extracellular matrices with predesigned macroporous architectures. *Journal of Biomedical Materials Research*, **52**, 430–438.

4

Understanding transport phenomena and degradation of bioresorbable medical polymers

F. ROSSI and G. PERALE, Politecnico di Milano, Italy

Abstract: The thermodynamic processes involved in degradation and drug release in resorbable polymeric drug loaded systems are explained in detail. To achieve a quantitative description of the thermodynamic movement to equilibrium in such systems presents some mathematical difficulties and the differing approaches are considered. The importance of irreversible thermodynamic processes is investigated by the analysis of phenomenological and kinetic mathematical approaches. The importance of mathematical models in investigating the transport phenomena that influence the design parameters and properties of drug release kinetics is discussed.

Key words: biodegradable polymers; controlled drug release; mathematical modelling; mass transport.

4.1 Introduction to transport phenomena in irreversible processes

Transport phenomena are the subject of more than half of chemical engineering research. All problems of determined physical quantity, such as the manner in which mass, energy or momentum is transferred from one point to another, are collected under this definition. (Beek *et al.*, 1999; Bird *et al.*, 2002). For example, the study of transport phenomena in industrial processes includes the evaluation of: (a) the fluid velocity profile along a pipeline, and (b) the contact surface between two phases for mass or heat transport. The study of transport phenomena began at the end of the 19th century, with the advent of engineering applications related to thermal machines and industrial plants. In general, the definition of *transport phenomena* concerns the transfer of physical units into a system or across its boundary. Its importance is well known to the modern scientific community and its criteria are applied to several different studies and topics. Whereas in classic thermodynamics equilibrium systems are studied, transport phenomena are used to investigate systems that are far from equilibrium and where gradients of quantities such as velocity, temperature or concentrations are present. Concentration gradients are typical of drug delivery systems (Cu and Saltzman, 2009). One system could be analysed according to different scales, each characterised by a typical magnitude. This approach is typical of a multiscale study and makes possible a good overview of the same system from a differing point of view, underlining the importance of each in respect to the others (Bird, 2004). In the macroscopic view, the study deals with finite dimensions where the control volume includes the whole system and the variation in the values of its properties is obtained by balanced equations that contain properties entering and exiting a time unit. The intermediate view of the same system implies analysis and description of phenomena occurring in a defined measurement between a micrometre and a centimetre. The same system studied on the microscopic scale considers transport mechanisms concerned with the molecular properties of that system. From a microscopic point of view, turbulent and chaotic movements of molecules and their clusters are sources of transport phenomena and consequently those systems evolve to equilibrium conditions. Dissipative processes are associated with a process that is phenomenologically identified with the resistances responsible for the dissipation. A thermodynamic system not in equilibrium undergoes a spontaneous irreversible transformation. The speed at which this occurs depends on the characteristics of the system and on its distance from the equilibrium state (X-X_{eq}). The driving force presented here is concentration.

4.1.1 Phenomenological approach

A spontaneous transformation in an isolated system is associated with the creation of entropy (Bird *et al.*, 2002). This entropy variation can be divided into two categories: (a) mass and heat exchange with the environment, and (b) irreversible entropy creation. The phenomenological hypothesis consists of the supposition that the speed of entropy creation, characterising the degree of irreversibility, is directly connected with the driving force of the transformation. The application of this theory is the starting point of several international studies that have attempted to evaluate an adequate mathematical scheme for the description of the characteristics of the process. It is practical to first consider systems constituted by a finite number of regions. In each region, the intensive variables are considered to have uniform values and discontinuities to be in proximity to surfaces which separate different subsystems, assuming appropriate divisions. A globally isolated system is considered, constituted by two subsystems that are divided by a movable wall permeable to a generic i component as presented in Fig. 4.1.

The entropy variation that the system undergoes in a generic infinitesimal transformation from subsystem 1 to subsystem 2, may be expressed as follows:

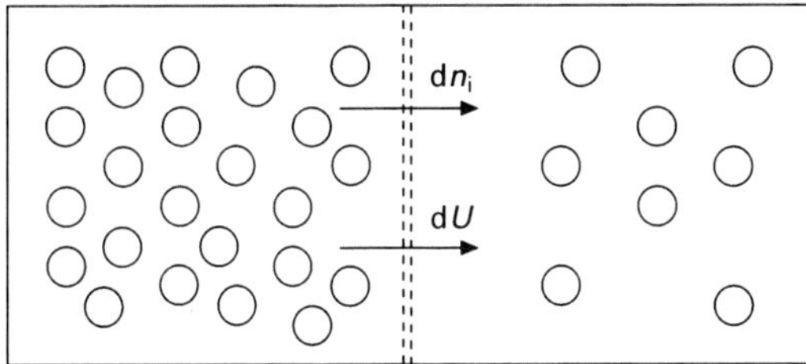

4.1 A globally isolated system, comprising two subsystems divided by a moveable wall permeable to a generic *i* component.

$$\mathrm{d}_{\mathrm{ir}}S = \left(\frac{1}{T^{(1)}} - \frac{1}{T^{(2)}}\right)dU^{(1)} + \left(\frac{P^{(1)}}{T^{(1)}} - \frac{P^{(2)}}{T^{(2)}}\right)\mathrm{d}V^{(1)} + \left(\frac{\mu_{\mathrm{i}}^{(1)}}{T^{(1)}} - \frac{\mu_{\mathrm{i}}^{(2)}}{T^{(2)}}\right)\mathrm{d}n_{\mathrm{i}}^{(1)} = X_{\mathrm{U}}\mathrm{d}U^{(1)} + X_{\mathrm{V}}\,\mathrm{d}V^{(1)} + X_{\mathrm{i}}\,\mathrm{d}n_{\mathrm{i}}^{(1)} \qquad [4.1]$$

where S is the irreversible entropy, T the temperature, P the pressure, U the internal energy, V the volume and μ the chemical potential. The X_{k} above are defined as thermodynamic forces. If the time unit is considered, it is possible to obtain:

$$\frac{\mathrm{d}_{\mathrm{ir}}S}{\mathrm{d}t} = X_{\mathrm{U}}\frac{\mathrm{d}U^{(1)}}{\mathrm{d}t} + X_{\mathrm{V}}\frac{\mathrm{d}V^{(1)}}{\mathrm{d}t} + X_{\mathrm{i}}\frac{\mathrm{d}n_{\mathrm{i}}^{(1)}}{\mathrm{d}t} = X_{\mathrm{U}}J_{\mathrm{U}} + X_{\mathrm{V}}\,J_{\mathrm{V}} + X_{\mathrm{i}}J_{\mathrm{i}} = \sum_{\mathrm{k}} X_{\mathrm{k}}J_{\mathrm{k}} \qquad [4.2]$$

where J_{k} indicates the flow of the different extensive quantities present. In particular, three different types of flows may be defined: J_{U} = internal energy flow, J_{V} = volume flow, J_{i} = *i* component flow.

Using a pure thermal energy flow (heat), J_{Q} expressed as follows could be advantageous:

$$J_{\mathrm{Q}} = J_{\mathrm{U}} - \bar{H}_{\mathrm{i}}J_{\mathrm{i}} \qquad [4.3]$$

The global flow of energy between two subsystems contains an associated contribution to the molecular flow, that for dn_{i} transferred moles are equal to H_{i}dn_{i}. So the flow of pure thermal energy can be obtained by the subtraction between the flows of global energy J_{U} and H_{i}dn_{i}. The speed of entropy creation is expressed by the addition of the products of existing flows in the system in respect to their associated thermodynamic forces. Equation [4.2], referring to a discontinuous system, is constituted of different subsystems, in each of which, the values of the intensive quantities are uniform. The extension to continuous systems in which variables differ in several points exhibits a considerable difficulty: the calculation of entropy in the non-equilibrium state. That difficulty may be overcome using a postulate of local equilibrium: 'To every infinitesimal region of a system is associated a value of entropy and its dependence from local parameters is equal to the correspondent equilibrium states'.

The calculation of the local velocity of entropy creation in a continuous system is a classic exercise of vector analysis. It is appropriate to employ the densities of the extensive quantities involved, reporting to the volume unit. Assuming S as the density of entropy and Y as the density of a generic physical quantity and starting from equation [4.2], the velocity of local creation of entropy could be written as follows:

$$\frac{\partial S}{\partial t} = \sum_{k} X_k \frac{\partial Y_k}{\partial t} \qquad [4.4]$$

The use of a partial differential equation (PD) is necessary because the quantities vary during time and along the space. The definition of flows also needs modification: they could be expressed using J_k vectors that correspond to the quantity transferred in a time and space unit in one direction. If we consider a generic closed surface A, that contains the system (Fig. 4.1), the conservation law of each quantity could be expressed by:

$$\int_V \frac{\partial Y_k}{\partial t} dV + \int_A J_k n \, dA = 0 \qquad [4.5]$$

where n is a unitary vector perpendicular to the surface. Using the Gauss theorem, the following continuity law may be obtained:

$$\frac{\partial Y_k}{\partial t} + \nabla J_k = 0 \qquad [4.6]$$

Substituting equation [4.6] in [4.4] gives:

$$\frac{\partial S}{\partial t} = - \sum_{k} X_k \nabla J_k \qquad [4.7]$$

However, if we consider:

$$X_k \nabla J_k = \nabla (X_k J_k) - J_k \nabla X_k \qquad [4.8]$$

equation [4.7] may be rewritten thus:

$$\frac{\partial S}{\partial t} + \nabla \sum_{k} (X_k J_k) = \sum_{k} J_k \nabla X_k \qquad [4.9]$$

The left side of equation [4.9] is the typical continuity law with the flow expressed by $\sum_{k} (X_k J_k)$, whereas on the right, there is the local velocity of entropy creation. It may be easily observed that the velocity is still expressed by a bilinear form of flows and forces represented by gradients of the X_k.

Researching the expression of forces and their corresponding flows in different physical situations presents a difficult problem. In Table 4.1 the expressions that correspond to particular interesting situations are summarised.

The analysis illustrated above appears to be very theoretical and far removed from its physical implications, as it establishes the definitions of flows and forces and expresses the velocity of entropy generation in a system prepared for an irreversible transformation. For a better understanding, it is necessary to examine evidence of the relationship between flows and the corresponding driving forces. Researching the appropriate laws that express the dependence of flows by the forces involved in a determined system goes back to the very beginning of thermodynamics. Flows may be written using a power series development:

$$J_k = \sum_l L_{lk} X_l + \frac{1}{2!} \sum_{m,l} L_{mlk} X_m X_l + \ldots \qquad [4.10]$$

The constant term of the development is omitted because every flow is cancelled out when the forces are equal to zero. The quantities L_{lk}, L_{mlk} ... are termed the phenomenological coefficient of first, second order etc. In equation [4.10], the existence of combined effects derived from the union of processes apparently independent of each other is included. Specific information about equation [4.10] has been obtained by historic experience. In 1811, Fourier observed that in the first approximation, a heat flow is linearly dependent on the temperature gap. Subsequently, Fick emphasised that the longitudinal mass flow is proportional to the difference of concentration. At the same time, Ohm established that an electric flow in a conductor depends linearly on the corresponding forces. All these observations are evidence that in a situation close to equilibrium, flows could be assumed to be proportional to the forces, so equation [4.10] could be approximated to:

$$J_k = \sum_l L_{lk} X_l \qquad [4.11]$$

The presence of coupled phenomena was emphasised by other experiences, as for example, electric current and heat transport in solid conductors. A

Table 4.1 Flows and conjugated forces in continuous and discontinuous systems

Flows	Forces	
	Discontinuous systems	Continuous systems
Chemical reactions $(1/v_i)dC_i/dt$	$-(1/T)(\partial G/\partial \lambda)_{P,T}$	$-(1/T)(\partial G/\partial \lambda)_{P,T}$
Heat flow J_Q	$\Delta(1/T) \cong \Delta T/T^2$	$\Delta(1/T) \cong \Delta T/T^2$
Mass flow J_i	$\Delta(\mu_i/T)$	$-\nabla(\mu_i/T)$
Volume flow J_V	$\Delta(P/T)$	$-\nabla(P/T)$
Electricity flow J_e	$\Delta\psi/T$	$-(1/T)\nabla\psi$

fluid is subject to convective motion when there is a temperature gap at its extremes. The phenomenology considered is more complex, as appears in Table 4.2.

The previous results justify the form of equation [4.11] as coupled phenomena have a specific role and their entity depends on the value of the mixed coefficient L_{lk}. However, a large number of coefficients is inconvenient and much experimental work would be necessary to estimate them independently. This may be avoided by using the symmetry law of Onsager: 'The entire set of phenomenological coefficients forms a matrix where reciprocity relations are valid'. In mathematical terms it can be expressed thus:

$$L_{lk} = L_{kl} \quad [4.12]$$

This law (1931) was the first attempt to use the thermodynamics of irreversible processes as a useful instrument for the rationalisation of physical–chemical systems. An example of the application of the above is the Seebeck effect in the thermoelectric field. If the extremities of a bimetallic couple reach different temperatures, there will be a flow of electrical current I caused by the potential difference. Considering Table 4.1 and the discontinuous system gives:

$$J_Q = L_{11}\frac{\Delta T}{T^2} + L_{12}\frac{\Delta \psi}{T} \quad [4.13]$$

$$I = L_{21}\frac{\Delta T}{T^2} + L_{22}\frac{\Delta \psi}{T} \quad [4.14]$$

From these relations, the following may be obtained:

$$\left(\frac{J_Q}{I}\right)_{\Delta T=0} = \frac{L_{12}}{L_{22}} \text{ and } -\left(\frac{\Delta \psi}{\Delta T}\right)_{I=0} = \frac{L_{21}}{L_{22}T}$$

Using the Onsager law defined above ($L_{12} = L_{21}$):

$$\left(\frac{J_Q}{I}\right)_{\Delta T=0} = -T\left(\frac{\Delta \psi}{\Delta T}\right)_{I=0} = \frac{L_{21}}{L_{22}} \quad [4.15]$$

There exists therefore, a well-defined proportional relation between the temperature and potential differences in the absence of an electric current.

Table 4.2 Phenomena involved for energy and mass flows

	ΔT	ΔC
Energy flow	Heat conduction (Fourier)	Thermo diffusion (Dufour)
Mass flow	Thermal diffusion (Soret)	Diffusion (Fick)

It is interesting to consider the mass and heat transfer processes in a fluid system constituted of a mixture of two non-reactant components with temperature and chemical potential gradients. Using equation [4.11] the following expressions of component and heat flows are obtained:

$$J_1 = L_{11}X_1 + L_{12}X_2 + L_{13}X_Q$$

$$J_2 = L_{21}X_1 + L_{22}X_2 + L_{23}X_Q$$

$$J_3 = L_{31}X_1 + L_{32}X_2 + L_{33}X_Q \qquad [4.16]$$

The system is in a steady state, thus:

$$J_1 + J_2 = 0 \qquad [4.17]$$

because the total molar flow should be equal to zero. This last relation is compatible with equation [4.11] only if $L_{11} = -L_{21}$, $L_{12} = -L_{22}$ and $L_{13} = -L_{23}$. Using the Onsager law explained as $L_{12} = L_{21}$, $L_{13} = L_{31}$, $L_{23} = L_{32}$, the phenomenological laws in equation [4.17] can be written in a more concise manner with only three parameters, L_{21}, L_{13} and L_{33}:

$$J_1 = -J_2 = -L_{21}(X_2 - X_1) + L_{13}X_Q$$

$$J_Q = L_{13}(X_1 - X_2) + L_{33}X_Q \qquad [4.18]$$

where the force expressions are summarised in Table 4.1. The above relations make possible the description of the four phenomena involved:

1. Diffusion: term $L_{21}(X_2 - X_1)$ flow of each component caused by concentration difference.
2. Heat conduction: term $L_{33}X_Q$ heat flow deriving from temperature difference.
3. Thermal diffusion or the *Soret effect*: term $L_{13}(X_1 - X_2)$ mass reflux caused by temperature difference.
4. Dufour thermodiffusive effect: term $L_{13}(X_1 - X_2)$ heat flow deriving from concentration difference.

The listed phenomena are only examples and there are many more in which it is possible to apply the thermodynamics of irreversible processes in a linear phenomenological setting, such as problems in the biophysics field. In cases where the knowledge of macroscopic mechanisms is limited, the use of thermodynamics in irreversible processes could be useful. However, it should be noted that this approach does not give any information about the nature of the coefficients involved and so could give rise to errors if the linearity hypothesis is not respected. So the thermodynamics of irreversible processes has a very large field of application, but its contribution is not as yet significant.

4.1.2 Kinetic approach

The evolution of a thermodynamic system towards the equilibrium condition may also be studied by a different approach (Hirschfelder *et al.*, 1954). The kinetic theory may be used to understand the behaviour of rarefied gases. Interactions involve pairs of molecules because collision with a larger number of molecules appears improbable. The motion of a molecule can be simulated with a zig-zag representing the mean free path between two consecutive collisions (Chapman and Cowling, 1939; Reid *et al.*, 1987). The mean value of that quantity is indicated as l. In low-density gases this is around 10^{-5} cm. This system may be described by a statistical approach in which referring to a space of phases is advantageous. This space has six dimensions which indicate the position $r(x_k, x_l, x_m)$ and the velocity $v(v_k, v_l, v_m)$ of a generic molecule. Moreover, if $dr = dx_k dx_l dx_m$ and $dv = dv_k dv_l dv_m$ is considered, the element with the volume of the geometric and velocity space, the product $d\Omega = dr dv$ indicates an element with the volume of the phases space. The insertion of a distribution function $f(r, v, t)$ is useful in such an expression, $f(r, v, t)\, dr\, dv$ supplies the number of molecules present in dr, having included the velocity between v and $v + dv$ at time t. In a more general setting, it would also be necessary to consider the variables relative to the external motion of molecules. However, in this phase, that effect is ignored so the treatment is only valid for monatomic gases. In addition, f is considered as a continuous function. This approximation is only valid if dr represents a physical volume having dimensions greater than l^3 and smaller than the system dimensions. It should be noted that $f(r, v, t)$ is essentially a function with the properties of molecules number/volume and velocity from which the average values of the observable quantities may be evaluated. Thus, the molecular density is:

$$\hat{n} = \int f(r,v,t)dv \qquad [4.19]$$

and the total number of molecules is:

$$N = \int \int f(r,v,t)drdv \qquad [4.20]$$

whereas, in general, for a quantity ψ, the flow of ψ in the k direction is:

$$<\psi_{vk}> = \int v_k f(r,v,t)\psi dv \qquad [4.21]$$

This last relation is particularly important in studying irreversible processes where different types of flows are involved. The mass flow in the z direction is:

$$J_k = \int v_k f(r,v,t)dv \qquad [4.22]$$

the momentum flow is:

$$P_{\mathrm{kl}} = \int (mv_{\mathrm{k}})v_{\mathrm{k}}\, f(r,v,t)\mathrm{d}v \qquad [4.23]$$

and the kinetic energy flow is:

$$q_{\mathrm{k}} = \int \left(\frac{mv}{2}\right) v_{\mathrm{k}}\, f(r,v,t)\mathrm{d}v \qquad [4.24]$$

In the definitions above, flows are considered to be vectorial quantities (energy and mass) which express the transport in time and surface units. In a non-uniform gas system which is in a condition of non-equilibrium, the velocity of molecules could be expressed by the addition of two terms: $v = u + c$. The first, u, is associated with an eventual convective motion of molecules, whereas c considers chaotic molecular motions. The balance of the molecules contained in a volume element $\mathrm{d}\Omega$ of phase space should be considered in a $\mathrm{d}t$ time interval. A molecule moving from r to $r+v\,\mathrm{d}t$ in the absence of collisions may be expressed as:

$$f(r + v\mathrm{d}t,\, v,\, t + \mathrm{d}t)\mathrm{d}\Omega = f(r,\, v,\, t)\mathrm{d}\Omega \qquad [4.25]$$

From this relation, it is easily established that molecules initially at point (r, v), arrive at $(r+\mathrm{d}r,\, v)$. If collisions are considered, the situation is very different:

$$\left| f(r + v\mathrm{d}t,\, v,\, t + \mathrm{d}t) - f(r,\, v,\, t)\right| \mathrm{d}\Omega = (\Gamma^{+} - \Gamma^{-})\mathrm{d}\Omega\mathrm{d}t \qquad [4.26]$$

The terms Γ^{+} and Γ^{-} indicate the number of molecules gained or lost during a time unit in $\mathrm{d}\Omega$ by the collision effect. If a development in the Taylor series is considered, the following is obtained:

$$f(r + v\mathrm{d}t,\, v,\, t + \mathrm{d}t) = f(r,\, v,\, t) + \left[v\nabla + \frac{\partial f}{\partial t}\right]\mathrm{d}t + \ldots \qquad [4.27]$$

The transport equation [4.28] is derived by substituting [4.26] in [4.27]:

$$\frac{\partial f}{\partial t} + v\nabla f = \Gamma^{+} - \Gamma^{-} = \Gamma \qquad [4.28]$$

This case is completely different as the molecular chaos may generate transport without the presence of a gradient.

4.1.3 Importance of mass transport: membrane for controlled drug delivery

During recent decades, the biomedical industry has developed a large number of devices able to control the delivery of drugs, growth factors or protein, and in particular, the well-known zero-order drug delivery, constant over time. Clearly, owing to the diffusion effect, the mass transfer becomes a decreasing trend. During drug diffusion, concentration decreases with the driving force. In order to counterbalance the Fick law effect, companies have proposed many alternatives such as double release through a patch. In these systems, the drug is highly concentrated within particles loaded in a larger matrix (the patch) (Mauri, 2005). The drug initially diffuses through the matrix where its concentration varies more slowly than in the particles. It can then be transported into the target tissue. However, this system is not always effective because the drug delivery decreases over time. Researchers have therefore explored many alternatives aiming to provide constant drug delivery in which diffusion is coupled with a transport phenomenon. An example of drug delivery controlled by enzymes is as follows. The decreasing trend of the diffusive drug flow is counterbalanced with an increase in porosity of the matrix, owing to enzymatic erosion. Therefore, the diffusion force decreases but the diffusion coefficient increases. It is possible to use a bio-artificial polymeric matrix composed of natural and synthetic polymers such as amide and polyvinyl alcohol. By entrapping amylase in the composite matrix, it is possible to manage and control the effects of the driving forces and diffusion coefficients. The most important physical properties of a membrane are its hydraulic permeability and effective diffusion coefficient. The permeability k measures the facility of crossing the membrane and may be approximated with Darcy's law:

$$V = \frac{k}{\mu L}\Delta P \tag{4.29}$$

where V is the flow velocity, ΔP the difference of pressure, μ the viscosity and L the membrane depth. Using the Blake–Kozeny semiempirical correlation, the permeability could be established as:

$$k = \frac{\delta^2 \varepsilon^3}{150(1-\varepsilon)^2} \tag{4.30}$$

where ε is the matrix porosity and δ the dimensions of the pores. In general, k increases as the porosity and dimensions increase. The other quantity involved is the effective diffusivity that measures solute diffusion through the composite material. It is assumed that on one side of the membrane there is a fluid with a solute at low concentration C_s, and a pure fluid on the other side. This is a common situation in drug delivery, where the clearance does not allow the formation of an equilibrium state. In the absence of ΔP (convection phenomena) the solute massive flow J_s is determined by Fick's law:

$$J_S = \frac{D}{L} C_S \tag{4.31}$$

where D is the effective diffusivity evaluated as the product between molecular diffusivity and a constant depending on the matrix microstructure. In a more complex example with convection, J_s can be described as:

$$J_S = cV - D\frac{dc}{dz} \qquad [4.32]$$

where z is the distance from the membrane surface (longitudinal coordination axis), $c = c(z)$ is the local solute concentration, V is the average velocity of the solvent fluid and is proportional to ΔP. It must be noted that D presented here is different from the effective diffusivity introduced above, owing to dependence on the convective motion. When considered at the microscopic level, convection ignores the diffusion phenomenon, therefore the microscopic Peclet number ($Pe_\delta = V\delta/D_m >> 1$) is very high and the effective diffusivity can be expressed by:

$$D = \alpha^{-1} D_m Pe_\delta = \alpha^{-1} V\delta \qquad [4.33]$$

where α represents the tortuosity which is highly dependent on the microstructure of the matrix. From this, it is evident that D could be very much higher than D_m. Under constant conditions, solving $dJ_s/dz = 0$ with boundary conditions $c\ (0) = c_s$ and $c(L) = 0$, it is evident that $Sh = Pe/(1 - e^{-Pe})$, where $Sh = J_s/(Dc_s/L)$ and $Pe = VL/D = L/\alpha\delta$. Here Sh indicates the Sherwood number, the ratio between the solute mass flow and its microscopic diffusion component; whereas Pe is the macroscopic Peclet number as the ratio between the convective macroscopic mass flow and the diffusive flow. Peclet represents the ratio between the macroscopic and the microscopic scales. Because here $Pe >> 1$:

$$\lim_{Pe>>1} Sh = Pe \rightarrow \lim_{Pe>>1} J_s = \frac{kc_s}{\mu L} \cdot \Delta P \qquad [4.34]$$

It is necessary to consider enzymatic erosion in any detailed discussion of this topic. This process takes place in two steps: firstly, amide penetration through the membrane (transported by water) and pore walls; secondly, the enzymatic reaction occurs and the amide reacts with the enzyme trapped within the matrix, producing maltose. The characteristic duration of this process is generally the sum of the penetration time (τ_p) and the reaction time (τ_r). Therefore, because the reaction velocity (R_s) is proportional to the amide concentration c_s, the following is obtained:

$$R_s = r_s c_s \quad \text{where} \quad r_s = \frac{1}{\tau_s} = \frac{1}{\tau_p + \tau_r} \qquad [4.35]$$

The slowest process determines the hydrolysis kinetic. Here $\tau_r << \tau_p$ and therefore:

$$R_s = r_s c_s \frac{c_s}{\tau_p} \quad [4.36]$$

Initially, the membrane is completely dry, so the water, containing amide, penetrates by capillary flow. Assuming the pore walls are wettable (contact angle = 0°), the flow velocity in the longitudinal direction (perpendicular to the membrane surface) into the matrix is:

$$\frac{dz}{dt} = V_\sigma = \frac{\sigma\delta}{4\mu\alpha^2 z} \quad [4.37]$$

where σ is the superficial tension, z the penetration depth and α the tortuosity coefficient. This last coefficient assumes that in this model, pores are open to small pipes with radius δ which cross the membrane with an average length of l and thus: $\alpha = l/L$. Therefore, the penetration depth and the average velocity may be expressed as:

$$z = \sqrt{\frac{\sigma\delta t}{2\alpha^2\mu}} \Rightarrow V_\sigma = \sqrt{\frac{\sigma\delta}{8\alpha^2\mu t}} \quad [4.38]$$

This stage continues until the penetration depth is equal to half of the membrane depth. Thus for time (Fig. 4.2):

$$t < t^* = \frac{\alpha^2 L^2 \mu}{2\sigma\delta} \quad [4.39]$$

The process is dominated by convection ($Pe >> 1$) and so the amount of amide that reacts during the time unit J_{tot}, is equal to the amount that enters the membrane and is represented by the sum of the entering mass flow of

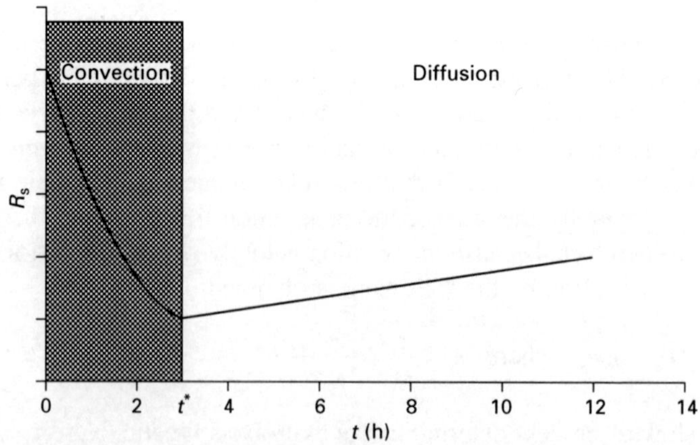

4.2 Kinetics of the hydrolytic reaction showing the respective dominant phenomena: convection for $t < t^*$ and diffusion for $t < t^*$.

the amide ($J_c = c_s V_\sigma$) and the wettable area εS, where ε is tortuosity and S is the membrane surface. Considering that the membrane volume is equal to LS, the velocity of the hydrolytic reaction (R_s), represented by the quantity of amide that reacts in the unit of time and membrane volume, is:

$$R_s = \frac{J_c(\varepsilon S)}{SL} = \frac{\varepsilon c_s}{\alpha L} \cdot \sqrt{\frac{\sigma\delta}{8\mu t}} \qquad [4.40]$$

Assuming that ε and δ are constant, R_s is decreasing as $t^{-1/2}$. For $t > t^*$, convective terms are absent and amide penetrates into the membrane only by diffusion. Thus, the characteristic penetration time is the diffusive one, $\tau_d = \alpha^2 L^2 / D_m$ and R_s may be expressed as:

$$R_s = r_s c_s \text{ where } r_s = \frac{1}{\tau_d} = \frac{D_m}{\alpha^2 L^2} \qquad [4.41]$$

At this stage, it is evident that as the enzymatic reaction occurs, the tortuosity α decreases and the speed of the hydrolytic reaction increases with time.

4.2 Introduction to mathematical modelling

Modelling may be viewed as a cognitive activity aimed at describing the behaviour of devices or objects in mathematical terms. Mathematical models are generally categorised as either empirical or theoretical. An empirical model is represented by a mathematical equation capable of describing the experimental trend of a quantity of interest, e.g. a drug or monomer concentration, as in the two following examples (4.2.1 and 4.2.2). Owing to the absence of a real mathematical analogy for the experimental evidence, its parameters have no physical meaning. For this reason, it does not draw on theoretical knowledge of the phenomena involved, but allows a more objective comparison between different experimental data on the basis of model parameter variations.

A theoretical model represents a possible mathematical schematisation of all the phenomena that are in agreement with the experimental evidence to be studied. In this case, the parameters possess physical meaning and so could be used to predict the experimental trend under different conditions. The theoretical model is therefore a better tool than the empirical model. However, owing to the high level of complexity of the biological factors, it is sometimes impossible to use a theoretical model. Although the reasons for using a mathematical model are implicit from the preceding discussion on empirical and theoretical models, it is worth emphasising the practical consequences of this approach. Indeed, in an industrial world increasingly interested in maximising earnings, the possibility of cutting expenses and experimental trials is very attractive.

In this context, mathematical modelling can be seen as a powerful tool, enabling a reduction in the number of experiments and their necessary assessments. Thus, many time-consuming experiments with a trial-and-error approach are replaced by the selection of a small number to confirm or reject hypotheses from the experimental evidence. Model building can be extremely difficult, especially in selecting the best model to describe a particular phenomenon. Figure 4.3 shows a schematic representation of the actions required to achieve a reliable model. Starting from the phenomenon analysis, the first step is the identification of the single mechanisms ruling the chosen phenomenon. Following that, validation of the hypothesis is translated into a mathematical equation. If the model is then able to fit the experimental data, its ability to predict new situations is tested to see if a reliable model has been obtained. Thus, we decided to focus our attention on two typical topics of biodegradable polymeric devices: modelling their ability to deliver the drugs loaded within them, and their biodegradability.

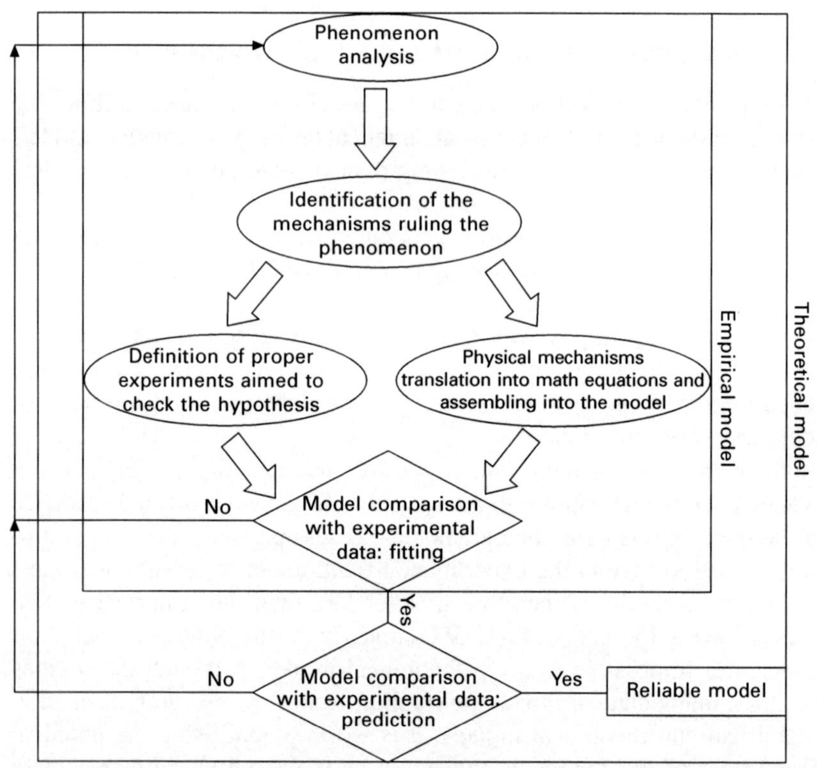

4.3 Schematic representation of the process for obtaining a reliable mathematical model.

4.2.1 Example of drug delivery model for suture threads

The following example, developed by Perale *et al.* (2009), was performed on a resorbable loaded polymeric device. The clarity of the mathematical model confirms the points underlined in this chapter when considering the irreversibility of drug delivery (Dantzig and Tucker, 2001). This assumption, in thermodynamic terms, is true in an *in vivo* context where the drug is immediately consumed by the body, and in fluid clearance. The concentration of the drug outside the device could be considered as always being equal to zero, and thus it cannot be treated as an equilibrium problem. A typical drug delivery scenario consists of three components: a matrix structure, which does not diffuse, thus having a diffusion coefficient of zero, water from the external environment which moves inside matrix structure, and the drug, which usually diffuses from the inner matrix to the external release environment. The drug is usually entrapped as solid particles within the volume of the porous polymer. Without loss of generality, drug particles are assumed to be uniformly scattered in the entire cross-section of the examined device. This hypothesis can be easily discarded when devices with non-uniform distribution of the drug particles are under consideration. In that framework, the drug release mechanism may be described through the following steps illustrated in Fig. 4.4:

1. Water diffuses through the polymeric matrix, wetting all its pores and activating the polymer swelling.
2. Solid drug particles are then wetted by water.

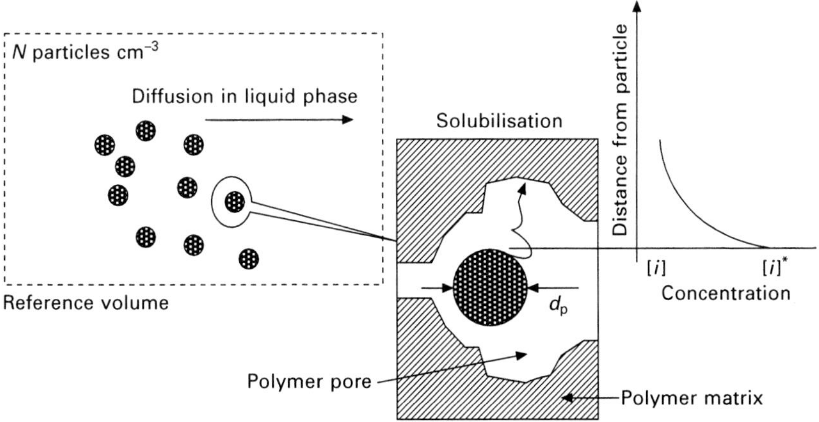

4.4 Schematic representation of the solubilisation of solid drug particles embedded in polymer matrix. Reprinted with permission from Elsevier (Perale *et al.*, 2009).

3. The drug in contact with the water starts to solubilise according to its thermodynamics and the kinetics of the process.
4. A solubilised amount of the drug diffuses through the polymer matrix.

The solubilisation of a solid drug particle placed in a generic location within the device and n_i moles of the examined drug can be expressed by the following equation:

$$\frac{\partial n_i}{\partial t} = -k_C([i]^* - [i])\pi d_p^2 \qquad [4.42]$$

where k_C, $[i]$, $[i]^*$ and d_p are the mass transport coefficients for the drug within a stagnant fluid layer, the drug molar concentration in the liquid phase surrounding the solid particle and its solubility value in water and the particle diameter, respectively. For sake of simplicity, equation [4.42] assumes solid particles of spherical shape. Because $n_i = \rho_i \pi d^3_p/6$, equation [4.42] can be written in terms either of n_i or d_p, where ρ_i is the molar density of the solid drug. The mass transfer coefficient k_C can be estimated by means of the penetration theory because the liquid phase surrounding the solid drug particles is stagnant, and thus $Sh = 8/\pi = k_C d_p/D_i$ is the relationship to be used (Crank, 1975; Crank and Park, 1968). In the unit polymer, volume N particles are present and consequently, assuming these particles to be a monodisperse size system, the overall drug dissolution rate in relation to the device volume can be evaluated as follows:

$$\Delta_i = N\rho_i k_C([i]^* - [i])\pi(6n_i/\pi\rho_i)^{2/3} \qquad [4.43]$$

Finally, the equation expressing the mass balance for the drug in the liquid phase is as follows:

$$\varepsilon\frac{\partial[i]}{\partial t} = D_i\nabla^2[i] + \Delta_i \qquad [4.44]$$

where ε is the polymer porosity after polymer swelling. Thus, the final conservation equations for the dispersed drug are expressed by the combination of equation [4.42] and equation [4.44]. The boundary conditions for equation 4.44 are the symmetry and drug concentration in the solution surrounding the device. As the released drug is effectively removed under actual *in vivo* conditions by the outer fluids, its concentration in the media surrounding the device may be safely assumed to be zero (Birkett, 2002). The initial conditions are the initial size of the uniformly dispersed solid drug particles and a zero concentration in the liquid phase within the device. After these assumptions, it seems evident that polymeric devices for drug delivery should be treated as irreversible thermodynamic systems and their study could be included in the classic engineering topic of transport phenomena.

4.2.2 Example of polymer degradation modelling in polyesters

The degradation model is based on the formal proposal by Arosio *et al.* (2008) for aliphatic polyesters, because the available experimental data relates to this kind of biopolymer. Polymer degradation results from the hydrolysis mechanism. Water penetrates into the device and breaks the polymer backbone, producing small oligomers. These chain fragments are unable to diffuse properly from the matrix and they also catalyse a depolymerisation reaction because of their acidic groups. These phenomena make it possible to adopt a shrinking core approach, in which the system can be roughly divided in two zones: a degraded inner core and an external shell of unbroken polymer as shown in Fig. 4.5.

Mass fluxes are expressed with an effective mass transport coefficient and a concentration difference between the polymeric phase and the external environment. It is assumed that only monomers are able to leave the matrix because of the low mobility of chain fragments. The adopted kinetic scheme is one of reversible polycondensation: $P_{n+m} + W \leftrightarrow P_n + P_m$. Polymer degradation can thus be described through three mass balances involving monomer, water and n-long polymer chains respectively:

$$\frac{dC_M}{dt} = k_{C,M}\frac{S_{EXT}}{V_M}(C_M^0 - C_M) - 2k_P C_M \sum_{n=1}^{\infty} C_n + 2\frac{k_P}{K_{EQ}} C_W \sum_{n=2}^{\infty} C_n \quad [4.45]$$

$$\frac{dC_W}{dt} = k_{C,W}\frac{S_{EXT}}{V_R}(C_W^0 - C_W) + k_P \sum_{n=1}^{\infty} C_n \sum_{m=1}^{\infty} C_m - \frac{k_P}{K_{EQ}} C_W \sum_{n=1}^{\infty} (n-1)C_n \quad [4.46]$$

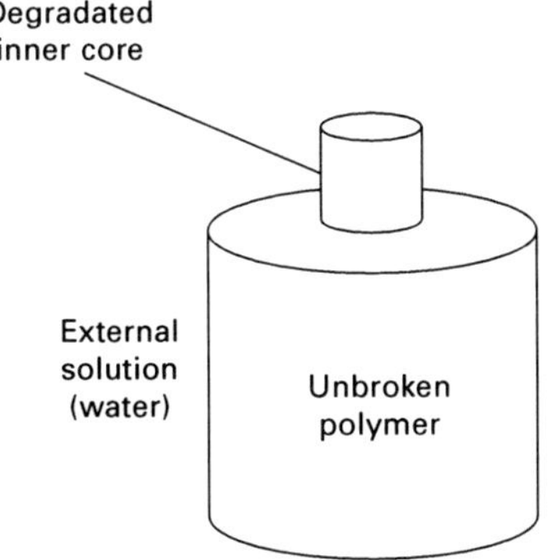

4.5 Schematic representation of shrinking core polymer degradation.

$$\frac{dC_n}{dt} = k_P \sum_{j=1}^{n-1} C_j C_{n-j} - 2k_P C_n \sum_{j=1}^{\infty} C_j$$

$$+2\frac{k_P}{K_{EQ}} C_W \sum_{j=n+1}^{\infty} C_j - \frac{k_P}{K_{EQ}} C_W (n-1) C_n \qquad [4.47]$$

where C_i, C_i^0 and $k_{C,i}$ are the molar concentration, the molar concentration in the external environment, and the effective mass transport coefficient for the *i*th species, respectively, k_P is the polymerisation kinetic constant, K_{EQ} is the polymerisation equilibrium constant, S_{EXT} is the external coating surface, V_R is the device volume and V_M is the volume of the degraded inner zone. In order to simplify the model, which would result in a large system of differential equations, the method of moments was applied. As the water and monomer mass balance equations (equations [4–45]–[4.47]) can be written in terms of statistical moments (μ_i), the following system is obtained:

$$\frac{dC_M}{dt} = k_{C,M} \frac{S_{EXT}}{V_M} (C_M^0 - C_M) - 2k_P C_M \mu_0 + \frac{k_P}{K_{EQ}} C_W (\mu_0 - C_M) \qquad [4.48]$$

$$\frac{dC_W}{dt} = k_{C,W} \frac{S_{EXT}}{V_R} (C_W^0 - C_W) + k_P \mu_0^2 - \frac{k_P}{K_{EQ}} C_W (\mu_1 - \mu_0) \qquad [4.49]$$

$$\frac{d\mu_0}{dt} = k_{C,M} \frac{S_{EXT}}{V_M} (C_M^0 - C_M) - k_P \mu_0^2 + \frac{k_P}{K_{EQ}} C_W (\mu_1 - \mu_0) \qquad [4.50]$$

$$\frac{d\mu_1}{dt} = k_{C,M} \frac{S_{EXT}}{V_M} (C_M^0 - C_M) \qquad [4.51]$$

$$\frac{d\mu_2}{dt} = k_{C,M} \frac{S_{EXT}}{V_M} (C_M^0 - C_M) + 2k_P \mu_1^2 + \frac{k_P C_W}{3K_{EQ}} \left(\mu_1 - 2\frac{\mu_2^2}{\mu_1} + \frac{\mu_2 \mu_1}{\mu_0} \right) \qquad [4.52]$$

Quantities such as average molecular weight and poly-dispersity can be directly computed from statistical moments.

4.3 Conclusions and future trends

The purpose of this chapter is to underline the importance of transport phenomena and mathematical modelling in biomedical applications where a thermodynamic system, not in an equilibrium condition, undergoes a spontaneous irreversible transformation, as in classic drug delivery systems. The irreversibility of thermodynamic processes was thoroughly investigated from a mathematical point of view, using phenomenological and kinetic approaches. Three biomedical examples were analysed in detail: membranes in controlled drug delivery, drug delivery from suture threads and the degradation of polyesters.

The recent highlighting of transport phenomena has focused research attention on its molecular aspects. The availability of high-level dynamic molecular codes has made possible the simulation of biological fluids similar to the actual conditions. Application to biological systems requires the inclusion of transport mechanisms that take into account the particular nature of cellular membranes and the phenomena of biological environments.

4.4 References

Arosio, P., Busini, V., Perale, G., Moscatelli, D. & Masi, M. 2008. A new model of resorbable device degradation and drug release – Part I: zero order model. *Polymer International*, **57**, 912.

Beek, W. J., Muttzall, K. M. K. & Van Heuven, J. W. 1999. *Transport phenomena*. New York, USA: J. Wiley & Sons.

Bird, R. B., Stewart, W. E. & Lightfoot, E. N. 2002. *Transport phenomena 2nd edition*. New York, USA: J. Wiley & Sons.

Bird, R. B. 2004. Five decades of transport phenomena. *AIChE Journal*, **50**, 273.

Birkett, D. J. (2002). *Pharmacokinetics made easy*. Australia: McGraw Hill.

Chapman, S. & Cowling, T. G. 1939. *The mathematical theory of non-uniform gases*. Cambridge, UK: Cambridge University Press.

Crank, J. 1975. *The mathematics of diffusion*. Oxford, UK: Oxford University Press.

Crank, J. & Park, G. S. 1968. *Diffusion in polymers*. New York, USA: Academic Press.

Cu, Y. & Saltzman, W. M. 2009. Mathematical modeling of molecular diffusion through mucus. *Advanced Drug Delivery Reviews*, **61**, 101.

Dantzig, J. A. & Tucker, C. L. 2001. *Modeling in materials processing*. Cambridge, UK: Cambridge University Press.

Hirschfelder, J. O., Curtiss, C. F. & Bird, R. B. 1954. *Molecular theory of gases and liquids*. New York: J. Wiley & Sons.

Mauri, R. 2005. *Elements of transport phenomena*. Pisa: PLUS.

Perale, G., Arosio, P., Moscatelli, D., Barri, V., Muller, M., Maccagnan, S. & Masi, M. 2009. A new model of resorbable device degradation and drug release: Transient 1-dimension diffusional model. *Journal of Controlled Release*, **136**, 196.

Reid, R. C., Prausnitz, J. M. & Poling, B. E. 1987. *The properties of gases and liquids*. New York, USA: McGraw Hill.

5 Synthetic bioresorbable polymers

R. E. CAMERON and A. KAMVARI-MOGHADDAM,
University of Cambridge, UK

Abstract: The main families of synthetic bioresorbable polymers, which find wide medical application as temporary mechanical supports such as sutures, as tissue engineering scaffolds, and as mediators of release rate for the controlled release of drugs are outlined. The physical and chemical mechanisms by which they degrade are discussed and the factors that can affect their rates of degradation are examined.

Key words: poly(alpha-hydroxy acids), degradation rate, polyglycolide, polylactide, degradation.

Note: This chapter was previously published as Chapter 3 'Synthetic bioresorbable polymers' by R. E. Cameron and A. Kamvari-Moghaddam, originally published in *Degradation rate of bioresorbable materials: predication and evaluation*, ed. F. J. Buchanan, Woodhead Publishing Limited, 2008 ISBN: 978-1-84569-329-9.

5.1 Introduction

Biomaterials are materials of natural or manmade origin that are used to direct, supplement, or replace the functions of tissues of the human body.[1] The use of biomaterials dates back to ancient civilisations; artificial eyes, ears, teeth and noses were found on Egyptian mummies, and waxes, glues and tissue were used by the Chinese and Indians in reconstructing missing or defective parts of the body.[2] Advances made in synthetic materials, sterilisation methods and surgical techniques have allowed progress to be made in the way biomaterials are used today. Biomaterials in the form of implants (such as sutures, screws, bone plates, joint replacements, heart valves, intraocular lenses and dental implants) and medical devices (such as pacemakers and biosensors) are regularly used to replace and restore damaged or dysfunctional tissues and organs within the body, thus helping to improve quality of life.

Polymer chemical structure can be tailored to control degradation behaviour, making them, under physiological conditions, bioinert or bioresorbable over a defined period. Polymer degradation is generally denoted by a deterioration in the functionality of the polymeric material caused by a change in its physical and/or chemical properties.[3] In this chapter, the different degradation mechanisms for synthetic bioresorbable polymers are presented and factors influencing their degradation are highlighted.

5.2 Bioresorbable polymers

Synthetic biodegradable polymers were first used commercially as medical implants in the late 1960s with the introduction of the biodegradable suture material Dexon®.[4] A steady progression in biodegradable polymer development has led to a growth in their experimental and clinical use in the fields of orthopaedics and traumatology as fracture fixation devices, in the pharmaceutical industry as drug delivery devices and, most recently, as scaffolds for tissue engineering.[2,5–7]

The terms biodegradable, bioabsorbable, and bioresorbable are often used interchangeably to represent natural or synthetic polymers that degrade over time. However, the terms can be more precisely defined.[8] Biodegradation can be thought of as the disintegration, erosion, dissolution, breakdown and/or chain scission of a polymer into metabolisable or excretable fragments in the human body, in animal models, or in *ex vivo* or *in vitro* test media, which represent, mimic or approximate the body environment. Williams[9] emphasised the biological agent (enzyme or microbe) as being the dominant component in the degradation process. Bioresorbable polymers however, can be defined as those classes of polymers whose degradation products 'resorb' in the body, i.e. can be metabolised and enter the general metabolic pathways.[8,9] These include poly(α-hydroxy acids) such as polyglycolide, polylactide and their copolymers. In contrast, bioabsorbable polymers are those that dissolve (or disperse) in biofluids, and are eliminated from the body without chain scission, as measured by molecular weight. Poly(vinyl alcohol) (PVAlc) and poly(ethylene glycol) (PEG) are examples of bioabsorbable polymers.[8,9] A list of common synthetic bioresorbable polymers is given in Table 5.1.[8]

What follows is a short overview of the properties and degradation mechanisms for the most widely used of the polymers listed in Table 5.1, with particular attention paid to the poly(α-hydroxy acids).

5.2.1 Poly(α-hydroxy acids)

Poly(α-hydroxy acids) are bioresorbable polyesters derived from α-hydroxy acids, HO–CHR–COOH, in particular glycolic acid (GA, R=H) and lactic acid (LA, R=CH_3).[10]

Poly(lactide) (PLA) and poly(glycolide) (PGA)

Poly(glycolic acid) is the simplest linear polyester and exists only in one form. Lactic acid on the other hand is a chiral compound, and thus exists

Table 5.1 List of common synthetic bioresorbable polymers

Poly(α-hydroxy acids)	Polyglycolide Polylactides Polycaprolactone Malates
Other polyesters	Poly[(benzyl malate)-malate]s Poly-*p*-dioxanone Polyesters of diacids and diols
Other polycondensates	Polyanhydrides Polyorthoesters Polycarbonates Polyaminoacids Poly(aminoesters) Poly(amidocarbonate)s Polyphosphazenes Polyethers
Vinylic polymers	Poly(alkyl cyanoacrylate)s Poly(vinyl alcohol) Polyvinylpyrrolidone

Source: Arshady, 2003[8]

under two enantiomeric forms, giving rise to different polymers, namely poly(L-lactic acid) (PLLA), and poly(D-lactic acid) (PDLA).The racemic mixture is signified by DL and is optically inactive (PDLLA).

The polymers are synthesised via two routes: direct polycondensation of lactic and glycolic acids or ring-opening polymerisation of the cyclic lactide and glycolide dimers.The nomenclature for polymers prepared by different routes is full of contradictions, but polymers prepared from lactic acid by polycondensation are strictly referred to by the acid, as in poly(lactic acid), and those prepared by ring-opening polymerisation by the dimer, as in polylactide (PLA).[11]

Direct polycondensation is the cheaper of the two routes, but the polymers produced have lower molecular weights and are more polydisperse than those produced by ring-opening polymerisation.

High molecular weight polylactide and polyglycolide can be obtained by ring-opening polymerisation of cyclic diesters using inorganic metal salts such as tin,[12] aluminium[13] and zinc[11,14] as catalysts in the process. The temperature, time, concentration of catalyst and concentration of the chain-length determining agent control the molecular weight of the final polymer. PGA synthesis is possible through simple polycondensation of glycolic acid with antimony trioxide,[15,16] but the resulting polymer has low molecular weight, and optimum properties are not obtained. Figure 5.1 shows the syntheses and chemical formulae for the poly(α-hydroxy acids).

LA-GA polymers are biocompatibile and bioresorbable, and wide ranges of physical, thermal, mechanical and biological properties can be covered by varying the chemical and configurational structures in the polyester chain.[2,11,15,17–19]

The homopolymer of the L-lactide (PLLA) exhibits high tensile strength (50–70 MPa) and low elongation (~4%), and consequently has a high modulus (3 GPa),[4,6,11] which makes it suitable for load-bearing applications such as orthopaedic fixation and sutures. PLLA is partially crystallisable with a melting temperature of 175–178 °C and a glass transition temperature

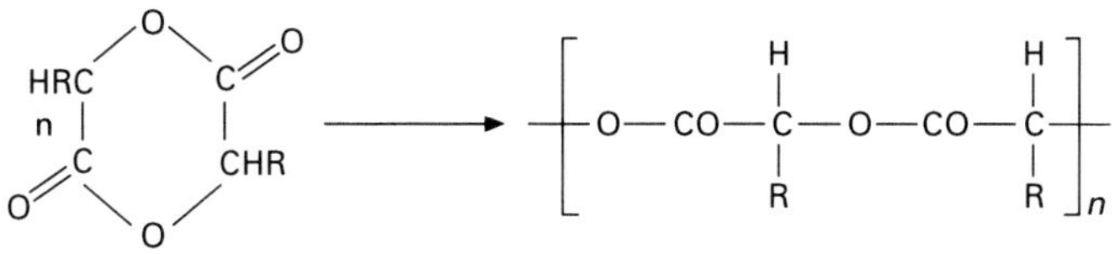

5.1 Chemical formula of polylactide and polyglycolide. (R = H, glycolide: R = CH_3, lactide)

Table 5.2 Summary of homopolymer properties for poly(α-hydroxy acids)

Polymer	Melting temperature (°C)	Glass transition temperature (°C)	Modulus (GPa)	Degradation time (months)
PGA	220–230	35–45	6.0–7.0	6 to 12
PLA	150–162	45–60	0.35–3.5	Several years
PLLA	170–200	55–65	2.7–4.14	>24
PDLLA	Amorphous	50–60	1–3.45	12 to 16
PCL	59–64	–60	0.2–0.4	Several years

Source: adapted from Van de Velde and Kiekens 2002[5] and Nakamura *et al.*, 1989[26]

of 60–65 °C.[6,20] It has the longest degradation time of the poly(α-hydroxy acids) requiring between 2 3 years to be completely absorbed.[21,22] However, extensive *in vitro* degradation studies[10,23–25] have shown that copolymerising PLLA with DL-lactide and glycolide results in considerably shorter degradation times.

Poly D,L-lactide, PDLLA, is an amorphous polymer exhibiting a random distribution of both isomeric forms of lactic acid, and accordingly is unable to arrange into an organised crystalline structure. This material has lower tensile strength, higher elongation, and a much more rapid degradation time (see Table 5.2), making it attractive as a drug delivery system.[10,27]

Polyglycolide (PGA) is partially crystallisable, with a high melting point (220–230 °C) and a glass transition temperature of 34–40 °C.[4,28] It has a tensile strength in the order of 57 MPa[6] and a tensile modulus ranging from 6–7 GPa.[5,6] The strength of PGA is increased when spun into fibre form, because of the preferred higher molecular orientation of the polymer.[29] It is not soluble in most organic solvents, except for extremely fluorinated organics such as hexafluoroisopropanol.[30]

Copolymers of PLA and PGA tend to be less crystalline and less hydrophobic than the homopolymer and subsequently have shorter degradation times.[31] Poly(lactide-co-glycolide) (PLGA) has been used extensively for drug delivery[32,33] and device manufacture.[4,31] Copolymers of glycolide with trimethylene carbonate (TMC), called polyglyconate, have been used as sutures (Maxon®) and as screws.[4]

Polycaprolactone

Polycaprolactone (PCL) was first synthesised in the 1930s by ring-opening polymerisation of ε-caprolactone. PCL is partially crystalline, with a melting point of 59–64 °C and a glass transition temperature of –60 °C.[4] It has a tensile strength of 16 MPa and tensile modulus of 0.4 GPa.[6] PCL is highly hydrophobic and thus has longer degradation times than PLA (2–5 years), which makes it suitable for applications where long degradation times are required.[7,8] Owing to its low melting temperature, PCL is easily processed by conventional melting techniques and can be filled with stiffer materials (particles or fibres) for better mechanical properties. PCL scaffolds have been used for tissue engineering of bone and cartilage.[7]

Table 5.2 summarises some of the properties of the poly(α-hydroxy acids) mentioned thus far.

5.2.2 Other polyesters

Of the common members of this group of polymers, poly-*p*-dioxanone and polyesters of diacids and diols are now discussed briefly.

Poly-p-dioxanone

Polydioxanone (PDS) is a colourless, partially crystalline, poly(ester ether), which is produced by ring-opening polymerisation of *p*-dioxanone monomers. The ring-opening polymerisation requires heat and an organometallic catalyst such as zirconium acetylacetone or zinc L-lactate.[8] PDS is crystallisable and has a glass transition temperature in the range –10 to 0° C.[4] PDS is also the trade name for the degradable suture made from poly-*p*-dioxanone.

Polyesters of diacids and diols

Poly(propylene fumarate) (PPF) is an unsaturated linear polyester which degrades via bulk hydrolysis. The products of its degradation are propylene glycol, poly(acrylic acid–fumaric acid), and fumaric acid which occur naturally as part of the Krebs cycle.[8]

5.2.3 Other polycondensates

Polyanhydrides hydrolyse to their constituent dicarboxylic acids in aqueous media. They have been used and investigated as an important biomaterial for short-term release of drugs for more than two decades.[34] They are produced by melt polycondensation of diacids and have glass transition temperatures in the range of 50–100 °C.[35] Owing to their highly hydrophilic nature, polyanhydrides are highly susceptible to hydrolysis and degrade by surface erosion. Poly(sebacic acid) (PSA) is the most prominent example, and degrades relatively quickly within 54 hours in saline.

Other polymers within the polycondensate group are also susceptible to hydrolysis and degrade predominantly via surface erosion. Polyorthoesters, polycarbonates and polyphosphazenes have been utilised on their own and as copolymers for drug delivery.[4,8]

5.3 Degradation of aliphatic polyesters

In vitro and *in vivo* degradation of aliphatic polyesters have been investigated[10,23–26] However, in many studies these experiments have been carried out with compounds of varying origins, for devices of various natures, shapes and sizes, and at various implantation sites, including various tissues and animals, making comparisons between studies difficult. Nonetheless, *in vitro* studies have been shown to be a good model for simulating polymer degradation in *in vivo* conditions.[36–38] The most widely adopted *in vitro* model is that of degradation in pH 6.9–7.4 phosphate buffer solution at 37 °C.

Once implanted in the body, mechanical bioresorbable devices should ideally maintain mechanical properties, allowing gradual transfer of load to the surrounding tissue before being fully degraded, absorbed and excreted by the body, leaving no trace. The micromechanisms of deformation are affected by changes within the microstructure occurring with degradation.[39]

Factors such as the size of the crystals within the polymer, pore size and pore volume within the implant, and the overall shape and size of the implant affect the mode of degradation within polymers, and these factors can thus be used to control the release profile in drug delivery applications.[40–44]

5.3.1 The chemistry of reaction mechanisms

Simple chemical hydrolysis of the hydrolytically unstable backbone is the prevailing mechanism for polyester degradation, which depends on the pH of the solution and may be catalysed by an acid or a base.The acid-catalysed reaction mechanism is given in Fig. 5.2.[45] The reaction is reversible and is displaced towards hydrolysis by an excess of H_2O. This mechanism is characterised by acyl-oxygen cleavage, and the removal of the alcohol is the slow stage of the reaction.

The base-catalysed ester hydrolysis reaction mechanism is outlined in Fig. 5.3.[45] This reaction has an irreversible acyl-oxygen cleavage mechanism, and the slow stage is the attack of the ester by the OH^-.

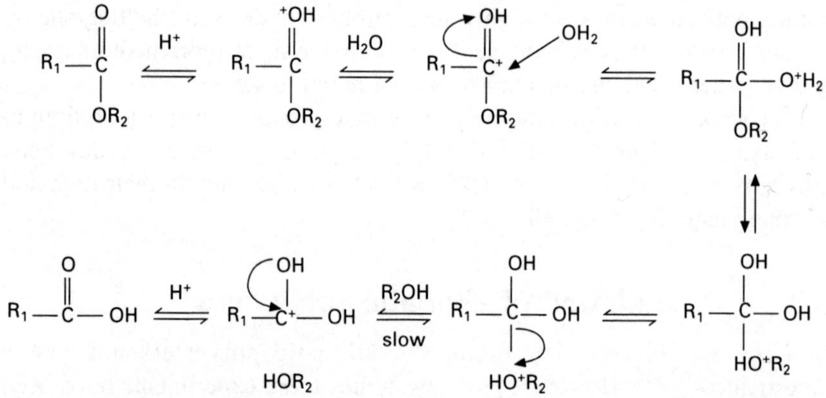

5.2 Acid-catalysed ester hydrolysis mechanism (based on Sykes, 1986[45]).

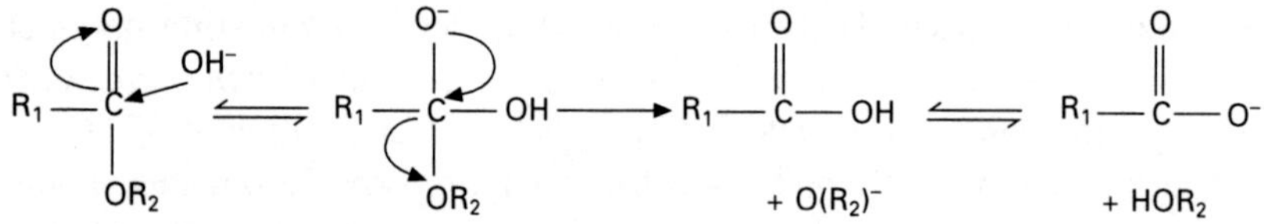

5.3 Base-catalysed ester hydrolysis mechanism (based on Sykes, 1986[45]).

5.3.2 Bulk and surface degradation

Hydrolytic degradation is commonly categorised under bulk and surface erosion, in which bulk erosion may be further split into homogeneous and heterogeneous degradation. In surface erosion, the rate at which water penetrates the device is slower than the rate of conversion of the polymer into water-soluble materials.[46] Surface erosion results in the device thinning over time while maintaining its bulk integrity. Hydrophobic polymers in which the chemical bonds are highly susceptible to hydrolysis undergo surface erosion (e.g. polyanhydrides and polyorthoesters). By contrast, in bulk erosion, degradation takes place throughout the whole of the sample and the rate of ingress of water into the sample is greater than the rate of degradation. Sample dimensions remain constant until a critical stage of degradation where there is dramatic mass loss. Homogeneous bulk erosion describes a gradual drop in molecular weight throughout the sample until a critical value is reached at which the material becomes soluble and erosion occurs. Heterogeneous erosion describes a situation where the central region of the polymer becomes more degraded than the surface over time.

The PLA/GA polymer system degrades through a mechanism of bulk heterogeneous degradation.The system can be subdivided into three classes of material, depending on the material's crystallisability (the notation PLA*X*GA*Y*, where *X* refers to the percentage of L-lactide, *Y* refers to the percentage of glycolide units and consequently 1-*X* refers to the percentage of D-lactide units, is used):[47]

(a) intrinsically amorphous PLA*X*GA*Y* that cannot crystallise with degradation;
(b) intrinsically amorphous PLA*X*GA*Y* that crystallises with degradation, or partially crystallisable PLA*X*GA*Y* that has been quenched to the amorphous state; and
(c) semicrystalline PLA*X*GA*Y*.

In category (a) the sample is considered to be completely amorphous and in a homogenous state. Water uptake is the first event that occurs upon implantation. The diffusion of water into the sample causes hydrolytic cleavage of the ester bonds throughout the sample. Initially, surface degradation exceeds the degradation in the centre of the sample as there is more water present at the surface. As hydrolysis proceeds, the molecular weight of the sample falls, and degradation products (monomers and oligomers) form. The degradation products at the surface are rapidly dissolved in the surrounding fluid and removed from the bulk polymer. The inability of large polymeric degradation products to diffuse away from the bulk device results in a local acidic environment in the interior of the implant. The increased acidic environment catalyses further degradation resulting in accelerated hydrolysis of the ester linkages in the interior, a process known as autocatalysis.[48] Meanwhile, the surface continues to degrade at its original rate, resulting in a surface–centre differentiation. Over time, the degradation at the centre continues and the inner material can become a viscous liquid of oligomers contained by an outer shell also known as a 'skin' layer. The hollow skin layer eventually degrades away at a reduced rate.

Li *et al.*[10,23,24] demonstrated that both *in vivo* and *in vitro*, large PLA/GA devices degrade heterogeneously, with the degradation being faster in the internal part than at the surface where a layer of less degraded material is formed. Studies carried out by Grizzi *et al.*[49] confirmed the formation of an outer skin layer as demonstrated in Fig. 5.4.

The thickness *t* of the skin depends on many factors such as the diffusion rates of the various species involved and the rate of ester bond cleavage. Diffusion coefficients of the soluble oligomers in PLA/GA depend on factors such as molar mass, degree of matrix swelling, and macromolecular conformation and rigidity. In the same way, degradation rates depend on the degree of swelling, and on the sequential distribution of chiral and achiral units along the polymer chains. Finally, the release of the soluble carboxyl-terminated oligomers depends on their solubility in the surrounding aqueous medium and thus on factors such as pH, ionic strength, temperature and buffering capacity.

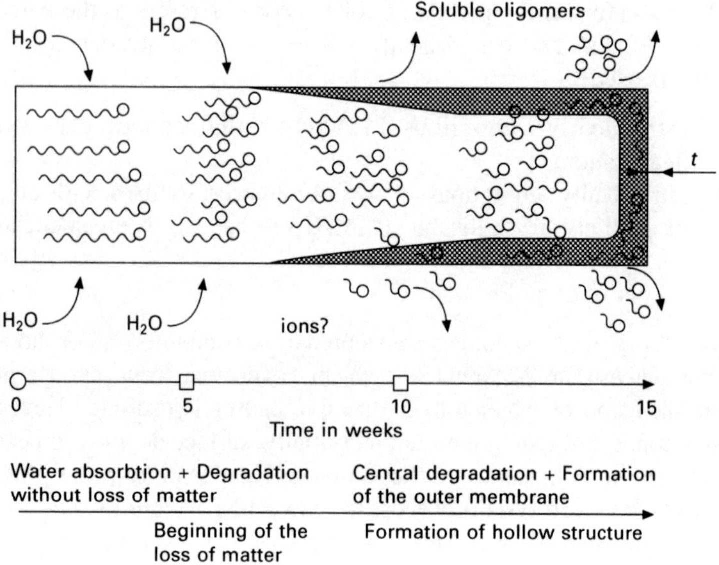

5.4 Schematic representation of the diffusion-reaction phenomena that occur during the hydrolytic degradation of implants, according to the model of heterogeneous degradation (modified from Grizzi *et al.*, 1995[49]).

The second class of materials considered, category (b), are those that are initially amorphous but crystallise with hydration and degradation. As before, once placed in an aqueous medium, water diffuses into the sample from the outside in and initially surface degradation exceeds the degradation in the centre of the sample. During the second step of degradation for this class of material, autocatalysis predominates in the centre of the sample. However, in this instance as molecular weight decreases, factors such as preferential degradation of some units, shorter chain length and plasticisation by water allow crystallisation to occur in the centre of the sample. As hydrolysis continues, the volume of crystalline material in the centre of the sample increases, while the surface degrades at a reduced rate, becoming only slightly crystalline. The centre of the sample reaches stable crystallinity and becomes very resistant to further degradation. Degradation occurs in the amorphous regions and, therefore, in the final stages, the centre is often found to be in the form of a white powder or a porous structure. A dense outer layer remains in which cracking may occur owing to shrinkage of the bulk sample on degradation.[24]

Li *et al.*[24] found this mechanism in initially amorphous PLLA samples, in which hydrolytic chain scission resulted in lower molecular weight and absorbed water acted as a plasticiser, both resulting in increased chain mobility, and the ability of the chain segments to crystallise, which in turn improved the material's resistance to degradation. Schwach *et al.*[38] also confirmed the ability of the PLA*X*GA*Y* polymers to crystallise with degradation.

In the third category (c), a PLA*X*GA*Y* polymer is fundamentally crystallisable and has a measure of crystallinity before degradation. When placed in an aqueous environment, water diffuses into the sample. Hydrolytic cleavage of ester bonds starts immediately where water is present and, thus initially, surface degradation exceeds degradation in the centre of the sample. Later on, a slight heterogeneity occurs as the outer surface remains resistant to degradation (because degradation products diffuse into the surrounding medium), while the central material undergoes autocatalysis with preferential degradation in the amorphous regions. Such samples are less likely to show a hollow structure. Li *et al.* found that crystalline PLLA degraded in this manner.[24]

It is important to note that in all these instances water diffuses into the amorphous regions first because they are less organised, allowing water to penetrate more easily than the highly ordered, densely packed crystalline regions.[25,50,51]

Commercially available polylactide and polyglycolide devices and sutures degrade by the bulk erosion mechanisms described above.[47] Knowledge of these mechanisms has been used to tailor the degradation rates of biodegradable polymers. For example, replacing carboxylic acid end groups with ester end groups (the end group being determined by the choice of initiator) on poly(D,L-lactide-co glycolide) (DLPLGA) polymers slows both water uptake and degradation rate *in vitro* as reported by Tracy *et al.*[52] The acid end groups add to the hydrophilicity of the polymer and catalyse degradation. A study conducted by Middleton *et al.*[53] in which the ester end groups in DLPLGA rods were replaced with methoxy poly(ethylene glycol) (mPEG) demonstrated enhanced water uptake without accelerated degradation.This was because the presence of ethylene glycol units enhanced polymer hydrophilicity without lowering the pH of the local environment. By increasing water uptake it may also have allowed the acidic degradation products to diffuse away from the interior of the rod more easily.

The incorporation of acidic and basic groups within the polymer matrix allows control of the local pH of the system during degradation.[54–59] In such cases, the control of the autocatalytic effect dominates over the effect of changing the reaction product concentration, and the effect of end-group neutralisation is to lower the reaction rate.

Renouf-Glauser *et al.*[60] observed an increase in the degradation rate of PLLA with the addition of lauric acid – an acid found in soaps, cosmetics and food additives. Lauric acid was found to catalyse the hydrolytic degradation, reducing the time to loss of tensile strength.

The addition of inorganic and ceramic fillers (such as $CaCO_3$, HA, TCP) to bioresorbable polymers has been widely reported in literature.[61–64] Both the basicity and the solubility of the inorganic phase play a role in degradation of the polymers. The presence of such fillers is generally thought to retard polymer degradation by neutralising the acidic degradation products during polymer hydrolysis. The autocatalytic effect associated with the accumulation of acidic products in the internal part of the polymer device is delayed if not hindered by the presence of ceramic fillers.[63]

5.3.3 Reaction erosion fronts

Work carried out by the Hurrell and Cameron group,[41,43,65] and Milroy *et al.*[66] extends the theories of Li *et al.*, by paying particular attention to polyglycolide degradation. This series of work suggest that in PGA reaction, erosion fronts contribute to a four-stage degradation process (Fig. 5.5). In stage I, small quantities of water diffuse rapidly into the sample, reaching an equilibrium level (less than 1 wt%). Little further water is absorbed in stage II but the hydrolysis causes the molecular weight of the polymer to decrease. Insertion secondary crystallisation, in which new crystals are inserted between existing crystals, takes place in this stage.[41,43] This is facilitated by both the presence of water molecules and the decrease in molecular weight, which causes the polymer chains to become more mobile. At the beginning of stage III, a critical molecular weight is reached where oligomers begin to diffuse from the surface of the sample. This creates space into which water molecules diffuse.

A co-operative diffusion of water molecules in and oligomers out gives rise to sharp reaction–erosion fronts close to the surface in a mechanism similar to that for the creation of the surface layer as proposed by Li *et al.*[10]

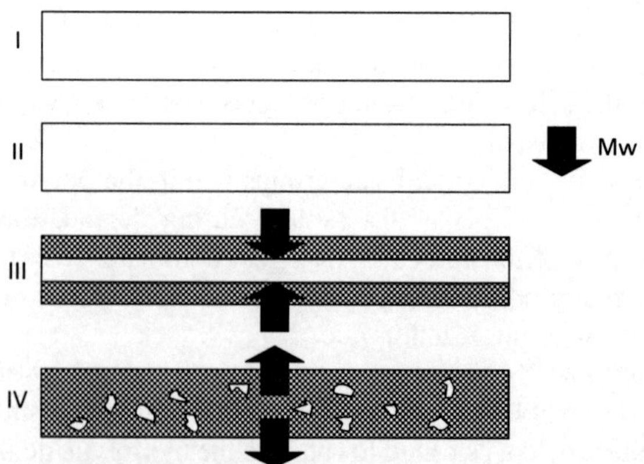

5.5 A schematic diagram illustrating the hypothesised water distribution in polymer samples during stages I–IV (modified from Hurrell *et al.*, 2003[43]).

and Grizzi *et al.*[49] for PLA/GA polymers. Behind the fronts, the polymer is hydrated and porous, whereas ahead of the fronts, oligomers have yet to diffuse out. During stage III, the fronts move linearly towards the centre of the sample. The front movement is a particular feature of PGA which seems to differ from other members of the PLA/GA family in which the division between layers is more static with time. Presumably the differences arise because of the particular balance of kinetics between diffusion and reaction rates within the system. Stage IV begins when the fronts meet at the centre of the sample. After this point, the degradation becomes more homogeneous throughout the now highly porous sample. The linear movement of fronts leads to the potential for zero-order drug release, because active agents embedded in the sample are released quickly from the porous regions behind the fronts and the kinetics of release are determined by front movement.[40,43,66]

5.4 Factors affecting aliphatic polymer degradation

The degradation rate of bioresorbable polymers depends on their intrinsic properties such as reactivity, hydrophilicity, molecular weight, degree of crystallinity, and glass transition temperature. However, other external factors such as the degradation media, sterilisation and sample size also play a role in the degree of degradation.

5.4.1 Polymer composition

There have been many studies in which the interplay between aliphatic polyester composition and degradation is considered.[19,23,30,67,68] Particular attention is given to PLA, PGA and their copolymers. Figure 5.6, shows the schematic variation in the degradation half-life of PGLA.[4]

PLA shows the longest degradation time of the PLA/PGA series, with the degradation time decreasing with increasing amounts of PGA, as random copolymerisation decreases the degree of crystallinity of the polymers and because of the faster hydrolysis rate and greater hydrophilicity displayed by PGA compared with PLA.[24] The half-life rises again when the copolymers contain mostly PGA as the polymer becomes more crystallisable with lower levels of copolymerisation. Amorphous regions are more accessible by water molecules than crystals, and this increases hydrolysis and chain degradation in these regions.

5.4.2 Degradation media

Media pH can affect polymer degradation, either directly, by altering the polymer chemistry involved during degradation, or indirectly, by interacting with degradation products and affecting consequent kinetics.

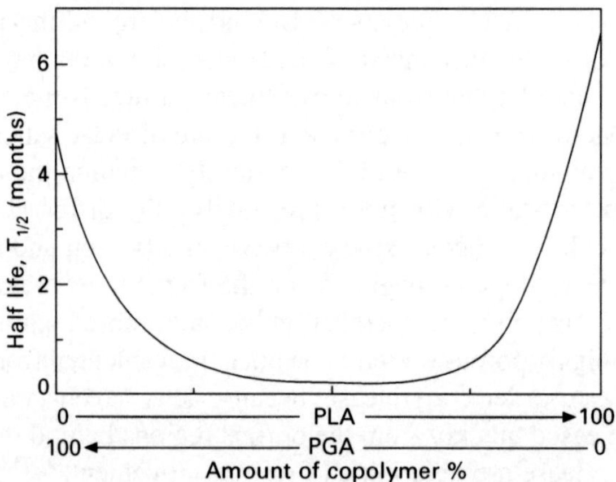

5.6 Half-life of PLA and PGA homopolymers and copolymers (from Middleton and Tipton[4]).

Chu[55] found there was a greater loss in the mechanical properties of PGA sutures in buffered than unbuffered solutions. Similarly, the presence of buffer ions increases the degradation rate of poly(α-hydroxy acid) copolymers as a result of the enhanced removal of degradation products through neutralisation of the end groups.[23,54,60]

Work carried out by King *et al.*[50] and Hurrell and Cameron[54] showed no significant change in PGA degradation rate for increases in ionic strength and for changes to phosphate salt concentration (from 0.01 to 0.1 M), but for an increase in pH (from 6 to 8) a small but significant increase was observed. Ginde and Gupta[69] also observed alkaline media (pH 9.2 and 10.6) to have a more drastic effect on the degradation and mechanical properties of PGA fibres than acidic or neutral media. Makino *et al.*[70] and Zaikov[71] also reported greater degradation in alkaline than in acidic conditions for homopolymers and copolymers of polylactide and polyglycolide. Their results imply that in alkaline conditions, surface erosion dominates over bulk erosion.

Hurrell and Cameron[54] concluded that the onset of reaction erosion fronts and the rate at which they move through the polymer depends on the rate at which acidic degradation products diffuse out, creating space for water in the structure. If the solution is made more alkaline or more concentrated, more of the acid is neutralised, driving the reaction forward. This hastens the onset of stage III, and encourages drug release from loaded drug releasing polymers.

Other authors[23,54,72,73] also observed that the presence of ions in solution initially decreases water uptake into the polymer compared with the uptake from distilled water, but, as degradation products are released from the polymer, the presence of ions increases the erosion rate.

5.4.3 *In vitro* and *in vivo* correlation

There is some contradiction between the results of previous studies concerning the extent of the effect of enzymes on polylactide and polyglycolide degradation. For example, Vert *et al.*[27] reported no difference in degradation between PLA50 (poly-DL-lactide) and PLA100 (100% L-lactide) in buffer and esterases solutions. However, Mason *et al.*[74] reported a degradation rate between two and six times higher for PLA50 in plasma that contains enzymes compared with simple buffers.

Despite these results, many studies found *in vitro* and *in vivo* degradation rates for a range of PGLA copolymers to be the same.[4,23,24]

5.4.4 Crystallinity and polymer morphology

Crystallinity has a significant effect on the degradation rate of aliphatic polyesters because it determines how easily water molecules can access the ester linkages to cause chain cleavage.

Aliphatic polyesters can be random copolymers which are amorphous and do not crystallise during degradation; homopolymers and block copolymers can be semicrystalline or amorphous depending on processing; and polymers in between are amorphous in the undegraded state but become more crystalline as they degrade. Crystallisable polymers can be given different morphologies by quenching or annealing before degradation.[15]

Li *et al.*[10,23] examined morphological changes of amorphous polymers during degradation. *In vitro* investigations of PLA50 (poly-D,L-lactic acid) and PLA37.5GA25 (75% D,L-lactide and 25% glycolide) demonstrated that the polymers started and remained amorphous throughout degradation. However, PLA75GA25 (75% L-lactide and 25% glycolide) samples were crystalline after 7 weeks degradation. H-NMR studies (proton-based nuclear magnetic resonance spectroscopy) suggested that PLA and PLA/PGA copolymers all degrade via the same mechanism but that the GA units on PLA/GA copolymers constitute vulnerable points on the macromolecular chains, so that degradation occurs preferentially on the GA bonds. This phenomenon was observed only up to 12 weeks degradation, after which point the lactide–glycolide ratio remained constant. Li *et al.* concluded that the glycolide removal caused crystallisation of the remaining lactide regions. The remaining glycolide was then incorporated into the new crystals protecting glycolide from hydrolysis after 12 weeks.

Gel permeation chromatography (GPC) and size exclusion chromatography (SEC) tests were carried out on 100% L-lactide (PLA100), 75% D,L-lactide and 25% glycolide (PLA37.5GA25) and 50% D,L-lactide and 50% glycolide (PLA25GA50) samples by Hakkarainen *et al.*[25] Results exhibited development of a multimodal distribution in molecular weight during degradation for the semicrystalline PLA100 samples, whereas the amorphous copolymers degraded smoothly with no additional peaks in the molecular weight distribution. This was attributed to the difference in degradation rates between the amorphous and crystalline micro-domains in the semicrystalline polymer. Li *et al.*[10,23] observed similar patterns for semicrystalline PLA. Gilding and Reed[15] also observed partial crystallisation of PGA and PLA/PGA copolymers after 3 days degradation.

It is clear that an increase in crystallinity during degradation need not be an indication of preferential amorphous material removal. Degrading PGA can show significant crystallinity increase in the early stages of degradation. Hurrell and Cameron[41] reasoned that removal of amorphous material from the polymer structure should result in a significant loss of mass, which was not observed. Further analysis using small-angle X-ray diffraction (SAXS) deduced that insertion of secondary crystals within the amorphous region was the cause of the increase in crystallinity and decrease in long period. A slowing down of insertion crystallisation with time caused the subsequent levelling off of crystallinity and the rise in long period.

5.4.5 Molecular weight

The molecular weight and molecular weight distribution of polymers affects the volume fraction of chain ends and hence the free volume of the polymer and, consequently, determines the chain mobility and crystallisation. It also determines the number of acidic end groups that can participate in hydrolysis and their possible catalytic effect. Overall, the molecular weight affects both the chemical and physical properties of a polymer.[44]

Zhu *et al.*[75] and Park[76] both report faster degradation of PGA, PLA and their copolymers with decreasing molecular weight. This is attributed to an increase in the free volume and number of acidic reactive end groups.

Processing techniques also affect the molecular weight of polymer samples. The thermal treatments experienced in processing cause thermal degradation, which in turn results in a lowering of the molecular weight. Hurrell and Cameron[65] concluded that for thermal degradation to occur, the thermal treatments in general need to be quite severe. They observed no molecular weight changes between PGA samples with no prior treatment and those treated at 160 °C for 5 min, and at 120 °C for 2 h.

5.4.6 Sample size

Some studies have addressed the possible interplay between sample size and degradation of aliphatic polyesters. Sample size is commonly interchanged with sample geometry. Production of variously shaped devices introduces a variety of processing routes, which results in further changes to polymer degradation.

Grizzi *et al.*[49] and Ginde and Gupta's[69] work suggested that the degradation rate of PLA and PGA devices was very much dependent on size, and the greater the thickness of the device, the faster the degradation.

In a separate experiment, Visscher *et al.*[77] investigated the effect of size on the release of drugs in microparticles made of a copolymer of 25% D-lactide, 25% L-lactide and 50% glycolide. The microparticles ranged in size from 45–177 μm and, in accordance with the surface layer hypothesis, the larger microparticles degraded first.

Tormala *et al.*[37] degraded SR-PGA rods with diameters ranging from 1.5–4.5 mm, which were prepared by sintering bundles of PGA sutures (Dexon) together. In these experiments, in contrast to those reported above, tensile measurements revealed that the larger rods degrade more slowly. This was attributed to the smaller surface area to volume ratio, which resulted in slower diffusion of water into the samples. Another factor that would have affected the degradation is a change in internal porosity of the rods with sample size.

Hurrell *et al.*[43] found that during PGA degradation the progression of reaction erosion fronts through the samples was linear and at the same rate irrespective of sample size. Stage I of the degradation is diffusion-controlled and is therefore strongly affected by the thickness of the sample. However, because this diffusion occurred quickly in comparison with the timescale of the degradation it did not have a strong effect. Once water had diffused through the bulk of the sample by the beginning of stage II, hydrolysis occurred at the same rate regardless of sample size, until the critical molecular weight was reached. The reaction–erosion fronts (whose appearance marks the onset of stage III) started at the same time in samples of different size. They concluded that it was only the onset of stage IV of degradation (explained in section 5.3.3), when the reaction erosion fronts meet in the centre of the sample, that showed size dependence, with the onset time increasing for thicker samples.

5.4.7 Sterilisation and packaging

It is necessary to sterilise all medical implants after fabrication and before their surgical placement to reduce the risk of infection and associated complications. The most common sterilisation techniques utilise heat, steam, radiation, or a combination of these methods.

PLA and PGA polymers, in addition to being susceptible to damage by moisture and radiation, are heat sensitive. Thus, selection of the correct sterilisation technique is of crucial importance to their physical and mechanical performance *in vivo*. Table 5.3 gives an overview of the sterilisation techniques commonly used and their advantages and disadvantages.[19] Sterilisation by γ-radiation is known to cause chain scission in PLA and PGA polymers. At

Table 5.3 Standard sterilisation techniques and their applicability to PLA–PGA

Sterilisation technique	Advantages	Disadvantages
Steam sterilisation (high steam pressure, 120–135 °C)	No toxic residues	Deformation/degradation owing to water attack, limited usage for PLA–PGA
Dry heat sterilisation (160–190 °C)	No toxic residues	Melting and softening of polymers, not usable for PLA–PGA
Radiation (ionising or γ)	High penetration, low chemical reactivity, rapid effect	Instability and deterioration, crosslinking/breakage of polymer bonds
Gas sterilisation (ethylene oxide)	Low temperature range	Lengthy process owing to degassing, residues are toxic

Source: Athanasiou *et al.*, 1996[19]

doses of 2.5 Mrad, Co^{60} γ-radiation causes deterioration of Dexon and Vicryl sutures.[78] Other studies have reported decreases in tensile strength of PLA and PGA polymers and an increased rate of degradation upon γ-radiation[79] as a result of a decrease in molecular weight.

The best method of sterilisation for polymers sensitive to heat and moisture, such as PLA and PGA, is chemical sterilisation by gases such as ethylene oxide (EO). However, this leaves residues in harmful quantities on the surface and within the polymers.[19] Hence, the polymeric implants must then be subjected to degassing or aeration so that residual EO concentrations are reduced to acceptable levels.[46]

A further point to note is that polymers and their composites are fully compatible with modern diagnostic methods such as computer tomography (CT) and magnetic resonance imaging (MRI) as they are non-magnetic. Their radio transparency can be adjusted by adding contrast medium to the polymer.[2] Peltoniemi *et al.*[51] reported no change in the mechanical properties of biodegradable implants as a result of postoperative radiation doses.

5.5 Processing and devices

There are many medical and surgical devices of various shapes and sizes made of aliphatic polyesters.These devices are made by various processing routes. In general, large-scale devices such as sutures [e.g. Dexon (100%PGA),Vicryl (copolymer of glycolide in combination with L-lactide), Monocryl (copolymer of ε-caprolactone) or Maxon (copolymer of trimethylene carbonate)] and macroscopic implants used for bone fixation can be manufactured by solvent- or melt-spinning processes.[11] The fibre forms can then be drawn under different conditions in order to orient the polymer chains. Fibres prepared by solvent-spinning usually have higher mechanical properties because of the thermal degradation during melt-spinning.

Micro and nano-particles used for oral administration of drugs are solvent cast using water or organic solvents. The stirring rate and temperature under which the particles are processed greatly affects their drug release rate and degradation properties.

Porous biodegradable polymer scaffolds have been used as matrices for bone regeneration in tissue engineering. Current approaches for their fabrication include fibre bonding, solvent casting and particulate leaching, melt modelling, phase separation, emulsion freeze drying, gas foaming, and combinations of these.[80]

5.6 Conclusions

Bioresorbable polymers are put to extensive use as medical materials because of their diverse biodegradability, good mechanical properties and biocompatibility. The ability to tailor their chemical structures to control their degradation behaviour and rate is a great advantage when it comes to designing implants with suitable mechanical and degradational properties for their intended use.

Poly(α-hydroxy acids) are the predominant group of polymers regarded as bioresorbable. Simple chemical hydrolysis of the ester backbone is the main chemical mechanism for their degradation whereas physical degradation is governed by a combination of homogeneous and heterogeneous degradation and the formation of reaction erosion fronts within the polymer systems.

The lactide/glycolide bioresorbable polymers are thermoplastics which can be processed by many methods, including fibre spinning, extrusion, and injection moulding, which means they can be fabricated into a variety of wound closure items (e.g. sutures), implantable devices (e.g. bone plates, bone screws), and drug delivery systems, which include microspheres, fibres, films, rods and others.

With the advancement of research, synthesis routes and implant manufacturing techniques, there is no doubt that bioresorbable polymers (PLA and PGA) will be used more and more as biomaterials to replace and/or augment damaged tissues within the body. The future for such polymers is bright and currently there is much attention being paid to the suitability of using these bioresorbable polymers in solving difficult orthopaedic problems such as osteotomy fixation, articular cartilage and meniscal repairs,[20] ligament and tendon reconstructions, and substitutes of autologous bone fills. Furthermore, a biodegradable implant system that provides a steady, controlled release of drugs or bioactive factors can be used as a delivery vehicle for substances that can enhance repair processes in the musculoskeletal system.

5.7 Sources of further information and advice

Encyclopedic handbook of biomaterials and bioengineering: Part A: Materials – eds.: Wise, D. L., Trantolo, D. J., Altobelli, D. E., Gresser, J. D. & Yaszemski, M. J. (Marcel Dekker, New York, USA, 1995).

The PBM series: biodegradable polymers: Volumes 1 & 2. ed: Arshady, R. (Citus Books, London, U.K., 2003).

The biomedical engineering handbook – ed: Bronzino, J. D. (CRC, USA, 2nd edition, 1999).

The Williams dictionary of biomaterials – ed: Williams, D. F. (Liverpool University Press, Liverpool, UK, 1999).

5.8 References

1. Black, J. *Biological performance of materials: fundamentals of biocompatibility* (Marcel Dekker, New York, 1998).
2. Ramakrishna, S., Mayer, J., Wintermantel, E. and Leong, K. W., Biomedical applications of polymer–composite materials: A review. *Composite Science and Technology* **61**, 1189–1224 (2001).
3. Schnabel, W. *Polymer degradation: principles and practical applications.* (Hanser International, German Democratic Republic, 1981).
4. Middleton, J. C. and Tipton, A. J., Synthetic biodegradable polymers as orthopaedic devices. *Biomaterials* **21**, 2334–2346 (2000).
5. Van De Velde, K. and Kiekens, P., Biopolymers: Overview of several properties and consequences on their applications. *Polymer Testing* **21**, 433–442 (2002).
6. Daniels, A. U., Chang, M. K. O., Andriano, K. P. and Heller, J., Mechanical properties of biodegradable polymers and composites proposed for internal fixation of bone. *Journal of Applied Biomaterials*, 57–78 (1990).
7. Mano, J. F., Sousa, R. A., Boesel, L. F., Neves, N. M. and Reis, R. L., Bioinert, biodegradable and injectable polymeric matrix composites for hard tissue replacement: State of the art and recent developments. *Composite Science and Technology* **64**, 789–817 (2004).
8. Arshady, R. *Biodegradable polymers* (ed. Arshady, R.) (Citus Books, London, 2003).
9. Williams, D. F. *The Williams dictionary of biomaterials* (Liverpool University Press, Liverpool, 1999).
10. Li, S. M., Garreau, H. and Vert, M., Structure property relationships in the case of degradation of massive aliphatic poly-(α-hydroxy acids) in aqueous media, Part 1: poly(DL-lactic acid). *Journal of Materials Science; Materials in Medicine* **1**, 123–130 (1990).
11. Sodergard, A. and Stolt, M., Properties of lactic acid based polymers and their correlation with composition. *Progress in Polymer Science* **27**, 1123–1163 (2002).
12. Kowalski, A., Duda, A. and Penczek, S., Kinetics and mechanism of cyclic esters polymerisation initiated with tin(II) octate. 3. Polymerisation of L,L-dilactide. *Macromolecules* **33**, 7359–7370 (2000).
13. Dubois, P., Jacobs, C., Jerome, R. and Teyssie, P., Macromolecular engineering

of polylactones and polylactides. 4. Mechanism and kinetics of lactide homopolymerisation by aluminum isopropoxide. *Macromolecules* **24** (1991).

14. Chabot, F., Vert, M., Chapelle, S. and Granger, P., Configurational structures of lactic acid stereocopolymers as determined by 13C-{1H} n.m.r. *Polymer* **24**, 53–59 (1983).
15. Gilding, D. K. and Reed, M. A., Biodegradable polymers for use in surgery – polyglycolic/polylactic acid homo- and copolymers 1. *Polymer* **20**, 1459–1464 (1979).
16. Ashammakhi, N. and Rokkanen, P., Absorbable polyglycolide devices in trauma and bone surgery. *Biomaterials* **16**, 3–9 (1997).
17. Vert, M., Christel, P., Chabot, F. and Leary, J., Bioabsorbable plastic material for bone in *Macromolecular biomaterials* ed. GW Hastings and P. Ducheyne, CRC Press, Boca Raton, Florida, 119, 1984.
18. Engelberg, I. and Kohn, J., Physico-mechanical properties of degradable polymers used in medical applications: a comparative study. *Biomaterials* **12**, 292–304 (1991).
19. Athanasiou, K. A., Neiderauer, G. G. and Agrawal, C. M., Sterilisation, toxicity, biocompatibility and clinical applications of polylactic acid/polyglycolic acid copolymers. *Biomaterials* **17**, 93–102 (1996).
20. Agrawal, C. M., Niederauer, G. G., Micallef, D. M. and Athanasiou, K. A. in *Encyclopedic handbook of biomaterials and bioengineering: Part A: materials* (eds. Wise, D. L., Trantolo, D. J., Altobelli, D. E., Gresser, J. D. and Yaszemski, M. J.) 1055–1089 (Marcel Dekker, New York, USA, 1995).
21. Michaeli, W. and Von Oepen, R., Processing of degradable polymers. *ANTEC-Conference Proceedings*, 796–804 (1994).
22. Rokkanen, P. U., Böstman, O., Hirvensalo, E., Mäkelä, E. A., Partio, E. K. and Pätiälä, H., Bioabsorbable fixation in orthopaedic surgery and traumatology. *Biomaterials* **21**, 2607–2613 (2000).
23. Li, S. M., Garreau, H. and Vert, M., Structure property relationships in the case of degradation of massive aliphatic poly(α-hydroxy acids) in aqueous media, Part 2: degradation of lactide–glycolide copolymers: PLA37.5 GA25 and PLA75 GA25. *Journal of Materials Science; Materials in Medicine* **1**, 131–139 (1990).
24. Li, S. M., Garreau, H. and Vert, M., Structure property relationships in the case of degradation of massive aliphatic poly-(α-hydroxy acids) in aqueous media, Part 3: Influence of the morphology of poly(L-lactic acid). *Journal of Materials Science; Materials in Medicine*, 198–206 (1990).
25. Hakkarainen, M., Albertson, A. and Karlsson, S., Weight loss and molecular changes correlated with the evolution of hydroxyacids in simulated *in vivo* degradation of homo and copolymers of PLA and PGA. *Polymer Degradation and Stability* **52**, 283–291 (1996).
26. Nakamura, T., Hitomi, S., Watanabe, S., Shimizu, Y., Janshidi, K., Hyan, S.-H. and Ikada, Y., Bioabsorption of polylactides with different molecular properties. *J. Biomed. Mater. Res.* **23**, 1115–1130. (1989).
27. Vert, M., Schwach, G., Engel, R. and Coudane, J., Something new in the field of PLA/PGA bioresorbable polymers. *Journal of Controlled Releases* **53**, 85–92 (1998).
28. Chu, C. C., Biodegradable polymeric biomaterials: an updated overview, in Biomedical *Engineering Handbook*, 2nd edition (ed. Bronzino, J. D.) CRC Press, Florida, 1999.

29. Tormala, P., Biodegradable self reinforced composite materials, manufacturing structures and mechanical properties. *Clinical Materials* **10**, 29–34 (1992).
30. Wu, X. S., Synthesis and Properties of Biodegradable lactic/glycolic acid polymers in *Encyclopedic handbook of biomaterials and bioengineering* (ed. Wise, D. L.) Marcel Dekker, New York, 1995.
31. An, Y. H., Woolf, S. K. and Friedman, R. J., Pre-clinical *in vivo* evaluation of orthopedic bioabsorbable devices. *Biomaterials* **21**, 2635–2652 (2000).
32. Loo, J. S. C., Ooi, C. P. and Boey, F. Y. C., Degradation of poly(lactide-co-glycolide) (PLGA) and poly(L-lactide)(PLLA) by electron beam radiation. *Biomaterials* **26**, 1359–1367 (2005).
33. Engwicht, A., Girreser, U. and Muller, B. W., Characterisation of co-polymers of lactic and glycolic acid for supercritical fluid processing. *Biomaterials* **21**, 1587–1593 (2000).
34. Uhrich, K. E., Cannizzaro, S. M., Langer, R. S. and Shakesheff, K. M., Polymeric systems for controlled drug release. *Chemical Reviews* **99**, 3181–3198 (1999).
35. Kumar, N., Langer, R. and Domb, A. J., Polyanhydrides: An overview. *Advanced Drug Delivery Reviews* **54**, 889–910 (2002).
36. Matsusue, Y., Yamamuro, T., Oka, M., Shikinami, Y., Hyon, S.-H. and Ikadi, Y., *In vitro* and *in vivo* studies on bioabsorbable ultrahigh-strength poly(L-lactide) rods. *Journal of Biomedical Materials Research* **26**, 1553–1567 (1992).
37. Törmälä, P., Vasenius, J., Vainionpää, S., Laiho, J., Pohjonen, T., Rokkanen P., Ultra-high-strength absorbable self-reinforced polyglycolide (SR-PGA) composite rods for internal fracture fixation of bone fractures: *in vitro* and *in vivo* study. *Journal of Biomedical Materials Research* **25**, 1–22 (1991).
38. Schwach, G. and Vert, M., *In vitro* and *in vivo* degradation of lactic acid-based interference screws used in cruciate ligament reconstruction. *International Journal of Biological Macromolecules* **25**, 283–291 (1999).
39. Ooi, C. P. and Cameron, R. E., The hydrolytic degradation of polydioxanone (PDSII) sutures. Part II: Micromechanism of deformation. *Journal of Biomedical Materials Research*, 291–298 (2002).
40. Braunecker, J., Baba, M., Milroy, G. E. and Cameron, R. E., The effects of molecular weight and porosity on the degradation and drug release from polyglycolide. *International Journal of Pharmaceutics* **282**, 19–34 (2004).
41. Hurrell, S. and Cameron, R. E., Polyglycolide: degradation and drug release. Part I: Changes in morphology during degradation. *Journal of Materials Sci.: Materials in Medicine*, **12**, 811–816 (2001).
42. Hurrell, S. and Cameron, R. E., Polyglycolide: degradation and drug release. Part II: Drug release. *J. Mater Sci; Mat. Med.* **12**, 817–820 (2001).
43. Hurrell, S., Milroy, G. E. and Cameron, R. E., The distribution of water in degrading polyglycolide. Part I: Sample size and drug release. *Journal of Materials Science: Materials in Medicine* **14**, 457–464 (2003).
44. Milroy, G. E. in *Degradation and drug release behaviour of polyglycolide* (PhD thesis, University of Cambridge, Cambridge, 2001).
45. Sykes, P., *Mechanisms in organic chemistry* (Longman, 1986).
46. Kohn, J. and Langer, R. in *Biomaterials science* (eds. Ratner, B. D., Hoffman, A. S., Schoen, F. J. and Lemons, J. E.) 64–72 (Academic Press, New York, 1996).
47. Renouf, A. C., *A degradation study of PLLA containing lauric acid; the effect of composition and microstructure*. p. 267 (PhD thesis, University of Cambridge, Cambridge, 2004).

48. Pitt, C. G., Gratzel, M. M., Kimmel, G.L., Surles, J. and Schindler, A., Aliphatic polyesters 2; The degradation of poly (DL-lactide), poly (ε-caprolactone) and their copolymers *in vivo*. *Biomaterials* **2**, 215–220 (1981).
49. Grizzi, I., Garreau, H., Li, S. M. and Vert, M., Hydrolytic degradation of devices based on poly (DL-lactic acid) size dependence. *Biomaterials* **16**, 305–311 (1995).
50. King, E., Robinson, S. and Cameron, R. E., Effect of hydrolytic degradation on the microstructure of quenched, amorphous, poly(glycolic acid): an X-ray scattering study of hydrated samples. *Polymers International* **48**, 915–920 (1999).
51. Peltoniemi, H., Ashammakhi, N., Kontio, R., Waris, T., Salo, A., Lindqvist, C., Grätz, K. and Suuronen, R., The use of bioabsorbable osteofixation devices in craniomaxillofacial surgery. *Oral Surgery, Oral Medicine, Oral Pathology, Oral Radiology and endodontics* **94**, 5–14 (2002).
52. Tracy, M. A., Firouzabadian, L. and Zhang, Y. in *Proceedings of the international symposium on controlled and related bioactive materials* 786–787 (1995).
53. Middleton, J. C. and Yarbrough, J. C., The effect of PEG end groups on the degradation of a 75/25 poly(DL-lactide-co-glycolide). *Transactions of the Society of Biomaterials 25th Annual Meeting* **22**, 535 (1999).
54. Hurrell, S. and Cameron, R. E., The effect of buffer concentration, pH and buffer ions on the degradation and drug release from polyglycolide. *Polymers International* **52**, 358–366 (2003).
55. Chu, C. C., An *in vitro* study of the effect of buffer on the degradation of poly(glycolic acid) sutures. *Journal of Biomedical Materials Research* **15**, 19–27 (1981).
56. Vert, M., Mauduit, J. and Li, S. M., Biodegradation of PLA/GA polymers: increasing complexity. *Biomaterials* **15**, 1013–1209 (1994).
57. Li, S. and Vert, M., Hydrolytic degradation of coral/poly(DL-lactic acid) bioresorbable material. *Journal of Biomaterials Science – Polymer Edition* **7**, 817–827 (1996).
58. Li, S., Girod-Holland, S. and Vert, M., Hydrolytic degradation of poly(DL-lactic acid) in the presence of caffeine base. *Journal of Controlled Release* **40**, 41–53 (1996).
59. Mauduit, J., Perouse, E. and Vert, M., Hydrolytic degradation of films prepared from blends of high and low molecular weight poly(DL-lactic acid)s. *Journal of Biomedical Materials Research* **30**, 201–207 (1996).
60. Renouf-Glauser, A. C., Rose, J., Farrar, D. and Cameron, R. E., A degradation study of PLLA containing lauric acid. *Biomaterials* **26**, 2415–2422 (2005).
61. Boccaccini, A. R., Blaker, J. J., Maquet, V., Chung, W., Jénôme, R., Nazhat, S. N., Poly(D,L-lactide) (PDLLA) foams with TiO_2 nanoparticles and PDLLA/TiO_2-Bioglass® foam composites for tissue engineering scaffolds. *Journal of Materials Science* **41**, 3999–4008 (2006).
62. Imai, Y., Fukuzawa, A. and Watannabe, M., Effect of blending tricalcium phosphate on hydrolytic degradation of a block polyester containing poly(L-lactic acid) segments. *Journal of Biomaterials Science – Polymer Edition* **10**, 773–786 (1999).
63. Maquet, V., Boccaccini, A. R., Pravata, L., Notingher, I. and Jérôme, R., Porous poly(α-hydroxy acids)/Bioglass® composite scaffolds for bone tissue engineering. I: Preparation and *in vitro* characterisation. *Biomaterials* **25**, 4185–4194 (2004).
64. Li, S. M. and Vert, M., Hydrolytic degradation of coral/poly(DL-lactic acid) bioresorbable material. *Journal of Biomaterials Science – Polymer Edition* **7**, 817–827 (1996).
65. Hurrell, S. and Cameron, R. E., The effect of initial polymer morphology on the degradation and drug release from polyglycolide. *Biomaterials* **23**, 2401–2409 (2002).

66. Milroy, G. E., Cameron, R. E., Mantle, M. D., Gladden, L. F. and Huatan, H., The distribution of water in degrading polyglycolide. Part II: Magnetic resonance imaging and drug release. *Journal of Materials Science: Materials in Medicine*, 465–473 (2003).
67. Chu, C. C., Degradation phenomena of two linear aliphatic polyester fibres used in medicine and surgery. *Polymer* **26**, 591–594 (1985).
68. Cutright, D. E., Hunsuck, E. E. and Beasley, J. D., Degradation rates of polymers and copolymers of polylactic and polyglycolic acids. *Oral Surgery*, 142–152 (1974).
69. Ginde, R. M. and Gupta, R. K., *In vitro* chemical degradation of poly(glycolic acid) pellets and fibres. *Journal of Applied Polymer Science* **33**, 2411 (1987).
70. Makino, K., Ohshima, H. and Kondo, T., Mechanism of hydrolytic degradation of poly(L-lactide) microcapsules: effects of pH, ionic strength and buffer concentration. *Journal of Microencapsulation* **3**, 203–212 (1986).
71. Zaikov, G. E., Quantitative aspects of polymer degradation in the living body. *Journal of Macromolecular Science, Part C: Polymer Reviews* **C25**, 551–597 (1985).
72. Schmitt, E. A., Flanagan, D. R. and Linhardt, R. J., Importance of distinct water environments in the hydrolysis of poly(DL-lactide-co-glycolide). *Macromolecules* **27**, 743–748 (1994).
73. Pratt, L., Chu, C., Auer, J., Chu, A., Kim., J., Zollweg, J. A. and Chu, C. C., The effect of ionic electrolytes on hydrolytic degradation of biodegradable polymers: mechanical and thermodynamic properties and molecular modeling. *Journal of Polymer Science: Part A: Polymer Chemistry* **31**, 1759–1769 (1993).
74. Mason, M. S., Miles, C. S. and Sparks, R. E., *Polymer Science Technology* **14**, 279 (1981).
75. Zhu, J. H., Shen, Z. R., Wu, L. T. and Yang, S. L., *In vitro* degradation of polylactide and poly(lactide-co-glycolide) microspheres. *Journal of Applied Polymer Science* **43**, 2099–2106 (1991).
76. Park, T. G., Degradation of poly(lactic-co-glycolic acid) microspheres: effects of copolymer composition. *Biomaterials* **16**, 1123–1130 (1995).
77. Visscher, G. E., Pearson, J. E., Fong, J. W., Argentieri, G. J. and Robinson, R. L., *Journal of Biomedical Materials Research* **22**, 733 (1988).
78. Kyriacos, A., Athanasiou, A., Gabriele, G., Neiderauer, G. and Agrawal, C., Sterilisation, toxicity, biocompatibility and clinical applications of polylactic acid/polyglycolic acid copolymers. *Biomaterials* **17**, 93–102 (1996).
79. Vainionpaa, S., Kilpikari, J., Laiho, J., Helevirta, P., Rokkanen, P. and Törmälä, P., Strength and strength retention *in vitro*, of absorbable, self reinforced polyglycolide (PGA) rods for fracture fixation. *Biomaterials* **8**, 46–49 (1987).
80. Lin, A. S. P., Barrows, T. H., Cartmell, S. H. and Guldberg, R. E., Microarchitectural and mechanical characterisation of oriented porous polymer scaffolds. *Biomaterials* **24**, 482–489 (2003).

6 Using synthetic bioresorbable polymers for orthopedic tissue regeneration

M. SANTORO, Politecnico di Milano, Italy and
G. PERALE, Industrie Biomediche Insubri SA, Switzerland

Abstract: The mechanical and biological properties and applicability of the most important polymers for bone regeneration are described. Fabrication techniques for improving applicability of the the polymers are examined with particular attention to tissue engineering, bone scaffold and drug delivery.

Key words: synthetic polymers, tissue engineering, bone scaffold, hydrogels, drug delivery.

6.1 Introduction

Overcoming diseases and providing worldwide medical care are high priorities. Materials science, in conjunction with biotechnology, can meet this challenge by developing artificial bones, organ implants and safe drug delivery systems. Bone has a vigorous potential to regenerate itself after damage; however, the efficacious repair for large bone defects resulting from resection or trauma or non-union fractures still requires the implantation of bone grafts.

Natural bone grafts possessing excellent osteoconduction and mechanical stability have been used extensively in clinical settings; depending on the relationship between the donor and the recipient, bone grafts are categorized into autografts, allografts, and xenografts. Autografts, considered the gold standard for bone implantation, have the advantage of immunocompatibility over allografts and xenografts.[1] However, problems such as donor-site morbidity, risk of infection and the availability of bone tissue of the correct size and shape, limit the use of autografts in orthopedic applications.

Every year, in the USA alone, hundreds of thousands of surgical cases of bone-grafting procedures are performed and the demand for bone grafts continues to rise and it is expected to be even greater over the next decades as the population ages. The efforts to address these problems and limitations of current available solutions have led to the development of new biomaterials and alternative therapies, among which a tissue engineering approach holds great promise.

Biomimetic scaffolds for bone engineering should be osteoconductive, osteoinductive, biocompatible, and biodegradable. Osteoconductivity refers to the ability of the graft to support the attachment of cells and allow new cell migration and vessel formation. The osteoinductive quality of scaffolds describes their ability to induce non-differentiated stem cells or progenitor cells along an osteogenic lineage. The scaffold should not elicit an immune response. Maximizing the porosity of the scaffold to promote cellular and neovascular ingrowth must be balanced by the need to maintain the structural integrity of the lattice (Table 6.1).[2]

Metals and ceramics are classically employed materials in bone engineering mainly because of their mechanical properties. Moreover, bone structure is very similar to that of many ceramics. Nevertheless, metal implants cannot perform as efficiently as a healthy bone, and metallic structures cannot remodel with time because they lack the capability of osteogenic regeneration. Most of these materials are not biodegradable, and therefore, might require subsequent surgical procedures. Recent advances in materials science have provided an abundance of innovations, which has led to the increasing importance of polymers in this field.

To help address the need for better bone substitutes, bone tissue engineers

Table 6.1 Synthetic and natural polymers for bone tissue engineering

Material	Characteristics
Poly(α-hydroxy acids)	Extensively studied aliphatic polyesters
	Degradation by hydrolysis
	Already approved for other health related applications
	Acidic by-products (e.g. lactic acid, glycolic acid), that enter the tricarboxylic acid cycle or alternatively (e.g. glycolic acid) are excreted in the urine
	Problems regarding biocompatibility and cytotoxicity in the surrounding area of the implantation site
Poly(ε-caprolactone)	Aliphatic polyester
	Degraded by hydrolysis or bulk erosion
	Slow degrading
	Degradation products incorporated in the tricarboxylic acid cycle
	Low chemical versatility
	Some problems related with withstanding mechanical loads
Poly(anhydrides)	Mainly developed as drug delivery carriers
	Biocompatible
	Support both endosteal and cortical bone regeneration
Poly(propylene fumarates)	Unsaturated polyester consisting of alternating propylene glycol and fumaric acids
	Main degradation products are fumaric acid and propylene glycol
	Satisfactory biological results

Adapted from Salgado *et al.*[2]

seek to create synthetic, three-dimensional bone scaffolds made from polymeric materials incorporating cells or growth factors to induce the growth of normal bone tissue. Polymeric materials show a great affinity for cell transplantation and differentiation, and their structure can be tuned in order to maintain an adequate mechanical resistance and be fully bioresorbable at the same time. In this chapter, the wide range of synthetic polymers used in tissue regeneration is described, in particular those used as bone scaffolds or drug delivery systems for osteogenic formation.

Specific features of these polymers, that are related to the many critical issues influencing effective scaffold design for bone repair, are here examined. The fabrication of tissue-engineered scaffolds and the use of polymer microspheres to deliver growth factors in bone tissue engineering applications are also described.

6.2 Poly (α-hydroxy acids)

The poly(α-hydroxy acids), specifically poly(lactic acid) (PLA), poly(glycolic acid) PGA, and related copolymers are the most widely used synthetic polymers in the tissue engineering field.[1,3–5] These polymers have gained popularity because they offer the typical synthetic polymer advantages of high purity, convenient processing, and good mechanical properties, in addition to their biodegradability. Their degradation products can be resorbed through the metabolic pathways in most cases, yielding CO_2 and water, and there is the potential to tailor their structure to alter degradation rates.[6]

However, Hollinger[7] has suggested that only lactic acid follows this pathway, and that glycolic acid is converted into glyoxylate (by glycolate oxidase), which is then transferred into glycine after reacting with glycine transaminase. Furthermore, since these materials have been used for over 25 years as resorbable sutures and fixation devices, they are already approved for human use in several forms and formulations by the FDA and EMEA. This class has been under intensive research in the development of osteosynthesis devices since the 1960s,[8–10] with the successful fabrication of several three-dimensional porous scaffolds,[11–13] craniofacial devices[14] and orthopedic implants,[15] such as pins and screws.

6.2.1 Poly(lactic acid) (PLA)

Poly(lactic acid) (PLA) is formed by the ring-opening polymerization of dilactide (Fig. 6.1), the dimerization product of lactic acid. As two enantiomeric isomers of lactide exist, PLA is available as the fully crystalline or the fully amorphous form, depending on the relative levels of the optical isomers present in the molecule. By tuning their relative amount it is also possible to mimic the mechanical properties of different tissues.

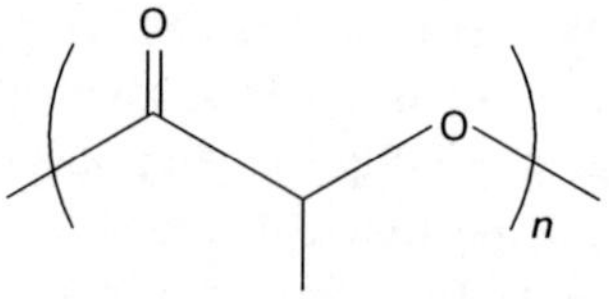

6.1 Poly(lactic acid) (PLA).

Poly(L-lactic acid) (PLLA) is a semicrystalline polymer with a crystallinity of about 37% and a melting temperature around 175 °C; it is therefore preferred in applications where high mechanical strength and toughness are required (e.g. for sutures and orthopedic devices). In contrast, the polymerization of racemic dilactide leads to poly(D,L-lactic acid) (PDLLA), which is an amorphous polymer used in, e.g., craniofacial fixation applications[16] and drug delivery systems. Further combinations have been employed to match stiffness and degradation kinetics, such as poly(L-lactide-co-D,L-lactide) (PLDL).

These scaffolds are bioresorbable, biocompatible and osteoconductive and can be easily molded to fit the individual defect.[17] These properties were demonstrated by implantation of PLLA membranes into New Zealand White rabbits to cover 1 cm mid-diaphyseal defects of the radii.[18] Untreated defects of a similar size on the contralateral limb served as controls. Results showed that within the experimental animals, cortical bone was seen spanning the defects with no adverse effects. In contrast, controls developed radial–ulnar synostosis without bone formation.

In practice, defect size limits the ability of lactide-based devices to promote bone formation. This was highlighted by Gugala and coworkers[19] when they attempted to treat tibial defects in sheep with PLLA. In the instances where only membranes were used, no osseous repair was noted. However, defects treated with both cancellous bone graft and synthetic PLLA membrane demonstrated significant bone repair.

Lin *et al.* tested the possibility of repairing large segmental bone defects (5 mm) in rats by developing a porous poly(L-lactide-*co*-D,L-lactide 7:3) (PLDL) scaffolds with a distinctive transversely isotropic oriented porosity.[20,21] Defects were created bilaterally in rats and either filled with a PLDL scaffold or left empty. Bone formation was observed in some of the control empty defects, indicating that 5 mm is not a critically sized long bone defect in the rat. However, scaffold-treated defects contained 30% more bone than empty ones.

6.2.2 Poly(glycolic acid) (PGA)

The other main polymer used in tissue engineering is poly(glycolic acid) (PGA) (Fig. 6.2), called also polyglycolide, as it is manufactured by ring

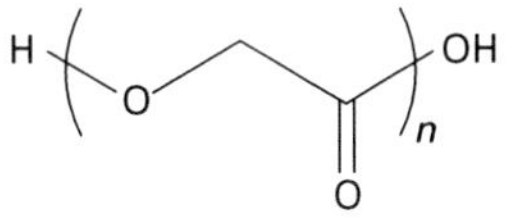

6.2 Poly(glycolic acid) (PGA).

opening of the dimer (glycolide). PGA of high molecular weight is a tough polymer melting at about 225 °C and, because of its high crystallinity, PGA unlike PLA is not soluble in most organic solvents.

Although it is possible to synthesize PGA by acid-catalyzed polycondensation in order to obtain longer chains, the resulting polymer generally has nevertheless a low molecular weight and often poor mechanical properties,[22] which compromise its employment in load-bearing applications.

Moreover, experimental studies showed that PGA had no specific osteostimulatory or osteoinhibitory properties compared with classical stainless steel implants.[23] No significant differences were noticed in biocompatibility between the implants and no adverse inflammatory foreign-body reactions. Research is, however, moving towards polymeric scaffolds, because of their easier processing and because of drawbacks related to metal devices, such as pseudomigration.[15] Attempts have been made to overcome these limitations by developing self-reinforced poly(α-hydroxy acids), polymer composites consisting of a polymer matrix and reinforcement elements, such as fibers, which have the same chemical composition as the matrix.

Studies on self-reinforced PGA (SR-PGA) rods assessed the suitability of these systems for fixation of cancellous bone fractures, osteotomies, and epiphyseal plate fractures where the fixation is not exposed to excessive mechanical stresses and where the loads are predominantly of a shear nature.[24]

Employment of SR-PGA devices in mechanical-loaded bones, such as the femur,[25] revealed that no permanent growth disturbance occurred in the operated femora compared with the control side. Unfortunately, SR-PGA implants lost a substantial part of their mechanical strength in approximately 2 weeks, confirming the problems of mechanical stability.

6.2.3 Poly(lactide-co-glycolide) (PLGA)

Copolymerization of different poly(α-hydroxy acids) is a way to tune the properties of the resulting polyester.[26] By varying the ratio of lactide to glycolide in poly(lactide-co-glycolide) (PLGA) (Fig. 6.3) it is possible to achieve the desired physical, chemical, surface and degradation properties.

The strength of the PLGA copolymer is maximal when healing of bone is just beginning, and it becomes less as bone healing advances.[27] This continuous decrease in integrity can, indeed be positive in some applications,

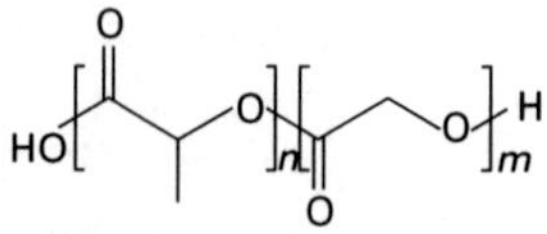

6.3 Structure of PLGA: n = number of units of lactic acid; m = number of units of glycolic acid.

as for example in bioabsorbable devices for cranial growth in children,[28] where compensatory bone lengthening (normalizing bone response) may take place, leading to maintained overall skeletal morphology.[29] For such purposes, more rapidly degrading materials such as PLGA are preferred because they soften with time and allow for device elongation without interfering with bone growth.[30]

Furthermore, implants made of PLGA devices have been demonstrated to represent excellent scaffolds for osseous ingrowth. *In vivo* bone formation mediated by PLGA foams seeded with rat marrow stromal cells was investigated into the rat mesentery.[12] As much as 11% of the foam volume penetrated by bone tissue was filled with mineralized tissue. The results proved that PLGA is capable of osteointegration for tissue-engineered surface modifications of cortical bone allografts.[31,32]

PLGA-based foam (PLGA 15:3) was also implanted in tibial defects created in male Sprague–Dawley rats, showing new woven bone formation in animals implanted with the PLGA-based foam after only one week.[33] Osteoclastic and osteoblastic activity and neovascularization was seen at the foam implantation site and it appeared that the foam served as a scaffold for new bone growth. Even if complete healing of the defect was not achieved, this study also confirmed that the bioresorbable PLGA-based foam was capable of serving as a scaffold for bony ingrowth.[33]

Despite the good performances of PLGA porous foams, some drawbacks arise as a consequence of the salt-leaching technique usually exploited for their fabrication. In salt-leaching, PLGA dissolved in an organic solvent with salt particles is placed in a mold to produce a polymer/salt mixture, which is immersed in water to remove salt particles and thus generate an open pore structure. It is claimed that scaffolds prepared by this method often exhibit a dense surface layer and poor interconnectivity between macropores, which reduces osteoblasts penetration so that tissue regeneration occurs only in the surface layer and not in the bulk.[11]

Other problems associated with PLGA scaffolds fabricated using the leaching techniques (particulate leaching) are: poor mechanical properties and the rapid decline of mechanical strength with increasing porosity, which is disadvantageous for structural tissue engineering applications.[34] These limitations have been overcome by means of the electrospinning technique, which allows polymeric ultrafine nanofibers to be produced in three-dimensional scaffolds.[35] The *in vitro* cell culture revealed that the resulting nanofiber provided an excellent osteoinductive and osteointegrative environment.

However, one of the major problems with PLGA scaffolds is the lack of osteoconductivity compared with the current gold standard of allograft.[36] The use of natural materials to coat the scaffolds used, is expected to increase osteoblast adhesion and to allow bone to express normal physiological function. To test this hypothesis, PLGA substrates were modified with coatings of collagen, chitosan, or *N*-succinylchitosan, and then used as scaffolds to evaluate their effects on osteoblast attachment, proliferation, and differentiation.[37] The results demonstrated that the pore size did not affect the osteoblast phenotype, but there was an increased cell attachment and proliferation owing to collagen, and an increase differentiation owing to chitosan and *N*-succinylchitosan.

These results promoted new strategies for modifying microenvironments to increase osteoblast adhesion, proliferation and differentiation on PLGA scaffolds, a strategy that might be useful for tissue regeneration. As a result, PLGA implants have proven to be versatile, support sufficient cell growth to be used commercially, and can be readily fabricated into highly porous scaffolds with different structures and sizes to fit anatomical bone defects.[38,39] Furthermore, devices made of amorphous PLGA have not caused clinically significant foreign body reactions.[15]

6.2.4 Comparing poly(α-hydroxy acids)

Copolymers, rather than homopolymers, are preferred for clinical application and they are thought to be associated with diminished risks of inflammatory reactions.[15] Polymers based on lactic and glycolic acids are still popular scaffold materials especially for orthopedic applications, such as bone, cartilage, and meniscus, as outlined in several reviews.[22,40,41] Each of these polymers, as well as various modifications or combinations of them, are capable of delivering cells or growth factors to target tissues while also providing a three-dimensional scaffold for cell function.[42,43]

Porous PLA/PGA copolymer has been proposed as a successful biodegradable matrix for tissue engineering for both bone and cartilage regeneration and osteoblasts are observed to adhere better to and produce more extracellular matrix proteins on PLA/PGA copolymer than on other osteocompatible bioresorbable materials.

Polyesters also have a major disadvantage. Most of them degrade by a bulk degradation mechanism,[44,45] which leads to the accumulation of acidic products within the polymer bulk that can cause late non-infectious inflammatory responses when released in a sudden burst upon structure breakdown.[46] An inflammatory response to poly(α-hydroxy acids) was also found to be triggered by the release of small particles during degradation that were phagocytized by macrophages and multinucleated giant cells.[47] This adverse reaction can occur weeks and months postoperatively and might need operative drainage. This is a major concern in orthopedic applications, where implants of considerable size would be required, thus resulting in release of degradation products with high local acid concentrations.

Furthermore, neither PGA nor PLA possess intrinsic bioactivity. Cellular responses to implants of these polymers are mediated mostly by surface adsorbed proteins, surface topography, and local acidity. Crystallinity seems to be another parameter affecting cell adhesion on PLA/PGA polymers.[48] The effects are believed to be a result of differences in protein conformation stemming from variations in binding to amorphous versus crystalline polymer surfaces. The chirality of crystalline regions may also play a role in controlling cellular response, but the detailed mechanisms of these effects are not fully understood.

Limitations of this class of materials include also insufficient mechanical properties with regard to load-bearing applications[49] and inflammatory or cytotoxic events owing to above-mentioned accumulation of acidic degradation products. The decrease of pH values in the tissues adjacent to degrading biodegradable polyesters may contribute to adverse effects. Consequently, one of the methods for the local re-establishment of physiological conditions could be incorporation of basic salts within the polymer. Promising results have already been presented in some *in vitro* studies.[50,51]

6.3 Polylactones

6.3.1 Poly(ε-caprolactone) (PCL)

The most prominent and thoroughly investigated polylactone is poly(ε-caprolactone) (PCL) (Fig. 6.4), an aliphatic, semicrystalline polyester with an interestingly low glass transition temperature (–60 °C) and melting temperature (59–64 °C). As a consequence, PCL is always in a rubbery state at room temperature and this unusual property undoubtedly contributes to the very high permeability of PCL for many therapeutic drugs[52] and to its high thermal stability.

PCL is prepared by the ring-opening polymerization of the cyclic monomer ε-caprolactone, and it can be copolymerized with numerous other monomers because of its high affinity with them.[53]

The discovery that PCL can be degraded by micro-organisms and by

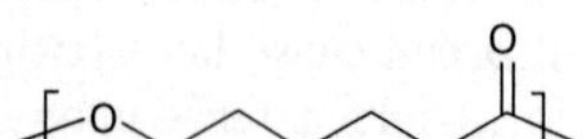

6.4 Poly(ε-caprolactone) (PCL).

hydrolysis under physiological conditions, led to the evaluation of PCL as a biodegradable material.[54] Several studies have revealed that bone marrow cells on caprolactone implants did not show alkaline phosphatase activity[55] and both PCL and its monomer are non-toxic and tissue-compatible,[56] as their degradation products are incorporated in the tricarboxylic acid cycle.

PCL retains mechanical properties for 5–6 months and then gradually loses its physical properties until completely metabolized over a period of 2 years,[57] and for this reason it is suitable for bone tissue engineering. Indeed, PCL degrades at a much slower rate than PLA and is therefore most suitable for the development of long-term implantable systems. By copolymerization of caprolactone with dilactide, it is also possible to tune the device degradation rates.[58]

Despite these advantages, in orthopedic applications the use of pure PCL is sporadic because considerable drawbacks arise from its low chemical versatility and ability to withstanding mechanical loads.[2] Examples are pure PCL pins implanted in rabbit humeri, which revealed minimal inflammation and abundant periosteal callus production.[59] Nevertheless, the feeble ossification rates indicated that these devices showed insufficient mechanical strength for load-bearing applications.[60]

Many efforts have been made to overcome these structural limitations and to develop PCL implants because it demonstrated excellent interactions with bone marrow cells[4] and an excellent compatibility with skeletal cell lines. Some studies investigated spiral-structured scaffolds, whose high porosity is pointed towards the improvement of nutrient transport and cell penetration, which is otherwise limited in conventional tissue-engineered scaffolds for large bone defects repair.[61] The resulting tool demonstrated enhanced cell proliferation, differentiation, and mineralization and allowed better cellular growth and penetration, owing to a porosity close to human trabecular bone. Unfortunately, significantly lower compressive modulus and strength than classical PCL scaffolds have been found, compromising the possibilities for these engineered devices.

Other attempts were made to synthesize solvent-free template arrays constituted of PCL nanowires,[62] which would be able to encapsulate active ingredients and enhance mesenchymal stem cell performances. Zein *et al.* created alternating ply designs of PCL using the fused deposition model (FDM) method.[63] Their results demonstrated that FDM could be used to produce scaffolds having adequate porosity for bone tissue engineering, while having mechanical properties just equal to soft trabecular bones.

Several studies followed another philosophy to solve mechanical problems in the use of PCL copolymer instead of changing the fabrication technique. Rat bone marrow cells were seeded and cultured on a porous polymeric system composed of cornstarch blended with PCL.[64] Results revealed that cells are well differentiated and form an extracellular matrix, while inducing an abundant formation of bone and bone marrow after one month. However, the polymers osteoconductive capacity is still lower than long-established bone graft implants.

Tricalcium phosphate (TCP) has also been incorporated into poly(ε-caprolactone), to tailor to the desired degradation and resorption kinetics of the polymer matrix.[65] This composite improves its biocompatibility and tissue integration. In addition, the basic resorption products of TCP would buffer the acidic by-products and help to avoid the formation of an unfavorable environment for cells.

Recently some biosynthetic composites have appeared, such as PCL/periosteum composites for osteochondral defect repair. *In vivo* studies on cylindrical defects created in 10 rabbits showed that PCL-based biocomposites promote excellent subchondral bone regeneration.[66] Research is currently focused on the synthesis of PCL composites, to combine the versatility of caprolactone together with the mechanical properties of other polymers. As poly(ε-caprolactone) is another FDA-approved polymer, PCL–PLA copolymers are primary items of investigation.

6.3.2 Poly(*p*-dioxanone) (PDS)

Poly(*p*-dioxanone) (PDS), another polylactone, is synthesized by catalyzed ring-opening polymerization of *p*-dioxanone and has gained increasing interest in the medical and pharmaceutical fields owing to its degradation to low-toxicity monomers *in vivo*.[67] This material (Fig. 6.5) has about 55% crystallinity with a glass transition temperature around –5 °C. PDS has a lower modulus than PLA or PGA, which have a higher degree of stiffness, and this allowed PDS to become the first degradable polymer to be used for monofilament sutures.

PDS demonstrated no acute or toxic effects on implantation, and thus has been used in a number of clinical applications ranging from suture materials to bone fixation devices.[68] Johnson and Johnson Orthopedics provides an absorbable pin for fracture fixation,[58] and bone pins have been introduced into the market under the names OrthoSorb and Ethipin, respectively, in the USA and Europe.[67] In craniofacial applications, the structure of PDS has been examined clinically in cranial vault procedures with promising results.[69] Advantages include the absence of observed intracranial translocation, acceptable aesthetic outcomes and low complication rates. Nevertheless,

6.5 Poly(*p*-dioxanone) (PDS).

absorbable suture fixation shows a critical lack of rigidity.[69] Therefore the most successful uses of poly(*p*-dioxanone) remain fixation of osteochondral fragments[70] and allografts,[71–73] and stabilization of osteotomies in the foot.[74,75] Distal chevron osteotomies fixed with a single PDS healed without evidence of infection, osteolysis, non-union, or necrosis.[76]

Furthermore, the use of PDS pins appears to be a reliable alternative to the use of metal in the fixation of unstable osteochondral fractures,[77] as no inflammation is observed. However, complete tissue restoration did not occur within the follow-up, even after complete degradation of PDS and, most importantly, PDS implants had no specific osteoinductive properties compared with metal pins.[23]

Despite the clinical potential of polydioxanone implants, a resorption rate in humans has not been fully elucidated. Studies indicated that PDS pin channels may persist at least 3 and 6 months after surgery in the human knee, without formation of marrow edema and with spontaneous cartilage healing.[78] In addition, although occasional cases of postoperative osteolytic and foreign-body reactions caused by polydioxanone pins[79] have been reported, the incidence and severity of adverse inflammatory reactions elicited by these devices have not been determined. PDS has also been used as an alternative to autologous tissues during reconstruction of the nasal septum. Although the use of this implant deserves further investigations, PDS foils have been shown to be useful in the correction of complex septal deformity, avoiding the risk of postoperative saddling.[80] Genuine poly(*p*-dioxanone) devices are mainly employed in pins and wires for defects repair, but a wide range of PDS-based copolymers are under investigation, in particular tools of PLA–DS–PEG (poly-D,L-lactic acid–*p*-dioxanone–polyethylene glycol block copolymer), owing to their dual applicability as defects filler and drug-carriers.[81,82]

6.4 Polyanhydrides

Polyanhydrides are among the most reactive and hydrolytically unstable polymers currently used as biomaterials. Their high chemical reactivity is an advantage, as polyanhydrides degrade by surface erosion without the need to incorporate various catalysts into the device formulation, the major drawback being the potential reactivity of the polymer matrix toward nucleophiles, which limits the drugs that can be successfully incorporated.

Owing to their pronounced hydrolytic instability, polyanhydrides have therefore been explored as degradable implant materials. Aliphatic polyanhydrides degrade within days whereas some aromatic polyanhydrides degrade over several years. Thus, aliphatic–aromatic copolymers, having intermediate rates of degradation, are usually employed.

A critical element in the development of polyanhydride biomaterials is controlling hydrolysis within a polymeric device. By tuning the relative hydrophobicity of the matrix, which can be achieved by an appropriate combination of monomers, the degradation rate can then be adjusted: as it is the case, for example, of copolymers of sebacic acid (SA), a hydrophilic monomer, with carboxyphenoxypropane (CPP), a hydrophobic monomer (Fig. 6.6).[83]

A comprehensive evaluation of their toxicity showed that, in general, the polyanhydrides possess excellent *in vivo* biocompatibility.[84] Their employment in load-bearing orthopedic applications, however, is restricted owing to inadequate mechanical properties.[85] Polyanhydrides-based devices for bone repair are limited to drug-release systems, as in the case of poly(sebacic anhydride) (PSA) and poly-D,L-lactide (PLA), for the treatment of chronic osteomyelitis and in the prophylaxis of bone infection.[42]

In order to overcome these structural limitations, several techniques were employed, among which photopolymerization is one of the most promising. Photopolymerizable polyanhydrides were synthesized with the objective of combining high strength, controlled degradation, and minimally invasive techniques for orthopedic applications and were shown to be osteocompatible.[86] Specifically, these monomers are photocurable, which allows for easy processing and *in situ* polymerization: hence they form highly crosslinked networks upon polymerization, which improve mechanical properties resulting in polymer networks that degrade controllably (and from the surface only) and allow maintenance of structural integrity with degradation. Depending on the chemical composition, these materials reached compressive and tensile strengths similar to those of cancellous bone.[3]

Initial mechanical studies with methacrylated monomers show that these polymers demonstrate enhanced mechanical integrity,[87] forming densely crosslinked networks. Moreover, they successfully polymerized *in situ* in a tibial bone defect, with good adhesion of the polymer to the cortical bone and medullary cavity, as well as minimal adverse tissue reaction to the photopolymerization reaction.[88]

Another strategy employed to enhance the mechanical strength, lies in the integration of aromatic imide bonds into the backbone of the polyanhydrides. This particular choice aims at combining the good mechanical properties of polyimides with the degradative properties of polyanhydrides.

Poly(anhydride-*co*-imides) matrices met compressive strengths similar to human bone,[89] displayed good osteocompatibility[90] and surface-eroding

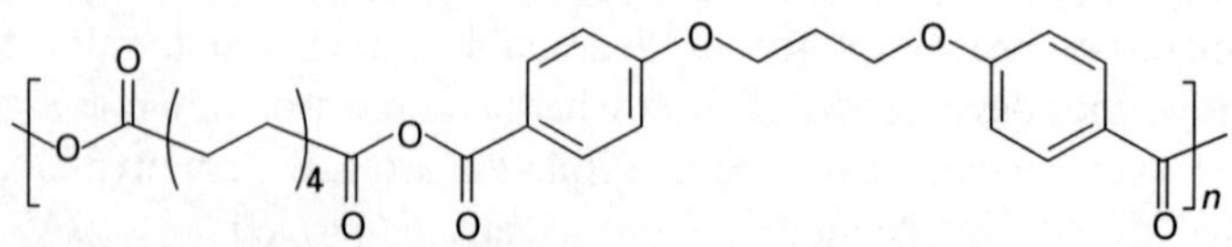

6.6 Polyanhydride SA-CPP.

properties.[91] Langer and coworkers[89–91] developed poly(anhydride-*co*-imides) (Fig. 6.7) that were compression-molded into circular discs, then implanted in rat subcutaneous tissues for nearly two months. The polymer matrices support endosteal and cortical bone regeneration and show minimal inflammation with dense fibrosis. Matrices degraded slowly and maintained their shapes over the period studied, displaying compressive properties similar to cancellous bone and thus being promising as devices for orthopedic applications.[90]

The main limitation of polyanhydrides is their lack of storage stability, requiring storage under refrigeration. These polymers undergo spontaneous depolymerization to low molecular weight polymers in organic solutions or upon storage at room temperatures and above.[93]

6.5 Fumarate-based polymers

The development of fumarate-based polyesters for biomedical applications started around 20 years ago. Fumaric acid is a natural metabolite involved in Krebs cycle, and is comprised of a reactive double bond available for chemically crosslinking reactions. These characteristics make fumaric acid a candidate building block for crosslinkable polymers. The first and most comprehensively investigated fumarate-based copolymer is the biodegradable copolyester poly(propylene fumarate) (PPF) (Fig. 6.8).[3]

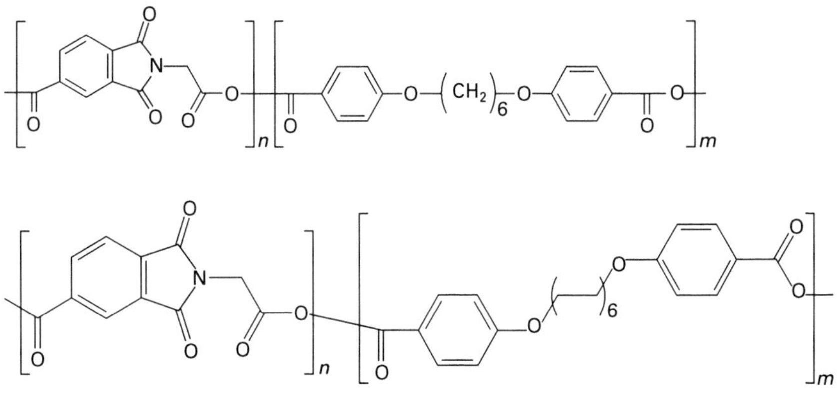

6.7 Poly[trimellitylimidoglycine-co-1,6-bis(*p*-carboxyphenoxy)hexane] developed for subcutaneous implantation.[92]

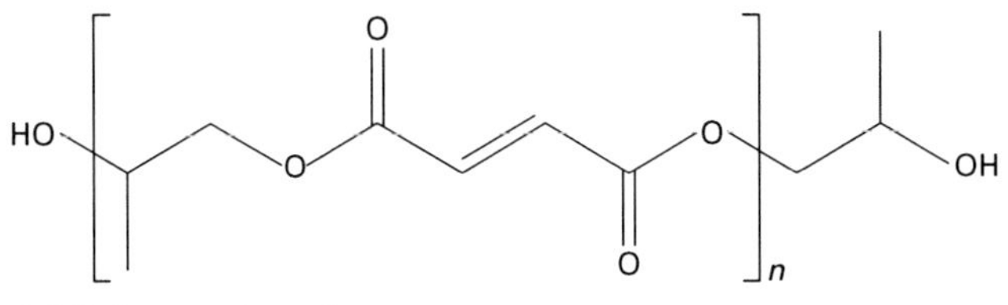

6.8 Polypropylene fumarate.

PPF-based materials are promising biodegradable scaffolds for filling skeletal defects, as their main advantage is the ability to cure *in vivo* into bone voids of any shape and size. The injectable nature of these materials makes them easy to be shaped into a desired interconnected porous structure, thus avoiding the use of severe invasive techniques.

Furthermore, these scaffolds have been shown to be both biodegradable and biocompatible *in vivo*. Results indicated that PPF is biocompatible within both soft and hard tissues, minimal fibrous encapsulation of the scaffolds occurred, and tissue response appeared to improve with implantation time. A progressive reduction in inflammatory cell density and a continued organization of connective tissue with the interstitial space was observed, even if scaffold microstructure did not seem to play a key role.[94]

By altering the molecular weight (e.g. by adding PPF–diacrylate), and varying the crosslinking reaction, the compressive strength of PPF-based networks can be tailored within a wide range (20–130 MPa), resulting in a biodegradable device with mechanical properties similar to human trabecular bone.[95] Additionally, PPF scaffolds with an interconnected pore network can be easily fabricated by incorporating a porogen during the crosslinking reaction, usually sodium chloride crystals.[96] Upon implantation, salt crystals are leached out leaving behind a highly porous polymeric implant. This method is quite simple, but leads to the formation of an unpredictable interconnectivity between pores, and generates a hypertonic environment around the polymeric implant. These shortcomings led to the development of an alternative method of creating a porous scaffold, called the foaming reaction. In this technique, PPF is combined with a weak acid and sodium bicarbonate, which react with water to produce carbon dioxide during polymerization, which causes foaming to occur thus producing an extremely porous material.[97] The effect of PPF-based cement produced by foaming was evaluated on the healing of critical size defects made in rat tibia.[98] At the site of the cortical drill hole defect, healing was noted to progress to complete closure by formation of mature bone, even in the absence of osteoinductive growth factors.

The use of PPF-based polymers as delivery vehicles has also been explored. Preliminary work investigating the repair of rabbit cranial defects demonstrated significant bone formation when defects were treated with PPF scaffolds to which osteogenic ingredients were adsorbed.[99] More sophisticated controlled delivery systems have also been developed using PPF. In particular, microparticles encapsulating the therapeutic peptide TP508 have successfully been integrated into both the pores and the polymer network of PPF scaffolds.[100,101]

Despite their advantages, PPF and other biodegradable polymers (e.g. oligo polyethylene glycol–fumarate), generally lack the mechanical properties required for regeneration of hard and dense cortical bone, and their utility is limited to soft tissue defects and non-load bearing bone defects.[100]

An innovative strategy to enhance the mechanical properties of biodegradable polymers is the incorporation of nanomaterials as fillers within polymer matrices. With the appropriate modifications to facilitate dispersion into polymers and to enhance interactions with the surrounding matrix, nanocomposites have demonstrated improved mechanical properties compared with unfilled polymers or polymers loaded with larger, micrometer-sized particles. A few studies have also shown enhanced cell function when bone cells are cultured on nanophase ceramic materials.[102]

6.6 Hydrogels

Hydrogels represent another class of polymer scaffolds, which are formed by polymerization and crosslinking of molecules such as acrylic acid, and *N*-isopropylacrylamide. Hydrogels are an attractive option because of their temperature-dependent physical properties. They can be designed to be gelatinous at room temperature, but they take on more rigid qualities at body temperatures.[103] This property could allow for the administration of tissue-engineering constructs via injection. Hydrogels also allow for relatively easy chemical manipulation of individual peptides. Incorporation of arginine–glycine–aspartate (RGD) peptide motifs on these polymers has been demonstrated to enhance osteoblast adhesion and proliferation.[104]

Polymeric hydrogels have the distinct advantage of being injectable, which allows the delivery of the construct to be less invasive and thereby reduces surgical risks. Employment of these types of polymers also ensures delivery of an even distribution of a precise number of cells. They can be configured to provide mechanical support to the cells to maintain their specific phenotype, without inhibiting migration. Common hydrogel substrates include the copolymers of poly(ethylene oxide) and poly(propylene oxide), known as pluronics, and natural polymers, including alginate and agarose. The delivery of a known concentration of cells is simplified when using a hydrogel, whereby 100% of the cells are encapsulated within the delivery system, compared with the fibers, for which cell delivery is dependent on cell attachment. The hydrogels also allow the suspended cells to be uniformly distributed throughout the volume of polymer delivered. In contrast, the distribution of cells in the polymer fiber system is not uniform and is difficult to predict.[3,84]

6.7 Future trends

Their similarity to the biological environment, and reduced likelihood of toxicity and inflammatory reactions, gives materials of natural origin a distinct advantage over synthetic ones. Despite this advantage, naturally derived polymers possess poor mechanical properties. It was concluded that

'Hydrogel scaffolds [typical natural manufactured materials] do not possess the mechanical strength to be used in load-bearing applications'.[105]

In contrast, synthetic biodegradable materials are easily formed into desired shapes with good mechanical strength, but their hydrophobic properties inhibit cell-binding properties and prevent formation of biomimetic scaffolds. Thus, these two kinds of biodegradable polymers have been hybridized to combine the advantageous properties of both constituents:[3] composite polymers are expected to be physically and biologically superior to single-material based scaffolds, and the properties of a composite may be varied by mixing different materials in various ratios.[106,107]

Ceramic nanoparticles, carbon nanotubes and hydroxyapatite are components that could potentially be incorporated to improve the structural properties of these polymers and, thus, play a key role in future developments of tissue-engineered composites.

Mechanical properties are of crucial importance for the regeneration of load-bearing tissues such as bone, to withstand stresses, to avoid scaffold fracture, and to maintain the structure to define the shape of the regenerated tissue. Inorganic nanoparticle fillers have been shown to add tensile strength, stiffness, abrasion resistance, crack resistance, and stability to polymer networks.[108] Furthermore, the presence of an osteoinductive mineral phase, e.g. bone-like apatite, provides the further benefit of increased stiffness and enhances and accelerates new bone formation. The significantly superior mechanical properties of these scaffolds create a better environment for bone healing and formation within the defect.

Nevertheless, although ceramic particles increase material stiffness and enhance creep behavior, the higher the particle content, the higher the number of interfaces between the polymer and the ceramic. This has to be taken into account because failure can preferentially occur at such interfaces when the scaffold is under mechanical loading. High density polyethylene (HDPE) reinforced with hydroxyapatite particles, for example, showed no enhancement of structural behavior, owing to the low degree of chemical interaction between the polymer matrix and the ceramic fillers.[109] It appears that this issue has been neglected in the context of bone engineering, although much effort has been made in the enhancement of the interfacial adhesion in conventional polymer matrix composites.[110]

The development of coupling methodologies that increase the adhesion of ceramic particles to the polymeric matrix is believed to be a possible route for the improvement of mechanical performance of these composites. From a materials point of view, a clear trend towards the development of composites can be detected. Hence, it can be predicted that composites will be the second and third generation of scaffold materials to enter the clinical arena in bone engineering applications.[110]

In addition, in studies presented so far, materials implanted into surgically created bone defects, and the out- and in-growth of new bone on their surfaces was examined. Under these conditions, it is believed that the bone is formed by osteoblasts that migrated from the adjacent original bone and marrow cavities, a mechanism that is referred to as osteoconduction.[111] Although this osteointegration is important and essential, it is not the only mechanism involved during bone healing. There are situations where the scaffolds, besides providing the template for tissue regeneration, need to be osteoinductive in order to stimulate the migration of undifferentiated cells and induce their differentiation into active osteoblasts, thus promoting *de novo* bone formation. To improve the osteoinductive properties of grafting materials, they have been combined with growth factors and various cells types with variable results depending on the host regenerative capability.[112] Therefore, osteoinductive approaches are crucial when the bone regenerative ability is diminished or lost.[113] Unfortunately, many of the above-mentioned composites, when employed as growth factors carriers, show limitations in terms of biodegradability, inflammatory reaction, immunological rejection, disease transmission and, most importantly, the inability to provide a sustained therapeutic factor level.[112,114]

The repair and regeneration of musculoskeletal tissues, particularly bone, where scaffolds need to have a high elastic modulus in order to provide temporary mechanical support without showing symptoms of fatigue or failure, to be retained in the space they were designated for and to provide the tissue with adequate space for growth, remains a demanding application.[110]

Next-generation biomaterials should combine bioactive and bioresorbable materials, which mimic the natural function of bone and activate *in vivo* mechanisms of tissue regeneration. However, to date, an injectable, bioactive, and strong scaffold for stem cell encapsulation and bone engineering is yet to be developed.

6.8 Conclusions

The rapidly emerging field of biomimetic materials will form one of the most important technologies of the 21st century. Biomimetic materials seek to replicate or mimic biological processes and materials, both inorganic and organic (e.g. synthetic spider silk, DNA chips, and nanocrystal growth within virus cages). Better understanding of how living organisms produce minerals and composites will open up new areas of research and applications. Materials will be able to be fabricated much more precisely and efficiently, resulting in new functionalities and increase performance (e.g. self-repairing, ultrahard, and ultralight composites for aircraft). To develop these materials, we will need new chemical strategies that combine self-assembly with the ability to form hierarchically structured materials.

6.9 References

1. Ma, P. X.; Elisseeff, J. H. *Scaffolding in tissue engineering*; Taylor & Francis: Boca Raton, 2005.
2. Salgado, A. J.; Coutinho, O. P.; Reis, R. L. *Macromol biosci* 2004, **4**, 743–765.
3. Atala, A.; Lanza, R. P.; Thomson, J. A.; Nerem, R. M. *Principles of regenerative medicine*; Academic Press: Burlington MA., 2008.
4. Hollinger, J. O.; Einhorn, T. A.; Doll, B. A.; Sfeir, C. *Bone Tissue Engineering*; CRC Press: Boca Raton FL., 2005.
5. Dumitriu, S. *Polymeric biomaterials*; 2nd ed.; Marcel Dekker, Inc.: New York, 2002.
6. Gunatillake, P. A.; Adhikari, R. *Eur Cell Mater* 2003, **5**, 1–16; discussion 16.
7. Hollinger, J. O. *J Biomed Mater Res* 1983, **17**, 71–82.
8. Kulkarni, R. K.; Pani, K. C.; Neuman, C.; Leonard, F. *Arch Surg* 1966, **93**, 839–43.
9. Rokkanen, P. U. *Ann Chir Gynaecol* 1998, **87**, 13–20.
10. Suuronen, R.; Kallela, I.; Lindqvist, C. *J Craniomaxillofac Trauma* 2000, **6**, 19–27; discussion 28–30.
11. Ishaug-Riley, S. L.; Crane, G. M.; Miller, M. J.; Yasko, A. W.; Yaszemski, M. J.; Mikos, A. G. *J Biomed Mater Res* 1997, **36**, 17–28.
12. Ishaug-Riley, S. L.; Crane, G. M.; Gurlek, A.; Miller, M. J.; Yasko, A. W.; Yaszemski, M. J.; Mikos, A. G. *J Biomed Mater Res* 1997, **36**, 1–8.
13. Robinson, B. P.; Hollinger, J. O.; Szachowicz, E. H.; Brekke, J. *Otolaryngol Head Neck Surg* 1995, **112**, 707–713.
14. Habal, M. B. *J Craniofac Surg* 1997, **8**, 121–126.
15. Yaszemski, M. J. *Biomaterials in orthopedics*; M. Dekker: New York, 2004.
16. Imola, M. J.; Schramm, V. L. *Laryngoscope* 2002, **112**, 1897–1901.
17. Oreffo, R. O.; Triffitt, J. T. *Bone* 1999, **25**, 5S–9S.
18. Meinig, R. P.; Rahn, B.; Perren, S. M.; Gogolewski, S. *J Orthop Trauma* 1996, **10**, 178–90.
19. Gugala, Z.; Gogolewski, S. *J Orthop Trauma* 1999, **13**, 187–195.
20. Lin, A. S. P.; Barrows, T. H.; Cartmell, S. H.; Guldberg, R. E. *Biomaterials* 2003, **24**, 481–489.
21. Guldberg, R. E.; Oest, M.; Lin, A. S.; Ito, H.; Chao, X.; Gromov, K.; Goater, J. J.; Koefoed, M.; Schwarz, E. M.; O'Keefe, R. J.; Zhang, X. *J Musculoskelet Neuronal Interact* 2004, **4**, 399–400.
22. Agrawal, C. M.; Athanasiou, K. A.; Heckman, J. D. *Mater Sci for Tissue Engineering* 1997, **250**, 115–128.
23. Pihlajamaki, H. K.; Salminen, S. T.; Tynninen, O.; Bostman, O. M.; Laitinen, O. *Calcif Tissue Int* 2010, **87**, 90–98.
24. Tormala, P.; Vasenius, J.; Vainionpaa, S.; Laiho, J.; Pohjonen, T.; Rokkanen, P. *J Biomed Mater Res* 1991, **25**, 1–22.
25. Lautiainen, I.; Miettinen, H.; Makela, A.; Rokkanen, P.; Tormala, P. *Clin Mater* 1994, **17**, 197–201.
26. Smith, M.; March, J. *March's advanced organic chemistry: reactions, mechanisms, and structure*; 6th ed.; Wiley–Interscience: Hoboken, N.J., 2007.
27. Habal, M. B.; Pietrzak, W. S. *J Craniofac Surg* 1999, **10**, 491–499.
28. Antikainen, T.; Pernu, H.; Tormala, P.; Kallioinen, M.; Waris, T.; Serlo, W. *Acta Neurochir Wien.* 1994, **128**, 26–31.

29. Eppley, B. L.; Sadove, A. M. *J Craniofac Surg* 1992, **3**, 190–196.
30. Eppley, B. L.; Sadove, A. M. *J Craniofac Surg* 1994, **5**, 110–114; discussion 115.
31. Bostman, O.; Paivarinta, U.; Partio, E.; Vasenius, J.; Manninen, M.; Rokkanen, P. *J Bone Joint Surg Am* 1992, **74**, 1021–1031.
32. Bostman, O.; Partio, E.; Hirvensalo, E.; Rokkanen, P. *Acta Orthop Scand* 1992, **63**, 173–176.
33. Wise, D. L. *Biomaterials and bioengineering handbook*; Marcel Dekker: New York, 2000.
34. Thomson, R. C.; Yaszemski, M. J.; Powers, J. M.; Mikos, A. G. *J Biomater Sci Polym Ed* 1995, **7**, 23–38.
35. Zhao, L.; He, C.; Gao, Y.; Cen, L.; Cui, L.; Cao, Y. *J Biomed Mater Res B Appl Biomater* 2008, **87**, 26–34.
36. Kanczler, J. M.; Oreffo, R. O. *Eur Cell Mater* 2008, **15**, 100–114.
37. Wu, Y. C.; Shaw, S. Y.; Lin, H. R.; Lee, T. M.; Yang, C. Y. *Biomaterials* 2006, **27**, 896–904.
38. Antonov, E. N.; Bagratashvili, V. N.; Whitaker, M. J.; Barry, J. J.; Shakesheff, K. M.; Konovalov, A. N.; Popov, V. K.; Howdle, S. M. *Adv Mater Deerfield* 2004, **17**, 327–330.
39. Borden, M.; Attawia, M.; Khan, Y.; El-Amin, S. F.; Laurencin, C. T. *J Bone Joint Surg Br* 2004, **86**, 1200–1208.
40. Hutmacher, D. W. *Biomaterials* 2000, **21**, 2529–2543.
41. Seal, B. L.; Otero, T. C.; Panitch, A. *Mater Sci Eng R-Rep* 2001, **34**, 147–230.
42. Chen, L. B.; Wang, H.; Wang, J.; Chen, M.; Shang, L. *J Biomed Mater Res Part B–Appl Biomater* 2007, **83B**, 589–595.
43. Yaszemski, M. J.; Payne, R. G.; Hayes, W. C.; Langer, R.; Mikos, A. G. *Biomaterials* 1996, **17**, 175–185.
44. Attawia, M. A.; Herbert, K. M.; Uhrich, K. E.; Langer, R.; Laurencin, C. T. *J Biomed Mater Res* 1999, **48**, 322–327.
45. Andriano, K. P.; Tabata, Y.; Ikada, Y.; Heller, J. *J Biomed Mater Res* 1999, **48**, 602–612.
46. Simon, J. A.; Ricci, J. L.; Di Cesare, P. E. *Am J Orthop Belle Mead NJ*. 1997, **26**, 754–762.
47. Xia, Z.; Triffitt, J. T. *Biomed Mater* 2006, **1**, R1–9.
48. Park, A.; Cima, L. G. *J Biomed Mater Res* 1996, **31**, 117–130.
49. Webb, A. R.; Yang, J.; Ameer, G. A. *Expert Opin Biol Ther* 2004, **4**, 801–812.
50. Agrawal, C. M.; Athanasiou, K. A. *J Biomed Mater Res* 1997, **38**, 105–114.
51. Bostman, O.; Pihlajamaki, H. *Biomaterials* 2000, **21**, 2615–2621.
52. Lee, P. I.; Good, W. R.; American Chemical Society. Division of Industrial and Engineering Chemistry.; American Chemical Society. Meeting *Controlled-release technology: pharmaceutical applications*; American Chemical Society: Washington, DC, 1987.
53. Yu, T.; Ren, J.; Gu, S. Y.; Yang, M. *Polym Adv Technol* 2010, **21**, 183–188.
54. Chasin, M.; Langer, R. S. *Biodegradable polymers as drug delivery systems*; M. Dekker: New York, 1990.
55. Calvert, J. W.; Marra, K. G.; Cook, L.; Kumta, P. N.; DiMilla, P. A.; Weiss, L. E. *J Biomed Mater Res* 2000, **52**, 279–284.
56. Matsuda, T.; Nagase, J.; Ghoda, A.; Hirano, Y.; Kidoaki, S.; Nakayama, Y. *Biomaterials* 2003, **24**, 4517–4527.

57. Hutmacher, D. W.; Schantz, T.; Zein, I.; Ng, K. W.; Teoh, S. H.; Tan, K. C. *J Biomed Mater Res* 2001, **55**, 203–216.
58. Middleton, J. C.; Tipton, A. J. *Biomaterials* 2000, **21**, 2335–2346.
59. Lowry, K. J.; Hamson, K. R.; Bear, L.; Peng, Y. B.; Calaluce, R.; Evans, M. L.; Anglen, J. O.; Allen, W. C. *J Biomed Mater Res* 1997, **36**, 536–541.
60. Agrawal, C. M.; Ray, R. B. *J Biomed Mater Res* 2001, **55**, 141–150.
61. Wang, J.; Valmikinathan, C. M.; Liu, W.; Laurencin, C. T.; Yu, X. *J Biomed Mater Res A* 2010, **93**, 753–762.
62. Porter, J. R.; Henson, A.; Popat, K. C. *Biomaterials* 2009, **30**, 780–788.
63. Zein, I.; Hutmacher, D. W.; Tan, K. C.; Teoh, S. H. *Biomaterials* 2002, **23**, 1169–1185.
64. Mendes, S. C.; Bezemer, J.; Claase, M. B.; Grijpma, D. W.; Bellia, G.; Degli-Innocenti, F.; Reis, R. L.; De Groot, K.; Van Blitterswijk, C. A.; De Bruijn, J. D. *Tissue Eng* 2003, **9**, S91–S101.
65. Nather, A. *Bone grafts and bone substitutes: basic science and clinical applications*; World Scientific: Hackensack, N.J., 2005.
66. Mrosek, E. H.; Schagemann, J. C.; Chung, H. W.; Fitzsimmons, J. S.; Yaszemski, M. J.; Mardones, R. M.; O'Driscoll, S. W.; Reinholz, G. G. *J Orthop Res* 2010, **28**, 141–148.
67. Makela, E. A.; Vainionpaa, S.; Vihtonen, K.; Mero, M.; Helevirta, P.; Tormala, P.; Rokkanen, P. *Clin Orthop Relat Res* 1989, 300–308.
68. Yang, K.-K.; Wang, X.-L.; Wang, Y.-Z. 2002, **42**, 373–398.
69. Fearon, J. A. *Plast Reconstr Surg* 2003, **111**, 27–38; discussion 39.
70. Matava, M. J.; Brown, C. D. *Arthroscopy* 1997, **13**, 124–128.
71. Convery, F. R.; Botte, M. J.; Akeson, W. H.; Meyers, M. H. *Contemp Orthop* 1994, **28**, 101–107.
72. Chu, C. R.; Convery, F. R.; Akeson, W. H.; Meyers, M.; Amiel, D. *Clin Orthop Relat Res* 1999, 159–168.
73. Bugbee, W. D.; Convery, F. R. *Clin Sports Med* 1999, **18**, 67–75.
74. Gill, L. H.; Martin, D. F.; Coumas, J. M.; Kiebzak, G. M. *J Bone Joint Surg Am* 1997, **79**, 1510–1518.
75. Winemaker, M. J.; Amendola, A. *Foot Ankle Int* 1996, **17**, 623–628.
76. Deorio, J. K.; Ware, A. W. *Foot Ankle Int* 2001, **22**, 832–835.
77. Plaga, B. R.; Royster, R. M.; Donigian, A. M.; Wright, G. B.; Caskey, P. M. *J Bone Joint Surg Br* 1992, **74**, 292–296.
78. Sirlin, C. B.; Boutin, R. D.; Brossmann, J.; Pathria, M. N.; Convery, F. R.; Bugbee, W.; Resnick, D. *Am J Roentgenol* 2001, **176**, 83–90.
79. Kalla, T. P.; Janzen, D. L. *J Foot Ankle Surg* 1995, **34**, 366–370.
80. Tweedie, D. J.; Lo, S.; Rowe-Jones, J. M. *Arch Facial Plast Surg* 2010, **12**, 106–113.
81. Matsushita, N.; Terai, H.; Okada, T.; Nozaki, K.; Inoue, H.; Miyamoto, S.; Takaoka, K. *J Orthop Sci* 2006, **11**, 505–511.
82. Eguchi, Y.; Wakitani, S.; Imai, Y.; Naka, Y.; Hashimoto, Y.; Nakamura, H.; Takaoka, K. *J Bone Miner Metabol* 2010, **28**, 157–164.
83. Saltzman, W. M. *Drug delivery: engineering principles for drug therapy*; Oxford University Press: Oxford [England]; New York, 2001.
84. Ratner, B. D. *Biomaterials science: an introduction to materials in medicine*; 2nd ed.; Elsevier Academic Press: Amsterdam; Boston, 2004.
85. Katti, D. S.; Lakshmi, S.; Langer, R.; Laurencin, C. T. *Adv Drug Deliv Rev* 2002, **54**, 933–961.

86. Anseth, K. S.; Shastri, V. R.; Langer, R. *Nat Biotechnol* 1999, **17**, 156–159.
87. Burg, K. J.; Porter, S.; Kellam, J. F. *Biomaterials* 2000, **21**, 2347–59.
88. Burkoth, A. K.; Anseth, K. S. *Biomaterials* 2000, **21**, 2395–2404.
89. Uhrich, K. E.; Laurencin, C.; Langer, R. S. *Polym Mater Sci Eng* 1993, **70**, 239–240.
90. Ibim, S. M.; Uhrich, K. E.; Bronson, R.; El-Amin, S. F.; Langer, R. S.; Laurencin, C. T. *Biomaterials* 1998, **19**, 941–951.
91. Staubli, A.; Ron, E.; Langer, R. *J Am Chem Soc* 1990, **112**, 4419–4424.
92. Uhrich, K. E.; Ibim, S. E.; Larrier, D. R.; Langer, R.; Laurencin, C. T. *Biomaterials* 1998, **19**, 2045–2050.
93. Kumar, N.; Langer, R. S.; Domb, A. J. *Adv Drug Deliv Rev* 2002, **54**, 889–910.
94. Fisher, J. P.; Vehof, J. W.; Dean, D.; van der Waerden, J. P.; Holland, T. A.; Mikos, A. G.; Jansen, J. A. *J Biomed Mater Res* 2002, **59**, 547–556.
95. Hedberg, E. L.; Kroese-Deutman, H. C.; Shih, C. K.; Crowther, R. S.; Carney, D. H.; Mikos, A. G.; Jansen, J. A. *Biomaterials* 2005, **26**, 4616–4623.
96. Fisher, J. P.; Holland, T. A.; Dean, D.; Engel, P. S.; Mikos, A. G. *J Biomater Sci Polym Ed* 2001, **12**, 673–687.
97. Kim, C. W.; Talac, R.; Lu, L. C.; Moore, M. J.; Currier, B. L.; Yaszemski, M. J. *J Biomed Mater Res Part A* 2008, **85A**, 1114–1119.
98. Lewandrowski, K. U.; Cattaneo, M. V.; Gresser, J. D.; Wise, D. L.; White, R. L.; Bonassar, L.; Trantolo, D. J. *Tissue Eng* 1999, **5**, 305–316.
99. Vehof, J. W.; Fisher, J. P.; Dean, D.; van der Waerden, J. P.; Spauwen, P. H.; Mikos, A. G.; Jansen, J. A. *J Biomed Mater Res* 2002, **60**, 241–251.
100. Holland, T. A.; Mikos, A. G. *Tissue Eng I: Scaffold Systems Tissue Eng* 2006, **102**, 161–185.
101. Hedberg, E. L.; Tang, A.; Crowther, R. S.; Carney, D. H.; Mikos, A. G. *J Control Release* 2002, **84**, 137–150.
102. Mistry, A. S.; Mikos, A. G.; Jansen, J. A. *J Biomed Mater Res A* 2007, **83**, 940–953.
103. Stile, R. A.; Healy, K. E. *Biomacromolecules* 2002, **3**, 591–600.
104. Bongio, M.; van den Beucken, J. J.; Nejadnik, M. R.; Leeuwenburgh, S. C.; Kinard, L. A.; Kasper, F. K.; Mikos, A. G.; Jansen, J. A. *Eur Cell Mater* 2011, **22**, 359–376.
105. Drury, J. L.; Mooney, D. J. *Biomaterials* 2003, **24**, 4337–4351.
106. Turhani, D.; Weissenbock, M.; Watzinger, E.; Yerit, K.; Cvikl, B.; Ewers, R.; Thurnher, D. *Int J Oral Maxillofac Surg* 2005, **34**, 543–550.
107. Arinzeh, T. L.; Tran, T.; McAlary, J.; Daculsi, G. *Biomaterials* 2005, **26**, 3631–3638.
108. Gleeson, J. P.; Plunkett, N. A.; O'Brien, F. J. *Eur Cell Mater* 2010, **20**, 218–230.
109. Wang, M.; Bonfield, W. *Biomaterials* 2001, **22**, 1311–1320.
110. Hutmacher, D. W.; Schantz, J. T.; Lam, C. X.; Tan, K. C.; Lim, T. C. *J Tissue Eng Regen Med* 2007, **1**, 245–260.
111. Mistry, A. S.; Mikos, A. G. *Adv Biochem Eng Biotechnol* 2005, **94**, 1–22.
112. Fischer, J.; Kolk, A.; Wolfart, S.; Pautke, C.; Warnke, P. H.; Plank, C.; Smeets, R. *J Cranio-Maxillofac Surg* 2011, **39**, 54–64.
113. Oliveira, S. M.; Mijares, D. Q.; Turner, G.; Amaral, I. F.; Barbosa, M. A.; Teixeira, C. C. *Tissue Eng Part A* 2009, **15**, 635–643.
114. De Laporte, L.; Cruz Rea, J.; Shea, L. D. *Biomaterials* 2006, **27**, 947–954.

Part II

Aspects of durability and reliability of non-bioresorbable medical polymers

7
Wear processes in polymer implants

D. E. T. SHEPHERD and K. D. DEARN,
University of Birmingham, UK

Abstract: Wear processes are discussed for polymers used in a wide variety of implants in the human body, such as in joint replacement implants for the hip and knee. The articulation of metal or ceramic components against a polymer component can lead to the generation of wear debris and the effect this debris may have in the body is examined.

Key words: debris, implants, polymer, wear.

7.1 Introduction

Wear is defined as the loss of material from a surface as the result of relative motion. In this chapter, the wear processes in polymer implants are discussed. Polymers are used in a wide variety of implants in the human body such as joint replacement implants, pacemakers, catheters and heart valves. Wear of polymer implants is almost exclusive to joint replacement implants, such as those used to replace the hip or knee. These implants involve the articulation of a metal or ceramic against a polymer. Typically these implants operate with a mixed or boundary lubrication regime and, therefore, there is contact between the bearing surfaces that can lead to the generation of wear debris. The chapter is divided into sections that cover implants, wear processes, polymers used in implants, the effect of wear debris on the body and, finally, likely future trends.

7.2 Implants

7.2.1 Surface articulating joint replacement

Human synovial joints, such as the hip and knee, can be affected by arthritis that results in damage to the natural articular cartilage joint surface. The diseased joint can be treated by replacing it with a joint replacement implant. The most common types of joint replacement implant are those for the hip and knee, although replacement implants also exist for other synovial joints such as the ankle, elbow, finger, shoulder and wrist. In addition to replacing synovial joints, there is a wide range of articulating implants available for replacing the intervertebral disc in the spine. However, for surface articulating joint replacement implants, we concentrate on hip and knee replacements, as they are the most commonly implanted joint replacements. In the UK in 2009 approximately 75 000 hip replacements and 80 000 knee replacements were performed.

The human hip joint consists of the articulation between the femoral head and the acetabulum. Forces acting on the hip joint during walking can be two to three times body weight (Bergmann *et al.* 2001). Thus, for a 75 kg person, the forces acting on the hip are between 1472 and 2207 N. The traditional hip replacement consists of femoral and acetabular parts that form a ball and socket joint (Fig. 7.1). The femoral component has a metal stem that fits into the femur and a spherical femoral head that articulates with the acetabular cup. Joint replacement surgery involves removing the natural femoral head, broaching the femur to create the shape of the femoral stem and reaming the acetabulum to create room for the acetabular component. The fixation of hip replacement implants can be with bone cement poly(methyl methacrylate) (PMMA) bone cement or an interference fit with the addition of a porous surface to encourage bone in-growth (Kapoor *et al.*, 2004; Kienapfel *et al.*, 1999).

There are a variety of bearing material combinations available for a hip replacement including metal against polymer, ceramic against polymer, metal against metal and metal against ceramic. The most commonly used

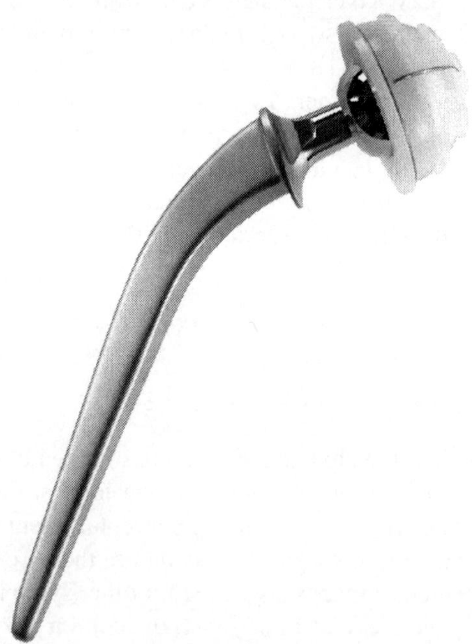

7.1 Stanmore hip system (reproduced with kind permission from Biomet. © by Biomet).

polymer is ultra high molecular weight polyethylene (UHMWPE) although increasingly crosslinked polyethylene is being used. The metal is CoCrMo alloy or stainless steel, with the ceramics being either alumina or zirconia (Dowson, 2001).

The main articulation in the human knee joint is between the femur and the tibia. The design of knee replacement implants comprises femoral and tibial components (Fig. 7.2). Bone is cut away from the natural femur and tibia in order to fit the knee replacement components. The femoral component is generally made from CoCrMo alloy. The tibial component is generally a two-piece design comprising a Ti alloy tibial tray and a polymer insert, made from ultra high molecular weight polyethylene. Although, the use of crosslinked polyethylene is increasing in knee replacement, there is great debate over its use and worry over possible failures owing to its poorer mechanical properties (Jacofsky, 2008; Rodriguez, 2008).

7.2.2 Soft layer joint replacement

Joint replacement implants have traditionally involved a metal against polymer or ceramic against polymer articulation, but these materials have a much

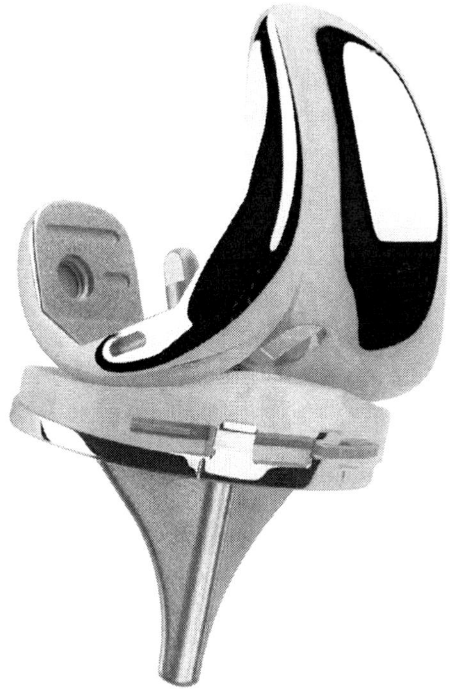

7.2 Vanguard complete knee system (reproduced with kind permission from Biomet. © by Biomet).

higher Young's modulus than that of the natural articular cartilage that is being replaced. It has been proposed that future designs of joint replacement implants may benefit from the use of a soft layer, which has mechanical properties similar to the natural articular cartilage (Fig. 7.3). This type of implant is known variously as compliant, cushion or soft-layer bearings. Over the years there has been much development in this area with designs proposed for replacement of the hip and knee (Dowson *et al.*, 1991; Auger *et al.*, 1995; Scholes *et al.*, 2007). Although there are promising results from laboratory studies, this type of implant has yet to be used in patients.

7.2.3 Single-piece elastomer joint replacement

Replacement of the finger and wrist joints commonly involves the use of single-piece implants manufactured from silicone. These implants do not have articulating bearing surfaces, as with most joint replacement implants, but consist of two stems joined to a central barrel (Fig. 7.4). The original design of implants for the finger and wrist were the Swanson designs. For the Swanson wrist implant, the proximal stem fits into a cavity created in the radius and the distal stem fits into a cavity created in the carpal bones and into the third metacarpal (Costi *et al.*, 1998; Shepherd and Johnstone, 2002). The implant stems are not fixed in position and the stems can move like a piston in and out of the bone during motion of the wrist. The Swanson finger implant is similar in design and there are a number of other designs of single-piece finger replacement joints such as the NeuFlex and Preflex (Joyce, 2004).

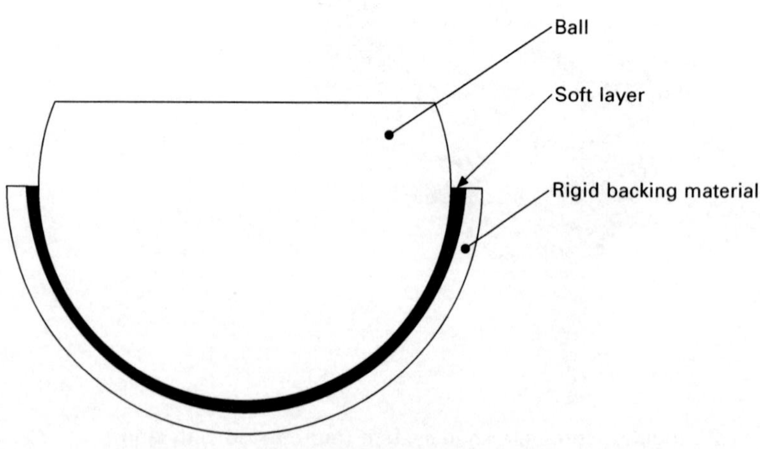

7.3 Cushion form joint for the hip.

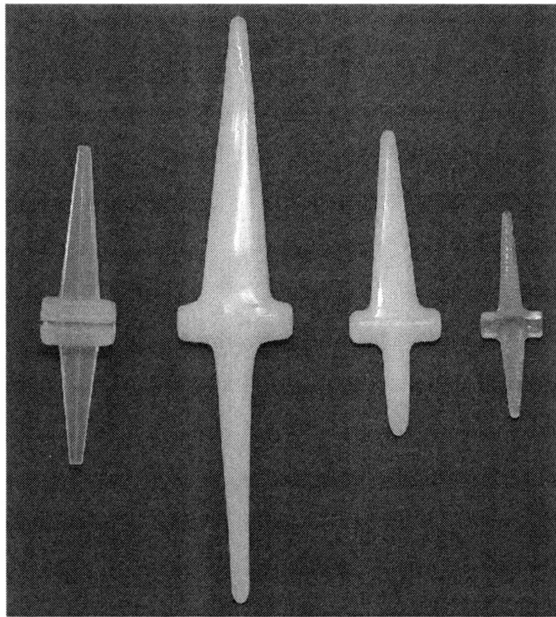

7.4 Various single-piece finger and wrist implants. From left to right; Avanta finger, Swanson wrist (large), Swanson wrist (small) and Swanson finger.

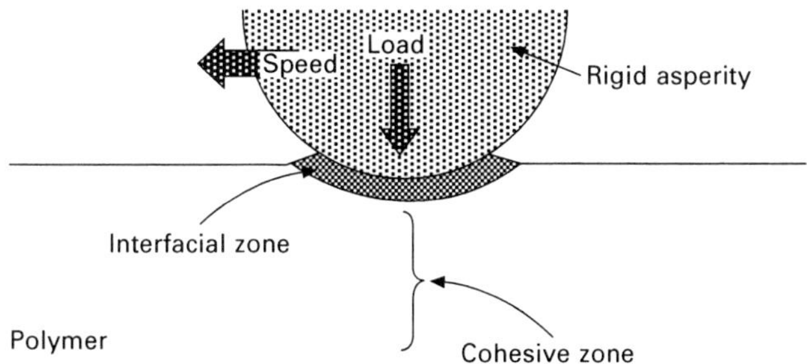

7.5 A schematic of the distinction between interfacial and cohesive wear in a polymer/rigid surface interface (after Briscoe and Sinha, 2002).

7.3 Wear processes and theory for polymer implants

There are two broad classifications of wear in polymers. These are interfacial wear that generally involves the surface and cohesive wear concerned with the subsurface. More specifically, the most prevalent form of surface induced wear is adhesion, whereas that below the surface occurs principally in the form of abrasion, fatigue and chemical/corrosive effects. Figure 7.5 shows schematically, the distinction between interfacial and cohesive wear processes at a polymer/rigid surface interface (Briscoe and Sinha, 2002). Strictly speaking corrosive wear generally involves a chemical reaction between a polymer and its environment, so is not a mechanism of wear, rather it can facilitate the onset of one or more of the other wear mechanisms and is not considered further here.

7.3.1 Adhesive wear

The mechanism of adhesive wear describes the transference between sliding surfaces that are in very close proximity, of a soft material to a harder mating counterface. It is caused by the solid-phase welding of asperities and when sliding is continuous, these junctions shear causing material to be transferred. The welded junctions between the surfaces occur through electrostatic forces (particularly van der Waals forces), the junction being stronger than the bulk properties of the polymer itself inducing failure in the bulk and the fragmented asperity detached. This can either be temporary (giving rise to free particles) or permanent in the form of a transfer film. The formation of the transfer film is governed by the counterface materials, surface roughnesses and the sliding conditions (Stachowiak and Batchelor, 2000).

The mechanisms of the formation of transfer layers are not uniform for all polymers. Certain polymers, including UHMWPE, are associated with low friction and wear rates that can be attributed to the formation of the transfer layer. At low sliding velocities and in the presence of a smooth mating surface, a thin layer of the polymer is deposited (approximately 10 nm thick). In this layer, long UHMWPE molecular chains are highly oriented in the direction of sliding. This provides a sound adherence to the counterface and allows further sliding to occur (Hutchings, 1992).

Polymers running under steady state conditions, display wear characteristics that are similar to those found in metals with the rate of material removal being proportional to normal load. This relationship is described by Archard's Equation (Archard, 1953):

$$Q = \frac{KW}{H}$$

This equation relates the volumetric material loss per unit sliding distance (Q) to the normal load (W) and hardness of the soft surface (H). The dimensionless constant K given above is an important property that provides a measure of the severity of the interaction between the asperities of two interacting surfaces and the likelihood of this interaction generating wear. However, in engineering applications, it is often more useful to use a dimensional wear coefficient, k (mm^3 N^{-1} m^{-1}), i.e. the volume of material lost to wear per unit distance slid, per unit normal load on the contact. The use of this coefficient means that *H*, which can be difficult to measure in some soft polymers and elastomers, can be eliminated. For the polymers, *k* is usually in the range 10^{-6} to 10^{-3} $mm^3 N^{-1} m^{-1}$ (Hutchings, 1992). Figure 7.6 shows a UHMWPE knee component removed after revision surgery displaying signs of both abrasive and adhesive wear.

7.3.2 Abrasive wear

Abrasion is a form of cohesive wear that can occur in two modes, viz. two-body and three-body abrasive wear. Two-body abrasion refers to a hard rough surface, of which the asperities 'plough' through the relatively stiffer counterface. The surface penetrations cause localised plastic displacement and indentations. Three-body abrasion refers to hard particles between two sliding surfaces, ploughing through at least one of the surfaces. The two are not mutually exclusive, as two-body abrasion can often lead to three-body when hard wear particles are detached from a surface. Abrasive wear is dependent on the bulk properties of the materials and the geometry of

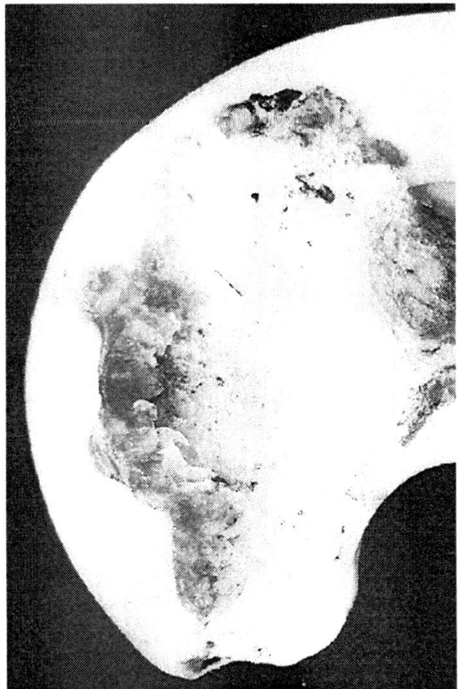

7.6 A UHMWPE knee component after revision surgery, owing to pain and instability, displaying signs of both abrasive and adhesive wear (Gomez-Barrena *et al.* 2008) (reprinted by permission of Taylor & Francis Group, http://www.informaworld.com).

the asperity or particle, although clearly this can be very difficult to define (Williams, 2005).

In its simplest form, an abrasive wear model can be defined by considering a hard conical asperity with a slope θ under a normal load W ploughing through a polymer surface, removing material and producing a groove. The amount of material lost by abrasive wear w is (where symbols have the same meaning as the previous equation):

$$w \approx \left(\frac{2\tan\theta}{\pi}\right)\frac{KW}{H}$$

Clearly this equation has a similar form to Archard's Equation for sliding wear and so several general laws of wear can be stated:

- wear increases with sliding distance;
- wear increases with normal applied load; and
- wear decreases as the hardness of the sliding surface increases.

The abrasive wear equation predicts that wear rate should be inversely proportional to hardness. This is not the case for the wear of polymers where the correlation is much worse than for metals. The reason for this lies in the difficulty of measuring the hardness of a polymer and separating it from time-dependent effects and the contribution of elastic and plastic effects. A much better correlation is found according to the Ratner–Lancaster correlation, which relates the inverse of the area under the stress–strain curve of a polymer (to the point of tensile failure) to abrasive wear rate (Hutchings, 1992).

7.3.3 Fatigue wear

Wear of the surface as a result of fatigue is perhaps one of the most difficult forms of wear to predict. Fatigue wear tends to be more prevalent in low modulus polymers, elastomers and, when running against a smooth counterface, harder glassy polymers. Its characteristic feature is the formation and development of cracks on, or in the region of the surface, as a result of cyclic loading. Wear occurs through material removal caused by the propagation and intersection of these cracks when they reach the surface. Whereas for abrasion, wear occurs by plastic deformation of the surface, fatigue wear occurs principally owing to elastic deformations. Hence, the overall mechanism is similar to and often leads to abrasive wear.

The fatigue wear rate is dependent on many different factors, including the mechanical and chemical properties of the surfaces, the operating and environmental conditions as well as the properties of the lubricant, if employed. However, it is possible that similar surfaces apparently subjected to identical conditions may exhibit wide variations in fatigue wear severity and failure. It is often necessary therefore to employ statistical methods for wear prediction (Bhushan, 2002).

The Paris law of crack propagation can be used to show that, once again, the fatigue wear rate is strongly dependent on normal load and to a lesser extent on surface roughness. It is worth considering, that all of the other wear mechanisms discussed above require not only a normal load but also physical contact between the surfaces. However, if the surfaces are separated by a lubricant film, adhesive and abrasive wear are virtually eliminated but fatigue wear can still occur (Hutchings, 1992).

7.4 Polymers

There are a variety of polymers used in joint replacement implants that can be subject to wear. In this section UHMWPE, crosslinked polyethylene, poly(ether ether ketone) (PEEK), silicone and polyurethan are discussed. Some of the mechanical properties for these polymers are shown in Table 7.1.

7.4.1 Ultra high molecular weight polyethylene

Ultra high molecular weight polyethylene (UHMWPE) has been the mainstay of joint replacement implants for over forty years. There are many studies that have undertaken laboratory investigations looking at the wear of UHMWPE against various counterface materials. Most screening work involves the use of a pin of UHMWPE that is loaded against a plate or disc made from stainless steel, CoCrMo alloy, alumina or zirconia. The plate or disc is then moved relative to the pin to create wear debris. The use of lubricants is crucial in the wear testing of materials used for joint replacement implants to attempt to simulate the synovial fluid found in the natural synovial joint. The lubricant used in wear testing is typically bovine serum that is diluted with distilled water (Pylios and Shepherd, 2008) although in some tests distilled water is used on its own.

Table 7.1 Typical mechanical properties of polymers used for joint replacement implants

Material	Young's modulus (GPa)	Ultimate tensile strength (MPa)	Reference
Crosslinked polyethylene	860	29.3	Lewis (2001)
PEEK	3.6	93	Brown (2006)
Polyurethan	0.02	10	Scholes *et al.* (2006)
Silicone	0.03	7	Brown (2006)
UHMWPE	915	48.7	Lewis (2001)

Wear factors for UHMWPE can be in the range 10^{-9} to 10^{-6} $mm^3 N^{-1} m^{-1}$, depending on factors such as the test apparatus, lubricant and speed (Fisher and Dowson, 1991; Fisher, 1994). The surface roughness of the plate or disc can affect the wear factor. Lancaster *et al.* (1997) investigated the wear of UHMWPE against stainless steel, CoCrMo, alumina and zirconia, using a pin-on-plate apparatus. The surface roughness values for the different materials were varied between 0.005 and 0.04 μm. The wear factor of UHMWPE was found to increase from 7.4×10^{-9} $mm^3 N^{-1} m^{-1}$ (R_a of 0.005 μm) to 16.5×10^{-9} $mm^3 N^{-1} m^{-1}$ (R_a of 0.04 μm). Multidirectional motion for pin-on-plate wear testing was shown to be crucial to produce more realistic wear rates to those seen *in vivo*. Using a multidirection apparatus, Saikko (1998) measured the wear factor for UHMWPE against stainless steel to be 0.8×10^{-6} $mm^3 N^{-1} m^{-1}$.

A pin-on-plate or disc-on-plate apparatus is useful for screening various material combinations or investigating factors such as the type of lubricant or surface roughness, but more realistic loads and motions are required to attempt to simulate use in the body. For this reason, hip and knee simulators were developed (Burgess *et al.*, 1997; Goldsmith and Dowson, 1999a) and international standards (BS ISO 14242-1, 2002; BS ISO 14243-1, 2009) published so that comparison can be made between the various designs and materials combinations available for the implants. For a hip replacement, the volume of wear generated from an UHMWPE acetabular cup when articulated against a CoCrMo alloy femoral head is about 48.2 mm^3 per million cycles (Smith *et al.*, 2000). A million cycles, on average, represents about one year in the human body (Shepherd and Azangwe, 2007). For zirconia against UHMWPE, the wear volume is much smaller at 6.3 mm^3 per million cycles (Goldsmith and Dowson, 1999b). The wear of total knee replacements using simulators shows the volume of wear to be between 1 and 10 mm^3 per million cycles (Ash *et al.*, 2000; Flannery *et al.*, 2008; Utzschneider *et al.*, 2009). Flannery *et al.* (2008) determined the mean wear to be 6.4 mm^3 per million cycles, which corresponds to a wear factor of 0.033×10^{-6} $mm^3 N^{-1} m^{-1}$, whereas a wear factor of 0.068×10^{-6} $mm^3 N^{-1} m^{-1}$ was found by Ash *et al.* (2000), with a mean volume of wear of 3.7 mm^3 per million cycles.

7.4.2 Crosslinked polyethylene

Crosslinked polyethylene was introduced for joint replacement because it has lower wear rates than conventional UHMWPE. However, there are some concerns that, although wear rates are reduced, the strength of the material also reduces, and this may lead to fracture of the polymer implant. The crosslinking of polyethylene is achieved through high-energy radiation, with the amount of crosslinking proportional to the absorbed radiation dose. The polymer is then subjected to a thermal processing step (Kurtz *et al.*, 2008).

Experimentally, wear was shown to be reduced following crosslinking. Using a pin-on-plate apparatus, the wear factor was found to decrease with increasing crosslinking of the polyethylene (Galvin *et al.*, 2006). Simulator studies also showed a reduction in wear when crosslinked polyethylene was used. Using a hip simulator, Estok *et al.* (2007) showed a reduction in wear from 3.8 mg per million cycles to 0.01 mg per million cycles when the radiation dose was increased from 5 to 9.6 Mrad. For hip implants with crosslinked polyethylene, Affatato *et al.* (2008) found the hip to generate about 1 mg per million cycles (0.96 mm^3 per million cycles) compared with about 20 mg per million cycles for conventional UHMWPE. Similar results were found when the wear of crosslinked polyethylene was investigated for knee replacement implants on simulators. Muratoglu *et al.* (2004) found that the volume of wear reduced from 9.6 mm^3 per million cycles for conventional UHMWPE to 0.7 mm^3 per million cycles for crosslinked polyethylene. A similar reduction was found by Utzschneider *et al.* (2009) who determined wear of about 9 mm^3 per million cycles for conventional UHMWPE and this decreased to 0.67 to 4.64 mm^3 per million cycles for crosslinked polyethylene.

7.4.3 Poly(ether ether ketone) (PEEK)

Poly(ether ether ketone) (PEEK), in various formulations, is found in a wide variety of applications as an alternative biomaterial to ceramic, metal and other polymer implants (such as UHMWPE). These applications include trauma fixation, as well as dental, orthopaedic and spinal implants and, as a result of ongoing research, the uses of PEEK as a biomaterial continue to grow (Toth *et al.* 2006). Research conducted by Morrison *et al.* (1995) emphasised the biocompatibility of PEEK and its composites. This may mean that the probability of adverse tissue reactions induced by wear debris may be minimised through the use of PEEK as an implant material.

From an engineering perspective, PEEK has preferential mechanical properties as well as all the characteristics that would be expected of an implantable polymer. Unfilled PEEK has a Young's modulus of approximately 5 GPa, and the inclusion of short-chopped and continuous carbon fibres as well as carbon particles can result in a Young's modulus ranging from 20–150 GPa. Such a wide range of stiffness means that PEEK formulations can be produced with modulus values similar to that of cortical bone and hence can minimise or prevent bone resorption (caused by the disparity between metallic implant and bone). This is perhaps one of the main reasons why PEEK is so abundantly employed in hard tissue applications (Kurtz and Devine, 2007).

Carbon fibre implants have not, as a rule, been successful. Connelly *et al.* (1984) and Busanelli *et al.* (1996) reported on the clinical use of carbon-fibre-reinforced (CFR) UHMWPE in both pelvic and tibial implants. They describe wide failure particularly in the tibial implants. This was attributed to poor bonding between the carbon fibres and UHMWPE matrix that was exacerbated by the poor creep resistance of UHMWPE. However, the high creep resistance of PEEK minimises the risk of de-bonding at the interface between carbon filler and matrix polymer.

The wear performance of PEEK and its composites was extensively reported in general tribological science terms. However, this is not the case when only biomedical applications are considered, with only a limited number of studies published relating to the biotribology of PEEK. Scholes and Unsworth (2009) reported wear rates of between 0.1 and 0.2×10^{-6} mm^3 N^{-1} m^{-1} for both polyacrylonitrile (PAN) and pitch PEEK composites against CoCr alloys. These wear rates were shown to be much lower than for unreinforced PEEK rubbing against a similar surface (wear rate approximately 7.5×10^{-6} mm^3 N^{-1} m^{-1}). Similar experiments were conducted using ceramic counterfaces, again demonstrating low rates of wear, trends and magnitudes that were similar to the results for metallic bearing surfaces (Scholes and Unsworth, 2007).

All polymer-bearing couplings were also examined. Both Austin *et al.* (2009) and Scholes and Unsworth (2010) tested unreinforced PEEK/PEEK and CFR PEEK (both PAN and pitch) rubbing against similar counterfaces. Wear rates reported agree that PAN CFR PEEK produced the lowest wear. The average steady-state wear rates for CFR PEEK, of various compositions, rubbing against metallic, ceramic and polymer counterfaces are summarised in Table 7.2. Finally, it should be noted that the results reported were generated using pin-on-plate apparatus, highly simplified from the loads and stress states that are found in the actual implants.

7.4.4 Silicone

Silicone was used to manufacture single-piece finger and wrist replacement implants. Because the number of finger and wrist implants is much less than that for lower limb joints, there has been little research investigating the wear of silicone for this use. Pylios and Shepherd (2008) investigated the wear of medical-grade silicone rubber against titanium and UHMWPE using a pin-on-disc apparatus. The lubricants used were Ringer's solution and bovine serum diluted with distilled water. The wear factors of the silicone rubber against titanium were 67×10^{-6} mm^3 N^{-1} m^{-1} (Ringer's solutions) and 40×10^{-6} mm^3 N^{-1} m^{-1} (diluted bovine serum). Against UHMWPE the wear factors were 88×10^{-6} mm^3 N^{-1} m^{-1} and 84×10^{-6} mm^3 N^{-1} m^{-1}, when lubricated with Ringer's solution and diluted bovine serum, respectively.

Finger joint simulators were used to test single-piece silicone implants, but there were no attempts to quantify the amount of wear debris generated

Table 7.2 A summary of the average steady-state wear rates of CFR PEEK against various counterface materials

Counterface material		CFR PEEK composition	Average steady-state wear rate (10^{-6} mm^3 N^{-1} m^{-1})	Reference
Metallic	CoCr (high carbon)	Pitch	0.123	Scholes and Unsworth (2009)
		PAN	0.176	Scholes and Unsworth (2009)
	CoCr (low carbon)	PAN	0.144	Scholes and Unsworth (2009)
Ceramic	Alumina (medical grade)	Pitch	0.134	Scholes and Unsworth (2007)
		PAN	0.194	Scholes and Unsworth (2007)
	Zirconia (medical grade)	Pitch	0.216	Scholes and Unsworth (2007)
		PAN	0.165	Scholes and Unsworth (2007)
Polymer	CFR PEEK (PAN)	–	0.921	Scholes and Unsworth (2010)
	CFR PEEK (pitch)	–	0.213	Austin *et al.* (2009)

during simulated use. Where simulators were used to test silicone implants, the studies successfully recreated the failure mechanisms seen *in vivo*, namely fracture of the implants (Stokoe *et al.*, 1990; Joyce and Unsworth, 2000, 2005).

7.4.5 Polyurethan

Polyurethan was proposed as the material for use in cushion-form joints. Jin *et al.* (1993) investigated the wear of polyurethan against stainless steel in a pin-on-disc apparatus, with a lubricant of distilled water. Wear factors were found to be 10^{-6} to 10^{-8} mm^3 N^{-1} m^{-1}. In simulators studies, both hip and knee cushion-form joints were investigated and there is evidence of fluid film lubrication occurring under some conditions. For cushion-form hips with a ceramic femoral head and a polyurethan acetabular cup, Bigsby *et al.* (1998) found negligible wear of polyurethan and no visible damage to the bearing surface. In a simulator study where a polyurethan acetabular cup was articulated against a CoCrMo alloy femoral head, the mean volume of polyurethan wear was 12 mm^3 per million cycles compared with 48.2 mm^3 for UHMWPE (Smith *et al.*, 2000). In the design of a polyurethan unicondylar knee replacement that was tested in a simulator, Scholes *et al.* (2007) determined the mean wear rate to be 1.12 mm^3 per million cycles.

7.5 Wear debris in the body

Polymer wear debris from implants interact with the human body and this interaction can cause an adverse cellular reaction leading to failure of the implant and revision surgery (Ingham and Fisher, 2000; Dowson, 2001; Fisher *et al.*, 2010). UHMWPE wear particles were shown to cause osteolysis, which leads to bone loss and loosening of the implant from the bone. It is not the overall volume of UHMWPE wear particles that causes the adverse cellular reaction, but the actual size of the particles. The critical size of particles was identified to be 0.2 to 0.8 μm (Ingham and Fisher, 2000). Although the size of wear particles is crucial, if the size of particles is normally distributed, the larger the volume of wear particles, the more wear particles there are in the crucial size range. Therefore, in the body it is crucial to determine wear. This is more typically done by measuring penetration rates rather than volume of wear.

Following hip joint replacement surgery, radiographs are taken at follow-up over a number of years and wear is thus determined. Typical penetration rates for a Charnley metal-on-UHMWPE hip replacement are 0.04 to 0.38 mm year^{-1} (Dowson, 2001). The tunneling expression can be used to estimate the volume of wear debris:

$$V = \pi r^2 p$$

where r is the radius of the femoral head and p is the depth of penetration. The Charnley femoral head has a radius of 11 mm, and, therefore, wear rates of 0.04 and 0.38 mm year^{-1} lead to wear volumes of 15 and 144 mm^3 year^{-1}, respectively.

Stilling *et al.* (2009) undertook a clinical comparison of penetration rates for femoral heads made from CoCrMo alloy and zirconia when articulated against UHMWPE, with a mean patient follow-up of 65 months. They found similar penetration rates for the femoral heads made from CoCrMo alloy (0.25 mm year^{-1}) and zirconia (0.23 mm year^{-1}).

With the introduction of crosslinked polyethylene in hip replacement implants, a number of recent clinical studies measured the wear rates in the human body. Ise *et al.* (2009) examined implants at a minimum follow-up of three years that had articulations of UHMWPE against zirconia, crosslinked polyethylene against zirconia and crosslinked polyethylene against stainless steel. The penetration rates were reduced when crosslinked polyethylene was used (Table 7.3). Similar results were found by Glyn-Jones *et al.* (2008), who found penetration rates for UHMWPE and highly crosslinked polyethylene of 0.1 mm year^{-1} and 0.06 mm year^{-1}, respectively.

A very effective method of analysing the wear of polymer parts in joint replacement implants is to make measurements on implants retrieved from patients. This typically happens where revision surgery is performed and

Table 7.3 Penetration rates and estimated volume of wear for hip replacements with bearing surfaces either UHMWPE or crosslinked polyethylene against zirconia or stainless steel

Acetabular material	Femoral head material	Penetration rate (mm year^{-1})	Volume of wear (mm^3 year^{-1})
UHMWPE	Zirconia	0.17	49
Crosslinked polyethylene	Zirconia	0.067	20
Crosslinked polyethylene	Zirconia	0.059	17
Crosslinked polyethylene	Stainless steel	0.068	20

Source: Ise *et al.*, 2009.

a joint replacement implant is replaced with a new one. Hall *et al.* (1996) measured the UHMWPE acetabular cup from retrieved Charnley hip systems and found the mean volume of wear was 55 mm^3 year^{-1}, with a mean penetration rate of 0.2 mm year^{-1}. In a major retrieval study of 128 polymer cups, Jasty *et al.* (1997) found that the mean volume of wear was in the range 8 to 284 mm^3 year^{-1}. The lowest volume of wear was found in implant retrievals from patients that had died (mean of 35 mm^3 year^{-1}), whereas, for patients having revision surgery, the wear was higher in retrievals (mean of 62 mm^3 and 94 mm^3 for polymer-only and metal-backed acetabular cups, respectively).

Roentgen stereophotogrammetric analysis is the only reliable method to measure wear in total knee replacements *in vivo*. Using this method, Gill *et al.* (2006) measured UHMWPE linear wear, at a mean follow-up of 6.4 years, to be 0.1 mm year^{-1} equating to a volume of about 100 mm^3 year^{-1}. The most common method for determining the wear of materials in total knee replacement is to measure components from retrieval studies. This typically involves measuring implants removed from the patient during revision surgery. Engh *et al.* (2009) investigated the UHMWPE inserts from mobile and fixed bearings and found the mean penetration for them to be 0.329 and 0.32 mm, respectively. Atwood *et al.* (2008) determined the wear volume from 100 retrieved mobile bearings to be 54 mm^3 year^{-1}, when the implants were implanted for more than two years.

The use of crosslinked polyethylene in knee replacements is still relatively new and there are few studies into the wear occurring *in vivo*. Iwakiri *et al.* (2009) measured the number of wear particles contained in synovial fluid removed from the knee joint of patients with a total knee replacement; the implants in each patient were the same design, but the bearing surface in four knees had a crosslinked polyethylene insert, whereas three knees had an insert made from conventional UHMWPE. The number of wear particles was less for the crosslinked polyethylene insert (0.28×10^6) compared with the conventional UHMWPE insert (6.87×10^6). Röhrl *et al.* (2007) measured the penetration of the femoral head into acetabular sockets manufactured from highly crosslinked polyethylene and conventional UHMWPE. The penetration rates were found to be less than 6 μm for the highly crosslinked polyethylene and 72 μm for the conventional UHMWPE.

With single-piece silicone implants for the finger and wrist, the stems of the implant are free to move and therefore silicone wear debris is generated as the silicone abrades against the bone. These silicone wear particles can cause an inflammatory response that results in pain, joint stiffness, loss of joint motion and soft tissue swelling (Shepherd, 2002; Shepherd and Johnstone, 2002).

7.6 Future trends

The use of polymers in joint replacement implants is unlikely to change in the near future. There are many concerns over the generation of polymer wear debris in the body, such as osteolysis, leading to alternative bearing combinations being sought. However, even 40 years after the take off of hip replacement, polymers are still used in the majority of designs. Crosslinked polyethylene was used as a replacement for UHMWPE in many designs. The addition of vitamin E to the crosslinked polyethylene was investigated as a way of preventing oxidation and this technique is likely to increase in use (Oral *et al.*, 2008). Many companies and researchers are currently looking at the potential of PEEK for use in joint replacement implants. Soft layer bearings for joint replacement that involve the use of a polyurethan bearing surface is likely to develop further in the future (Dowson, 2001). Although the design has not been implanted into patients yet, animal studies have shown positive results. Hip arthroplasty with a compliant bearing surface was implanted into sheep (Khan *et al.*, 2005; Carbone *et al.*, 2006). The retrieved implants after up to three years of implantation show no significant macroscopic damage to the compliant layer. The future use of polymers in the body will include tissue engineering, where polymer scaffolds are used to support cells as they lay down extracellular matrix (Shepherd and Azangwe, 2007). These polymers (such as polycaprolactone) are bioresorbable, meaning that over a period of time they break down in the body.

7.7 Sources of further information and advice

There are a number of peer-reviewed journals that specialise in biomaterials, biomedical engineering, joint replacement and wear. The main ones are: *Biomaterials*; *Journal of Arthroplasty*; *Journal of Biomechanics*; *Journal of Bone and Joint Surgery*; *Journal of Engineering in Medicine*; *Medical Engineering and Physics*; *Wear*.

Professional bodies that engage in polymers for use in implants include: European Society of Biomechanics; Institution of Mechanical Engineers;

Institute of Materials, Minerals and Mining; Institute of Physics and Engineering in Medicine; Society for Biomaterials.

Recommended web pages include:

UHMWPE lexicon http://www.uhmwpe.org

7.8 References

Affatato S, Zavalloni M, Taddei P, Di Foggia M, Fagnano C, Viceconti M (2008), 'Comparative study on the wear behaviour of different conventional and cross-linked polyethylenes for total hip replacement', *Tribol Int*, **41**, 813–822, DOI: 10.1016/j.triboint.2008.02.006.

Archard, JF (1953), 'Contact and rubbing of flat surfaces', *J Appl Phys*, **24**, 981–988, DOI: 10.1063/1.1721448.

Ash HE, Burgess IC, Unsworth A (2000), 'Long-term results for Kinemax and Kinematic knee bearings on a six-station wear simulator', *Proc Inst Mech Eng*, **214**, 437–447.

Atwood SA, Currier JH, Mayor MB, Collier JP, Van Citters DW, Kennedy FE (2008), 'Clinical wear measurement on low contact stress rotating platform knee bearings', *J Arthroplasty*, **23**, 431–440, DOI: 10.1016/j.arth.2007.06.005.

Auger DD, Dowson D, Fisher J (1995), 'Cushion form bearings for total knee joint replacement. Part 1: Design, friction and lubrication', *Proc Inst Mech Eng H*, **209**, 73–81.

Austin H, Powell M, Medley J, Langohr D (2009), 'Exploring the wear of a PEEK all-polymer articulation for spinal applications' *Transactions of the Society for Biomaterials*.

Bergmann G, Deuretzbacher G, Heller M, Graichen F, Rohlmann A, Strauss J, Duda GN (2001), 'Hip contact forces and gait patterns from routine activities', *J Biomech*, **34**, 859–871.

Bhushan B (2002), *Introduction to tribology*, New York, John Wiley, pp 732.

Bigsby RJA, Auger DD, Jin ZM, Dowson D, Hardaker CS, Fisher J (1998), 'A comparative tribological study of the wear of composite cushion cups in a physiological hip joint simulator', *J Biomech*, **31**, 363–369.

Briscoe BJ and Sinha SK (2002), 'Wear of polymers', *Proc Inst Mech Eng J*, **216**, 401–413.

Brown SA (2006), Synthetic biomaterials for spinal applications. In: Kurtz SM, Edidin AA (eds.) *Spine Technology Handbook*, London, Elsevier, pp. 11–33.

BS ISO 14242-1 (2002), Implants for surgery. Wear of total hip joint prostheses. Loading and displacement parameters for wear-testing machines and corresponding environmental conditions for test, London, British Standards Institute.

BS ISO 14243-1 (2009), Implants for surgery. Wear of total knee-joint prostheses. Loading and displacement parameters for wear-testing machines with load control and corresponding environmental conditions for test, London, British Standards Institute.

Burgess IC, Kolar M, Cunningham JL, Unsworth A (1997), 'Development of a six station knee wear simulator and preliminary wear results', *Proc Inst Mech Eng H*, **211**, 37–47.

Busanelli L, Squarzoni S, Brizio L, Tigani D, Sudanese A (1996), 'Wear in carbon fiber-reinforced polyethylene (poly-two) knee prostheses' *Chir Organi Mov*, **81**, 263–267.

Carbone A, Howie DW, Mcgee M, Field J, Pearcy M, Smith N, Jones E (2006), 'Aging performance of a compliant layer bearing acetabular prosthesis in an ovine hip arthroplasty model', *J Arthroplasty*, **21**, 899–906. DOI: 10.1016/j.arth.2005.07.023.

Connelly GM, Rimnac CM, Wright TM, Hertzberg RW, Manson JA (1984), 'Fatigue crack propagation behavior of ultrahigh molecular weight polyethylene' *J Orthop Res*, **2**, 119–125.

Costi J, Krishnan J, Pearcy M (1998), 'Total wrist arthroplasty: a quantitative review of the last 30 years'. *J Rheumatol*, **25**, 451–458.

Dowson D (2001), 'New joints for the Millennium: wear control in total replacement hip joints', *Proc Inst Mech Eng H*, **215**, 335–358.

Dowson D, Fisher J, Jin ZM, Auger DD, Jobbins B (1991), 'Design considerations for cushion form bearings in artificial hip joints', *Proc Inst Mech Eng H*, **205**, 59–68.

Engh GA, Zimmerman RL, Parks NL, Engh CA (2009), 'Analysis of wear in retrieved mobile and fixed bearing knee inserts', *J Arthroplasty*, **24**, 28–32, DOI: 10.1016/j.arth.2009.03.010.

Estok DM, Burroughs BR, Muratoglu OK, Harris WH (2007), 'Comparison of hip simulator wear of 2 different highly cross-linked ultra high molecular weight polyethylene acetabular components using both 32-and 38-mm femoral heads', *J Arthroplasty*, **22**, 581–589, DOI: 10.1016/j.arth.2006.07.009.

Fisher J (1994), 'Wear of ultra high molecular weight polyethylene in total artificial joints', *Curr Orthop*, **8**, 164–169.

Fisher J, Dowson D (1991), 'Tribology of total artificial joints', *Proc Inst Mech Eng H*, **205**, 73–79.

Fisher J, Jennings LM, Galvin AL, Jin ZMM, Stone MH, Ingham E (2010), '2009 Knee Society presidential guest lecture polyethylene wear in total knees', *Clin Orthop Relat Res*, **468**, 12–18, DOI: 10.1007/s11999-009-1033-1.

Flannery M, McGloughlin T, Jones E, Birkinshaw C (2008), 'Analysis of wear and friction of total knee replacements. Part I. Wear assessment on a three station wear simulator', *Wear*, **265**, 999–1008, DOI: 10.1016/j.wear.2008.02.024.

Galvin A, Kang L, Tipper J, Stone M, Ingham E, Jin ZM, Fisher J (2006), 'Wear of crosslinked polyethylene under different tribological conditions', *J Mater Sci Mater Med*, **17**, 235–243, DOI: 10.1007/s10856-006-7309-z.

Gill HS, Waite JC, Short A, Kellett CF, Price AJ, Murray DW (2006), '*In vivo* measurement of volumetric wear of a total knee replacement', *Knee*, **13**, 312–317, DOI: 10.1016/j.knee.2006.04.001.

Glyn-Jones S, Saac S, Hauptfleisch J, McLardy-Smith P, Murray DW, Singh H (2008), 'Does highly cross-linked polyethylene wear less than conventional polyethylene in total hip arthroplasty?', *J Arthroplasty*, **23**: 337–343, DOI: 10.1016/j.arth.2006.12.117.

Goldsmith AAJ, Dowson D (1999a), 'Development of a ten-station, multi-axis hip joint simulator', *Proc Inst Mech Eng H*, **213**, 311–316.

Goldsmith AAJ, Dowson D (1999b), 'A multi-station hip joint simulator study of the performance of 22 mm diameter zirconia-ultra-high molecular weight polyethylene total replacement hip joints', *Proc Inst Mech Eng H*, **213**, 77–90.

Gomez-Barrena E, Puertolas JA, Munuera L, Konttinen YT (2008), 'Update on UHMWPE research: from the bench to the bedside' *Acta Orthop*, 79, 832–40, DOI: 10.1080/17453670810016939.

Hall RM, Unsworth A, Siney P, Wroblewski BM (1996), 'Wear in retrieved Charnley acetabular sockets', *Proc Inst Mech Eng H*, **210**, 197–207.

Hutchings, IM (1992), *Tribology – friction and wear of engineering materials*, London, Edward Arnold, pp 122–131.

Ingham, E and Fisher, J (2000), 'Biological reactions to wear debris in total joint replacement', *Proc Inst Mech Eng Part H*, **214**, 21–37.

Ise K, Kawanabe K, Tamura J, Akiyama H, Goto K, Nakamura T (2009), 'Clinical results of the wear performance of cross-linked polyethylene in total hip arthroplasty prospective randomized trial', *J Arthroplasty*, **24**, 1216–1220, DOI: 10.1016/j.arth.2009.05.020.

Iwakiri K, Minoda Y, Kobayashi A, Sugama R, Iwaki H, Inori F, Hashimoto Y, Ohashi H, Ohta Y, Fukunaga K, Takaoka K (2009), '*In vivo* comparison of wear particles between highly crosslinked polyethylene and conventional polyethylene in the same design of total knee arthroplasties', *J Biomed Mater Res Part B: Appl Biomater*, **91B**, 799–804, DOI: 10.1002/jbm.b.31458.

Jacofsky DJ (2008), 'Highly cross-linked polyethylene in total knee arthroplasty: in the affirmative', *J Arthroplasty*, **23**, 28–30. DOI: 10.1016/j.arth.2008.06.017.

Jasty M, Goetz DD, Bragdon CR, Lee KR, Hanson AE, Elder JR, Harris WH (1997), 'Wear of polyethylene acetabular components in total hip arthroplasty – an analysis of one hundred and twenty-eight components retrieved at autopsy or revision operations', *J Bone Joint Surg Am*, **79A**, 349–358.

Jin ZM, Dowson D, Fisher J (1993), 'Wear and friction of medical grade polyurethane sliding on smooth metal counterfaces', *Wear*, **162**, 627–630.

Joyce TJ (2004), 'Currently available metacarpophalangeal prostheses: their designs and prospective considerations', *Expert Rev Med Dev*, **1**, 193–204, DOI: 10.1586/14734440.1.2.193.

Joyce TJ and Unsworth A (2000), 'The design of a finger wear simulator and preliminary results', *Proc Inst Mech Eng H*, **214**, 519–526.

Joyce TJ and Unsworth A (2005), 'NeuFlex metacarpophalangeal prostheses tested *in vitro*', *Proc Inst Mech Eng H*, **219**, 105–110, DOI: 10.1243/095441105X9192.

Kapoor B, Datir SP, Davies B, Wynn-Jones CH, Maffulli N (2004), 'Femoral cement pressurisation in hip arthroplasty: a laboratory comparison of three techniques', *Acta Orthop Scand*, **75**, 708–712.

Kienapfel H, Sprey C, Wilke A, Griss P (1999), 'Implant fixation by bone ingrowth', *J Arthroplasty*, **14**, 355–368.

Khan M, Smith N, Jones E, Finch DS, Cameron RE (2005), 'Analysis and evaluation of a biomedical polycarbonate urethane tested in an *in vitro* study and an ovine arthroplasty model. Part II: *in vivo* investigation', *Biomaterials*, **26**, 633–643, DOI: 10.1016/j.biomaterials.2004.02.064.

Kurtz S, Medel FJ, Manley M (2008), 'Wear in highly crosslinked polyethylenes', *Curr Orthop*, **22**, 392–399, DOI: 10.1016/j.cuor.2008.10.011.

Kurtz SM and Devine JN, (2007), 'PEEK biomaterials in trauma, orthopedic, and spinal implants', *Biomaterials*, **28**, 4845–4869, DOI: 10.1016/j.biomaterials.2007.07.013.

Lancaster JG, Dowson D, Isaac GH, Fisher J (1997), 'The wear of ultra-high molecular weight polyethylene sliding on metallic and ceramic counterfaces representative of current femoral surfaces in joint replacement', *Proc Inst Mech Eng H*, **211**, 17–24.

Lewis G (2001), 'Properties of crosslinked ultra-high-molecular-weight polyethylene', *Biomaterials*, **22**, 371–401.

Morrison C, Macnair R, MacDonald C, Wykman A, Goldie I, Grant MH (1995), '*In vitro* biocompatability testing of polymers for orthopaedic implants using cultured fibroblasts and osteoblasts', *Biomaterials*, **16**, 987–992.

Muratoglu OK, Bragdon CR, Jasty M, O'Connor DO, Von Knoch RS, Harris WH (2004), 'Knee-simulator testing of conventional and cross-linked polyethylene tibial inserts', *J Arthroplasty*, **19**, 887–897, DOI: 10.1016/j.arth.2004.03.019.

Oral E, Beckos CG, Malhi AS, Muratoglu OK (2008), 'The effects of high dose irradiation on the cross-linking of vitamin E-blended ultrahigh molecular weight polyethylene', *Biomaterials*, **29**, 3557–3560, DOI: 10.1016/j.biomaterials.2008.05.004.

Pylios T and Shepherd DET (2008), 'Wear of medical grade silicone rubber against titanium and ultrahigh molecular weight polyethylene', *J Biomed Mater Res Part B: Appl Biomater*, **84B**, 520–523, DOI: 10.1002/jbm.b.30899.

Rodriguez JA, (2008) 'Cross-linked polyethylene in total knee arthroplasty: in opposition', *J Arthroplasty*, **23**, 31–34, DOI: 10.1016/j.arth.2008.06.031.

Röhrl SM, Li MG, Nilsson KG, Nivbrant B (2007), 'Very low wear of non-remelted highly cross-linked polyethylene cups', *Acta Orthop*, **78**, 739–745, DOI: 10.1080/17453670710014509.

Saikko V (1998), 'A multidirectional motion pin-on-disk wear test method for prosthetic joint materials', *J Biomed Mater Res*, **41**, 58–64.

Scholes SC, Burgess IC, Marsden HR, Unsworth A, Jones E, Smith N (2006), 'Compliant layer acetabular cups: friction testing of a range of materials and designs for a new generation of prosthesis that mimics the natural joint', *Proc Inst Mech Eng H*, **220**, 583–596, DOI: 10.1243/09544119H06404.

Scholes SC and Unsworth A (2007), 'The wear properties of CFR-PEEK-OPTIMA articulating against ceramic assessed on a multidirectional pin-on-plate machine', *Proc Inst Mech Eng H*, **221**, 281–289, DOI: 10.1243/09544119JEIM224.

Scholes SC and Unsworth A (2009), 'Wear studies on the likely performance of CFR-PEEK/CoCrMo for use as artificial joint bearing materials', *J Mater Sci Mater Med*, **20**, 163–170, DOI: 10.1007/s10856-008-3558-3.

Scholes SC and Unsworth A (2010), 'The wear performance of PEEK-OPTIMA based self–mating couples', *Wear*, **268**, 380–387, DOI: 10.1016/j.wear.2009.08.023.

Scholes SC, Unsworth A, Jones E (2007), 'Polyurethane unicondylar knee prostheses: simulator wear tests and lubrication studies', *Phys Med Biol*, **52**, 197–212, DOI: 10.1088/0031-9155/52/1/013.

Shepherd DET (2002), 'Risk analysis for a radio-carpal joint replacement', *Proc Inst Mech Eng H*, **216**, 23–29.

Shepherd DET, Azangwe G (2007), 'Synthetic versus tissue engineered implants for joint replacement', *Appl Bionics Biomech*, **4**, 179–185, DOI: 10.1080/11762320701816966.

Shepherd DET and Johnstone AJ (2002), 'Design considerations for a wrist implant', *Med Eng Phys*, **24**, 641–650.

Smith SL, Ash HE, Unsworth A (2000), 'A tribological study of UHMWPE acetabular cups and polyurethane compliant layer acetabular cups', *J Biomed Mater Res (Appl Biomater)*, **53**, 710–716.

Stachowiak GW and Batchelor AW (2000), 'Engineering tribology', London, Butterworth–Heinemann, pp. 744.

Stilling M, Nielsen KA, Soballe K, Rahbek O (2009), 'Clinical comparison of polyethylene wear with zirconia or cobalt–chromium femoral heads', *Clin Orthop Relat Res*, **467**, 2644–2650, DOI: 10.1007/s11999-009-0799-5.

Stokoe SM, Unsworth A, Viva C, Haslock I (1990), 'A finger function simulator and the laboratory testing of joint replacements', *Proc Inst Mech Eng H*, **204**, 233–240.

Toth JM, Wang M, Estes BT, Scifert JL, Seim HB, Turner AS (2006), 'Polyetheretherketone as a biomaterial for spinal applications', *Biomaterials*, **27**, 324–334, DOI: 10.1016/j.biomaterials.2005.07.011.

Utzschneider S, Harrasser N, Schroeder C, Mazoochian F, Jansson V (2009), 'Wear of contemporary total knee replacements – a knee simulator study of six current designs', *Clin Biomech*, **24**, 583–588, DOI: 10.1016/j.clinbiomech.2009.04.007.

Williams, JA (2005) '*Engineering tribology*', Oxford, Oxford University Press, pp. 487.

8
Ageing processes of biomedical polymers in the body

A. MAHOMED, University of Birmingham, UK

Abstract: The chemical and biochemical degradation and calcification are investigated as processes that alter the physical and mechanical properties of implanted polymers. The principles of oxidative, hydrolytic and enzymatic degradation and calcification of polymers in the body are discussed and the natural ageing of polymers *in vivo* and *in vitro* and the accelerated ageing of polymers are examined. The use of accelerated ageng is described as a method to predict changes in the physical and mechanical properties of polymers *in vivo*.

Key words: chemical degradation, biochemical degradation, oxidative degradation, hydrolytic degradation, enzymatic degradation, calcification, accelerated ageing, polymer implants.

8.1 Introduction

Although the physiological environment of the human body may be perceived as being mild (37 °C, neutral pH and low salt concentration), it is in fact an aggressive medium (Coury *et al.*, 2004; Tanzi *et al.*, 1997). Retrieval studies (Doležel *et al.*, 1989a; Naidu, 2007; Swanson and Lebeau, 1974) have shown that over a period of time, these harsh conditions can lead to the degradation of the chemical and mechanical properties of polymers that are implanted in the body as substitutes for the natural human tissue. Examples of polymers commonly used in the human body for reconstructive or replacement surgery are medical-grade silicone elastomers, polyurethan (PU) and polylactide (Colas and Curtis, 2004; Coury *et al.*, 2004; Madhavan Nampoothiri *et al.*, 2010; Stokes *et al.*, 1995; Swanson *et al.*, 1973). Degradation and calcification of polymers can occur as a result of various processes including, initiation and propagation of cracks on the materials surface, swelling and the uptake of lipids and hydrolysis (Coury *et al.*, 2004). However, the properties of polymers that are suitable to be implanted into the body should not deteriorate unacceptably during their intended period of use *in vivo* (Hukins *et al.*, 2008).

This chapter consists of five main sections. Following on from the Introduction, section 8.2 outlines the principles of chemical and biochemical degradation and calcification of polymers in the body. Section 8.3 reviews previous literature on the effect of natural ageing on polymers *in vivo* and *in vitro* and in section 8.4, the concept of using accelerated ageing to predict the behaviour of polymers *in vivo* is discussed. Finally, section 8.5 presents conclusions and a summary.

8.2 Principles of chemical and biochemical degradation and calcification

Biodegradation of polymers in the human body can be described as the chemical breakdown of a material by the physiological environment of the body, implying that it is host-induced (Coury *et al.*, 2004). Before a polymer is classified as being suitable to be implanted in the body, it is subjected to rigorous and extensive laboratory testing and goes through a careful selection process (Coury *et al.*, 2004). Hence, in most instances, it is generally found that the polymer performs satisfactorily when it is first implanted (Coury *et al.*, 2004). However, problems may arise over time, as it is virtually impossible to predict precisely the behaviour of the materials after a period of extended use in the body (Coury *et al.*, 2004). Prediction techniques employed in the laboratory, such as accelerated ageing (Coury *et al.*, 2004; Hukins *et al.*, 2008), cannot identify all the factors that may cause the material to deteriorate unacceptably during their intended period of use *in vivo*. Consequently, many previously unknown factors are only identified from retrieval studies after an extended period of use *in vivo* (Coury *et al.*, 2004).

8.2.1 Polymer degradation

Biomedical-grade polymers degrade because the body constituents attack the materials, either directly or indirectly through other parts attached to the polymer in the medical device (Coury *et al.*, 2004). For example, some biological processes which should only become active to attack foreign organisms invading the human body attack and break down polymers implanted in the body (Coury *et al.*, 2004). After implantation, polymers absorb soluble components (proteins, lipids, water and ions) and adsorb proteinaceous components and as a result, cells attach to the surface of the materials and initiate chemical processes that may result in a change in their mechanical properties (Coury *et al.*, 2004). Furthermore, joints in the human body are loaded cyclically, i.e. subjected to cyclic stresses, and various joint implant testing standards are recommended (BS-ISO-14242-1:2002; BS-ISO-18192-1:2008). Joints also experience other forms of deformation such as abrasion, flexion, extension and bending, in an aqueous ionic environment which can be electrochemically active and cause the polymer to soften (Coury *et al.*, 2004). Biological processes that are activated, as a result, can allow cells to secrete oxidising agents and enzymes that digest the implant material (Coury *et al.*, 2004; Griesser, 1991).

Another factor to consider is that, before being implanted in the body, polymers undergo a treatment process that can degrade the properties of the material (Coury *et al.*, 2004). For example, it has been shown that gamma irradiation sterilisation of ultra high molecular weight polyethylene (UHMWPE) in hip implants can generate free radicals in the materials that react with oxygen in the body and result in undesirable oxidation products (Coury *et al.*, 2004). This, in turn, over the short and long term, causes oxidation and scission of the polymer chains, leading to embrittlement and reduced strength of the material (Coury *et al.*, 2004).

Table 8.1, which has been adapted from Coury *et al.* (2004), lists the chemical and physical processes that can lead to the degradation of polymers in the body.

8.2.2 Hydrolytic degradation

Hydrolysis is a chemical reaction which involves the splitting of molecules because of a reaction with water (Coury *et al.*, 2004). The likelihood of hydrolysis of a polymer occurring in the human body depends on several factors, including the physiological environment, the chemical structure, the length of time since implantation, the morphology and the dimensions (Coury *et al.*, 2004). For example, urethans, esters, amides, anyhydrides and carbonates are polymers that are highly hydrolysable in the body, i.e. they consist of carbonyls bonded to heterochain elements (O, N, S) (Coury *et al.*, 2004). The process of hydrolysis of polymers in the body creates more hydrophilic species, thus causing the polymer to swell. Swelling of polymers allows degrading species to enter the bulk of the material and thus both swelling and the uptake of water increases the number of reaction sites

Table 8.1 The chemical and physical processes that can lead to the degradation of polymers in the body

Chemical	Physical
Thermolysis e.g. radial scission	Swelling
Oxidation	Softening
Solvolysis e.g. hydrolysis	Sorption
Photolysis e.g. visible, ultraviolet	Impact fracture
Radiolysis e.g. X-rays, gamma rays	Fatigue fracture
Fracture-induced radical reactions	Stress cracking
	Dissolution
	Extraction
	Crystallisation

Source: adapted from Coury *et al.*, 2004. Reproduced with permission from Elsevier.

that can cause degradation of the material (Coury *et al.*, 2004). The rate of degradation as a result of hydrolysis depends on intrinsic properties, such as the functional groups and the morphological and molecular characteristics of the polymer (Coury *et al.*, 2004). Examples of factors that reduce the likelihood of hydrolysis include crosslinking, crystallinity and thermal annealing (Coury *et al.*, 2004).

8.2.3 Oxidative degradation

Oxidative degradation (Coury *et al.*, 2004; Griesser, 1991) in polymers occurs as a result of a chemical reaction that takes place when the material is exposed to oxygen, for example hydrogen peroxide can degrade polymers oxidatively (Griesser, 1991). Such a degradation process can be initiated by the physiological environment of the body or by the external environment (Coury *et al.*, 2004). Stress cracking is an example of oxidative degradation (Coury *et al.*, 2004; Griesser, 1991). This form of degradation attacks the surface of the polymer and causes chemical changes that occur *in vivo* or *in vitro* oxidising conditions (Coury *et al.*, 2004). For example, stress cracking in polyether urethans elastomers has been reported and common characteristics found in these elastomers include presence of oxidative aliphatic ether groups (Coury *et al.*, 2004; Griesser, 1991).

8.2.4 Enzymatic degradation

Oxidative and hydrolytic enzymes have been reported to attack polymers (Griesser, 1991). Examples of such enzymes include papain, urease, leucine aminopeptidase, esterase and trypsin, and trypsin derivatives, ficin and bromelain (Griesser, 1991). It is likely that different enzymes degrade the polymer through different mechanisms (Griesser, 1991). The major result of enzymatic degradation is that it alters the mechanical properties of the polymer and it is possible that it could release potentially harmful degradation products into the body fluid and tissue (Griesser, 1991).

8.2.5 Calcification

Deposits of calcium-containing compounds, such as calcium phosphate, can form on biomaterials in the human body (Coury *et al.*, 2004). This process is known as calcification and, although it is normal and desirable for deposits of calcium to form on teeth and bones, in the human body and on some biomaterials [e.g. osteoconductive materials used in dental and orthopaedic applications (Begley *et al.*, 1995)], it is not desirable for other medical devices such as silicone breast implants and heart valves to calcify because this can cause the devices to fail (Coury *et al.*, 2004). Incidences of failure because of calcification have been reported in several medical devices including, urinary prostheses, contact lenses, breast implants and cardiovascular applications (Coury *et al.*, 2004; Griesser, 1991). Furthermore, formation of cracks on the surface of the polymer increases the surface area and consequently the number of reaction sites that can lead to degradation of the material and can initiate calcification sites (Coury *et al.*, 2004).

8.3 Effect of natural ageing of medical polymers

Previous studies have investigated the effect that natural ageing has on the physical and mechanical properties of polymers *in vivo* and *in vitro*.

8.3.1 Hydrolytic and oxidative degradation

Polyurethans have been suggested for use in biomedical applications since 1967 (Boretos and Pierce, 1967). Biomedical applications of polyurethans include catheters, reconstructive surgery materials, blood bags and cardiovascular applications (Chandy *et al.*, 2009; Greil *et al.*, 2005; Gunatillake *et al.*, 2003; Gunatillake *et al.*, 2000; Hernandez *et al.*, 2008; Kanyanta and Ivankovic, 2010; Tanzi *et al.*, 1997; Wu *et al.*, 1999). However, it has been reported that adverse effects such as calcification and polymer degradation (hydrolytic, oxidative, and enzymatic) have limited the use of PU *in vivo* (Griesser, 1991; Stokes *et al.*, 1995; Tanzi *et al.*, 1997). For example, polyether urethans have shown signs of substantial oxidative surface degradation after ageing *in vivo* and *in vitro* (Schubert *et al.*, 1995; Schubert *et al.*, 1997; Wu *et al.*, 1992; Wu *et al.*, 1999). Furthermore, studies on polyurethans used in various medical applications including catheters (Chandy *et al.*, 2009), blood bags (Wu *et al.*, 1999), cardiovascular applications (Stokes *et al.*, 1990) and in various other medical applications (Hergenrother *et al.*, 1993; Sato *et al.*, 1995; Stokes *et al.*, 1995; Tanzi *et al.*, 1997; Xi *et al.*, 1994; Zhao *et al.*, 1990; Zhao *et al.*, 1991) have shown that the *in vivo* oxidative degradation in polyurethans manifests itself in the form of environmental stress cracking (ESC), autooxidation (AO) and metal ion oxidation (MIO). Polyester urethans have been known to undergo hydrolytic and enzymatic degradation, which is undesirable if the PU is to be used in the body for long periods of time (Griesser, 1991; Santerre *et al.*, 1994; Tanzi *et al.*, 1997; Zhang *et al.*, 1994).

In vitro, Tanzi *et al.* (1997) has shown that two polyurethans (Pellethane and Corethane) degrade in hydrolytic and oxidative (HOC, water, hydrogen peroxide, and nitric acid) environments. The degradation was affected by the ageing media; degradation was most evident when the polyurethans were immersed in nitric acid. Furthermore, lipid absorption was also evident in Corethane, after being immersed in bile, resulting in molecular changes to the surface of the polymer and it was suggested that lipid-induced long-term degradation should be considered as a possible adverse effect.

Silicone elastomers are another polymer commonly used in the body. Biomedical applications of silicone elastomers include orthopaedic implants (finger and wrist implants), aesthetic implants, cardiovascular applications, catheters, tubing, drains and cannulas (Colas and Curtis, 2004). Various studies have investigated the long-term performance of silicone elastomers *in vivo*. A study (Naidu, 2007) on the oxygen level of silicone elastomer finger implants which had been implanted over a period of time between 5 and 10 years, concluded that over time silicone elastomers oxidise *in vivo*. Furthermore, the implants had changed in colour with ageing and six of the oxidised implants had fractured, suggesting that oxidative degradation could contribute to the fracture of the implant and such fractures can initiate calcification sites. Studies (Goldfarb and Stern, 2003; Kay *et al.*, 1978; Swanson, 1972; Trail *et al.*, 2004; Wilson and Carlblom, 1989) on the long-term behaviour of silicone finger implants have reported that one of the major complications of the implant after ageing *in vivo* is the incidence of fracture at the stem-hinge junction. Varying fracture rates have been reported including: 67% after a 17 year follow-up (Trail *et al.*, 2004); 67% after a 14 year follow-up (Goldfarb and Stern, 2003); 82% after a 5 year follow-up (Kay *et al.*, 1978); 10.4% after a 8.5 year follow-up (Kirschenbaum *et al.*, 1993); and 0.7% after a 5.8 year follow-up (Swanson *et al.*, 1997).

8.3.2 Changes in the mechanical properties

Previous studies have also shown that the mechanical properties of polymers may change as a result of ageing *in vivo*. For example, it has been reported (Doležel *et al.*, 1989a) that polyethylene pacemaker leads that were implanted *in vivo* over a period of time between 7 days and 11 years, showed a structural change, resulting in a decrease in their mechanical properties. Furthermore, the failure of the leads were attributed to: (a) the degradation of the polyethylene in the physiological environment, resulting in chemical composition change and polymer embrittlement and (b) abrasion of the inner surface of the tubing resulting in pitting. Another study (Doležel *et al.*, 1989b) on silicone rubber pacemaker lead insulations, that were implanted over a period of time between 3 days and 11 years, concluded that the mechanical properties (tensile strength and elongation at break) of the tubing decreased, the crosslink density increased, and surface/structural changes (colour change, depositions, deformations in the inner surface of the tubing) and hydrolytic degradation were observed after ageing in the physiological environment.

Other studies have reported that the Young's modulus of Elast-Eon™, a PU with poly(dimethylsiloxane) and poly(hexamethylamine oxide) segments, increased after implantation in sheep for either six (Simmons *et al.*, 2008) or twelve (Simmons *et al.*, 2004) months. Naidu *et al.* (1997) measured the viscoelastic properties (storage and loss modulus) of unimplanted and retrieved silicone elastomer Silastic® HP-100 finger implants, which had been implanted in rabbits for four months and concluded that the moduli did not change significantly after implantation.

8.3.3 Calcification

Calcification of polyurethans has been reported, whereby calcium deposits have been detected on the surface of implanted polyurethans (Griesser, 1991). For example, several studies have reported calcification of PU heart valves (Bernacca *et al.*, 1995; Bernacca *et al.*, 1997; Mackay *et al.*, 1996; Wheatley *et al.*, 2000) and blood pumps (Golomb *et al.*, 1993) and a PU acetabular bearing surface for a hip joint (Khan *et al.*, 2005a; Khan *et al.*, 2005b) *in vivo* and *in vitro*. It has been suggested that the calcification plays an important role in the degradation of the properties of polyurethans because it leads to changes in the physical properties (for example, elasticity) (Griesser, 1991) and is attributed to be the leading cause of failure in bioprosthetic heart valves (Golomb *et al.*, 1993). However, in recent studies, it has been reported that polyurethans grafted with polydimethylsiloxane (silicone) were less likely to show signs of calcification after six months in an ovine model (Soldani *et al.*, 2010) or *in vitro* (Dabagh *et al.*, 2005), suggesting that surface modification of the PU can affect the likelihood of calcification. Another recent study on PU stent valves (Metzner *et al.*, 2010) concluded that there was no evidence of calcification after implanting seven stents into sheep for four weeks.

Furthermore, in silicone implants, calcification of silicone breast implant capsules has been reported in previous studies (Bantick and Taggart, 1995; Gümüs, 2009; Peters and Smith, 1995; Peters *et al.*, 2001; Siggelkow *et al.*, 2003) and is suggested as an important factor for implant failure. A long-term study on silicone toe implants (Smetana and Vencalkova, 2003) also reported evidence of calcification in fifteen of its cases. Encrustation of silicone, PU and latex urinary catheters with evidence of calcium and magnesium deposits on the surface of the material has also been reported (Cox *et al.*, 1988; Desgrandchamps *et al.*, 1997; Hukins *et al.*, 1983; Talja *et al.*, 1990).

8.3.4 Degradation as an intended consequence

For some medical applications, polymer degradation may be an intended consequence of the medical application, where a permanent device is not required. When a biodegradable device is implanted in the body, a general requirement is that the mechanical properties of the material should not alter while the device is in use (Middleton and Tipton, 2000). Once it is no longer in use, then it is expected that the device will degrade, be absorbed, and excreted by the body, with no further operations required to remove the device (Middleton and Tipton, 2000).

For example, polylactide (PLA) (Bergsma *et al.*, 1995; Madhavan Nampoothiri *et al.*, 2010; Middleton and Tipton, 2000; Zhu *et al.*, 2010) is a biodegradable polymer used in drug delivery, bone surgery and in medical devices such as implants, screws and sutures (Madhavan Nampoothiri *et al.*, 2010; Peng *et al.*, 2010; Van de Velde and Kiekens, 2002; Viljanen *et al.*, 1995; Zhu *et al.*, 2010), where degradation is an intended consequence. Degradation of PLA is dependent on a number of factors, including temperature, molecular weight, crystallinity, purity, pH, presence of terminal carboxyl or hydroxyl groups, location and size of device and water permeability (Middleton and Tipton, 2000; Park and Xanthos, 2009).

An example of where degradation of the polymer is an intended consequence of the medical application is in spinal fusion cages (Lazennec *et al.*, 2006). Fusion cages have previously been manufactured from titanium alloys, stainless steel and bone grafts, but it has been reported (Lazennec *et al.*, 2006) that complications such as extrusion, subsidence, corrosion, wear and stress shielding arose with these cages. Hence, more recently, it has been suggested that the use of bioresorbable cages manufactured from PLA would avoid these complications as they would degrade after fusing with the bone (An *et al.*, 2000; Lazennec *et al.*, 2006). Furthermore, a study on PLA bioresorbable cages (Lazennec *et al.*, 2006) that were implanted in sheep for 3 years, reported that the cages had degraded and calcified after 36 months, as intended. In a similar manner, a study (Viljanen *et al.*, 1995) on poly(L-lactide) (PLLA) screws for bone fractures, concluded that degradable PLLA screws encouraged more rapid healing and prevented weakening of the bone, when compared with metallic screws. Furthermore, an *in vivo* study (Peng *et al.*, 2010) on degradable PLA plugs for drug delivery, reported that the plugs were able to release the drug as required, into the eye, without major complications such as infections experienced previously with needles, and was recommended for future use.

8.4 Principles of accelerated ageing

Polymers that are suitable to be implanted in the body should not deteriorate unacceptably during their shelf-life or while *in vivo*; in addition, neither they nor any packaging materials should deteriorate before implantation (Hukins *et al.*, 2008). One method that can be used to study the material's ageing properties is from retrieval studies in the human body (Doležel *et al.*, 1989a), where implants are retrieved, after many years inside the human body, and the properties of their constituent materials investigated, or to implant it into animals (Martin *et al.*, 2000; Simmons *et al.*, 2004; Simmons *et al.*, 2006; Simmons *et al.*, 2008). However, necessary approval is required for this and the period of implantation (usually two years) used in these studies may not be sufficient.

8.4.1 A common approach used to express the rate of ageing of polymers

A method that can be used to determine whether deterioration is likely to occur over long timescales, is to subject materials to elevated temperatures, a process known as 'accelerated ageing' (Hemmerich, 1998; Hukins *et al.*, 2008; Mahomed *et al.*, 2010a). This is particularly useful to study the ageing of materials that are regarded as potential implant material.

A common approach is to assume that the rate of ageing is increased by a factor of (ASTM-WK4863, 2005; Hemmerich, 1998; Hukins *et al.*, 2008):

$$f = 2^{\Delta T/10} \qquad [8.1]$$

where $\Delta T = T - T_{ref}$. T is the elevated temperature used to accelerate the ageing process and T_{ref} is the reference temperature, at which to study the effects of ageing. For example, for studies involving materials suitable to be implanted in the body, T_{ref} is 37 °C (body temperature). Therefore, maintaining a material at 70 °C for 38 days is the same as ageing it for 38 $\times\ 2^{(70-37)/10} = 380$ days, i.e. ageing for $\approx$ 13 months, at 37 °C.

Further inspection of equation [8.1], shows that when ΔT = 10 °C is substituted, then $f = 2$ (Hukins *et al.*, 2008). This result is a mathematical expression of the empirical observation that increasing the temperature by about 10 °C roughly doubles the rate of many polymer reactions, the '10-degree rule' suggested by Hemmerich (1998). Furthermore, Hukins *et al.* (2008), also shows that by using the principles of chemical kinetics, this is equivalent to assuming that the ageing process is a first-order chemical reaction with an activation energy of $10R/\log_e 2$, where R is the universal gas constant. Hukins *et al.* (2008) based this on the fact that, for a first-order chemical reaction:

$$k = K \exp(-E_{act}/RT) \qquad [8.2]$$

where E_{act} is the activation energy for the ageing reaction, R is the universal gas constant (8.314 J mol^{-1}), K is an empirical factor and T the temperature.

If k_{ref} is the value of k when $T = T_{ref}$, equation [8.2] can be manipulated to define:

$$f' = \frac{k}{k_{ref}} = \exp\left(\frac{R\Delta T}{E_{act}}\right) \qquad [8.3]$$

This can be expressed as:

$$\log\left(\frac{k}{k_{\text{ref}}}\right) = \frac{R\Delta T}{E_{\text{act}}} \quad [8.4]$$

Hukins *et al.* (2008) show that, substituting $f' = 2$ and $\Delta T = 10$ °C (the 10-degree rule), into equation [8.4], gives an activation energy of $10R/\log_e 2$, which if substituted into equation [8.3] yields a value for f that is identical to the predictions of f with the empirical 10-degree rule.

Hukins *et al.* (2008) identified that the main weakness of equation [8.1] is that it assumes that increasing the temperature by 10 °C doubles the rate of ageing and they went on to suggest that this can be overcome if E_{act} for the ageing process is calculated using the first-order chemical reaction approach. However, it may not always be feasible or practicable to adopt this approach. Furthermore, both equation [8.1] and the first-order chemical kinetics approach are not valid if the ambient temperature is increased to a value that initiates other physical or chemical processes in the material that are unlikely to be involved in normal ageing processes (Hukins *et al.*, 2008). For example, it has been suggested that equation [8.1] is only valid for $T \leq 60$ °C (Hemmerich, 1998); it has also been recommended that the maximum value of T should be 70 °C (ASTM-WK4863, 2005).

Hukins *et al.* (2008) conclude that rather than assuming that a temperature increment of 10 °C increases polymer reaction rates by a factor of two, it may be more useful to identify that if a temperature increment θ were to increase a given polymer reaction rate n times, then an elevated temperature would increase the rate of ageing by a factor of $n^{\Delta T/\theta}$. Using the first-order chemical kinetics approach this would then correspond to an activation energy of $\theta R/\log_e n$, which is a better approach to use because it is based on experimental measurements specific to the process being investigated rather than an empirical observation (Hukins *et al.*, 2008; Verdu *et al.*, 2007).

8.4.2 Applications of accelerated ageing in polymers

Several studies investigated the accelerated ageing of silicone elastomers. A study by Ghanbari-Siahkali *et al.* (2005), where silicone elastomers were maintained in water at a temperature of 100 °C for two years, showed that the surface chemistry of the materials were significantly modified and there was some modification of the surface layer, although only to a thickness of about 100 μm. In another study by Konkle *et al.* (1947), silicone elastomers that were aged at 150 °C for 50 days retained their mechanical properties. Patel and Skinner (2001) maintained silicones in a moist inert gas atmosphere at temperatures of up to 190 °C and reported the loss of volatile products and some softening.

Several studies (Dootz *et al.*, 1993; Dootz *et al.*, 1994; Wagner *et al.*, 1995; Yu *et al.*, 1980) investigated the effect of light (using a xenon source to mimic natural sunlight) and increased temperature (exposure to air at a high relative humidity at 43 °C for 600–900 h) on maxillofacial implant materials and soft denture liners. Using equation [8.1] the harshest of these conditions corresponds to 57 days of ageing at 37 °C. It was reported (Dootz *et al.*, 1993; Dootz *et al.*, 1994; Wagner *et al.*, 1995; Yu *et al.*, 1980) that the tensile strength of some silicones was unaffected but that of the others decreased, whereas the tensile strength of poly(vinylchloride) (PVC) and poly(phosphazine) did not change considerably, however, a PU showed considerable signs of degradation. Yu *et al.* (1980) found that the tear resistance of silicones did not decrease as much for silicones as for PVC or PU; although the tear resistance of one silicone was found to increase. Furthermore, Dootz *et al.* (1993) found that the tear resistance of plasticised polymers increased and this was attributed to increased polymerisation and/or loss of plasticisers. In the second study by Dootz *et al.* (1994), the hardness of two out of the three silicones increased with ageing. Wagner *et al.* (1995) found that the viscoelastic properties of silicones and a poly(phosphazine) were affected by exposure to increased temperature. Furthermore, in two other studies (Craig *et al.*, 1980; Goldberg *et al.*, 1978), accelerated ageing degraded the mechanical properties of simple polyurethans, used for maxillofacial implants and dental liners.

Other ageing studies (Mahomed *et al.*, 2010b; Saber-Sheikh *et al.*, 1999) concluded that accelerated ageing of silicone is not likely to cause the silicone to degrade or greatly affect its viscoelastic properties or change its appearance. Wilson and Tomlin (1969) concluded that the appearance of two silicones for dental liners, Molloplast-B and Silastic 390, did not change after being immersed in water at 37 °C for six months.

Kennan *et al.* (1997) investigated the effect of accelerated ageing of medical-grade silicones at 100 °C for 45 h in saline solution. Using equation [8.1], these conditions simulate ageing at 37 °C, for approximately 59 days. The tensile strength remained unaffected, but there was a change in the contact angle of a liquid drop on the surface of the silicones before and after heat treatment, which suggested a change in surface properties. Furthermore, in a more recent study (Leslie *et al.*, 2008), it was reported that maintaining at least some silicones in saline solution at an elevated temperature may reduce their mechanical strength.

Simmons *et al.* (2006) investigated the shelf-life of Elast-Eon™ (AorTech, Melbourne, Australia), a PU with silicone segments which has been suggested as a possible material for making flexible finger and wrist joints (Shepherd and Johnstone, 2005). For the specimens that underwent accelerated ageing at 70 °C for two weeks (using equation [8.1], this corresponds to 138 days of ageing at 37 °C) and were sterilised by γ-irradiation or with ethylene oxide, it was reported that accelerated ageing showed no signs of degradation or surface cracking of Elast-Eon™ but led to microcrack formation in an unmodified PU, which could weaken its mechanical properties. However, signs of degradation or surface cracking of Elast-Eon™ were observed on the specimens that were autoclaved and underwent accelerated ageing at 70 °C for two weeks.

A more recent study (Mahomed *et al.*, 2010a) investigated the effect of accelerated ageing Elast-Eon™, at 70 °C in physiological saline solution for up to 114 days, (using equation [8.1] this simulates ageing at 37 °C, for 1, 2 and 3 years, respectively). Mahomed *et al.* (2010a) concluded that accelerated ageing affected the viscoelastic properties (E' and E'') and the appearance of Elast-Eon™ 3. Values of both E' and E'' increased significantly, as a result of accelerated ageing, although the effect was greater for E' values. Furthermore, in this study, discolouration was observed in Elast-Eon™ after accelerated ageing; discolouration has also been observed in simple polyurethans after immersion in cow blood at 37 °C for 28 days (Yu *et al.*, 1980).

8.5 Conclusions and summary

In this chapter, the oxidative, hydrolytic and enzymatic degradation and calcification processes that alter the physical and mechanical properties of implanted polymers have been examined. These forms of polymer degradation in the human body are of importance because they alter the mechanical and physical properties of the polymer (Coury *et al.*, 2004; Griesser, 1991). For example, physical polymer degradation can manifest itself in the form of cracks on the surface of the polymer, referred to as environmental stress cracking (Coury *et al.*, 2004; Griesser, 1991), and the mechanical properties of a polymer may decrease after ageing in the human body (Doležel *et al.*, 1989a; Doležel *et al.*, 1989b). Furthermore, retrieval studies that have reported polymer degradation and calcification in various *in vivo* and *in vitro* medical applications ranging from PU heart valves (Bernacca *et al.*, 1995), catheters (Chandy *et al.*, 2009; Cox *et al.*, 1988; Desgrandchamps *et al.*, 1997) and blood bags (Wu *et al.*, 1992; Wu *et al.*, 1999) and pumps (Golomb *et al.*, 1993) to silicone implants (Naidu, 2007; Peters *et al.*, 1998; Siggelkow *et al.*, 2003; Smetana and Vencalkova, 2003).

For some medical applications, polymer degradation may be an intended consequence. For example, PLA is a biodegradable polymer used in medical applications, such as bone surgery (Viljanen *et al.*, 1995; Zhu *et al.*, 2010), implants (Lazennec *et al.*, 2006), screws (Viljanen *et al.*, 1995), sutures (Zhu *et al.*, 2010) and in drug delivery (Peng *et al.*, 2010) where degradation is an intended consequence.

Furthermore, often it is not feasible or practical to study the degradation mechanisms of polymers using only retrieval studies or by implanting them into animals, because of the timescales involved of the projected lifetime of the polymer, possibly of the order of 20 years (Mahomed *et al.*, 2010a). One other method that has been suggested is the concept of accelerated ageing of polymers, which involves subjecting polymers to elevated temperatures as a method of simulating the ageing process (Hukins *et al.*, 2008). It has been shown that ageing of a material can be accelerated by a factor of $2^{\Delta T/10}$ by increasing the temperature by an increment ΔT (Hemmerich, 1998; Hukins *et al.*, 2008). Previous studies (Craig *et al.*, 1980; Goldberg *et al.*, 1978; Mahomed *et al.*, 2010a; Simmons *et al.*, 2006) reported that accelerated ageing of polymers resulted in mechanical and physical degradation of its properties.

In conclusion, polymers degrade and calcify while in the body and the likelihood and resistance of polymer degradation are important areas for further future research in medical polymer science (Griesser, 1991).

8.6 Sources of further information and advice

The following texts are recommended for further reading:

- Coury, A. J., Levy, R. J., Ratner, B. D., Schoen, F. J., Williams, D. F. & Williams, R. L. (2004) Degradation of materials in the biological environment in: *Biomaterials science: an introduction to materials in medicine*, edited by Ratner, B. D., Hoffman, A. S., Schoen, F. J. & Lemons, J. E., pp. 411–453, California; London, Elsevier Academic Press.
- Griesser, H. J. (1991) Degradation of polyurethanes in biomedical applications: a review. *Polymer Degradation and Stability*, **33**, 329–354.
- Middleton, J. C. & Tipton, A. J. (2000) Synthetic biodegradable polymers as orthopedic devices. *Biomaterials*, **21**, 2335–2346
- Stokes, K., Mcvenes, R. & Anderson, J. M. (1995) Polyurethane elastomer biostability. *Journal of Biomaterials Applications*, **9**, 321–354.

8.7 Acknowledgements

I would like to thank Professor David Hukins (University of Birmingham) for his guidance on writing this chapter and for proofreading.

8.8 References

An, Y. H., Woolf, S. K. & Friedman, R. J. (2000) Pre-clinical *in vivo* evaluation of orthopaedic bioabsorbable devices. *Biomaterials*, **21**, 2635–2652.

ASTM WK4863: Standard practice/guide for the mechanical characterization of lumbar nucleus devices. Draft standard edition (2005). American Society for Testing and Materials.

Bantick, G. L. & Taggart, I. (1995) Mammography and breast implants. *British Journal of Plastic Surgery*, **48**, 49–52.

Begley, C. T., Doherty, M. J., Mollan, R. A. B. & Wilson, D. J. (1995) Comparative study of the osteoinductive properties of bioceramic, coral and processed bone graft substitutes. *Biomaterials*, **16**, 1181–1185.

Bergsma, J. E., Rozema, F. R., Bos, R. R. M., Boering, G., De Bruijn, W. C. & Pennings, A. J. (1995) *In vivo* degradation and biocompatibility study of *in vitro* pre-degraded as-polymerized polylactide particles. *Biomaterials*, **16**, 267–274.

Bernacca, G. M., Mackay, T. G., Wilkinson, R. & Wheatley, D. J. (1995) Calcification and fatigue failure in a polyurethane heart valve. *Biomaterials*, **16**, 279–285.

Bernacca, G. M., Mackay, T. G., Wilkinson, R. & Wheatley, D. J. (1997) Polyurethane heart valves: fatigue failure, calcification, and polyurethane structure. *Journal of Biomedical Materials Research*, **34**, 371–379.

Boretos, J. W. & Pierce, W. S. (1967) Segmented polyurethane – a new elastomer for biomedical applications. *Science*, **158**, 1481–1482.

BS ISO 14242-1:2002: Implants for surgery: Wear of total hip-joint prostheses. British Standards Institution.

BS ISO 18192-1:2008: Implants for surgery: Wear of total intervertebral spinal disc prostheses. British Standards Institution.

Chandy, T., Van Hee, J., Nettekoven, W. & Johnson, J. (2009) Long-term *in vitro* stability assessment of polycarbonate urethane micro catheters: Resistance to oxidation and stress cracking. *Journal of Biomedical Materials Research Part B–Applied Biomaterials*, **89B**, 314–324.

Colas, A. & Curtis, J. (2004) Medical application of silicones In: *Biomaterials science: an introduction to materials in medicine*, edited by: Ratner, B. D., Hoffman, A. S., Schoen, F. J. & Lemons, J. E. pp. 697–707. California; London: Elsevier Academic Press.

Coury, A. J., Levy, R. J., Ratner, B. D., Schoen, F. J., Williams, D. F. & Williams, R. L. (2004) Degradation of materials in the biological environment In: *Biomaterials science: an introduction to materials in medicine*, edited by: Ratner, B. D., Hoffman, A. S., Schoen, F. J. & Lemons, J. E. pp. 411–453. California; London: Elsevier Academic Press.

Cox, A. J., Hukins, D. W. L. & Sutton, T. M. (1988) Comparison of *in vitro* encrustation on silicone and hydrogel-coated latex catheters. *British Journal of Urology*, **61**, 156–161.

Craig, R. G., Koran, A. & Yu, R. (1980) Elastomers for maxillofacial applications. *Biomaterials*, **1**, 112–117.

Dabagh, M., Abdekhodaie, M. J. & Khorasani, M. T. (2005) Effects of polydimethylsiloxane grafting on the calcification, physical properties, and biocompatibility of polyurethane in a heart valve. *Journal of Applied Polymer Science*, **98**, 758–766.

Desgrandchamps, F., Moulinier, F., Daudon, M., Teillac, P. & Leduc, A. (1997) An *in vitro* comparison of urease-induced encrustation of JJ stents in human urine. *British Journal of Urology*, **79**, 24–27.

Doležel, B., Adamírová, L., Náprstek, Z. & Vondráček, P. (1989a) *In vivo* degradation of polymers. I. Change of mechanical properties in polyethylene pacemaker lead insulations during long-term implantation in the human body. *Biomaterials*, **10**, 96–100.

Doležel, B., Adamírová, L., Vondráček, P. & Náprstek, Z. (1989b) *In vivo* degradation of polymers. II. Change of mechanical properties and cross-link density in silicone rubber pacemaker lead insulations during long-term implantation in the human body. *Biomaterials*, **10**, 387–392.

Dootz, E. R., Koran, A. & Craig, R. G. (1993) Physical property comparison of 11 soft denture lining materials as a function of accelerated aging. *Journal of Prosthetic Dentistry*, **69**, 114–119.

Dootz, E. R., Koran, A. & Craig, R. G. (1994) Physical properties of 3 maxillofacial materials as a function of accelerated aging. *Journal of Prosthetic Dentistry*, **71**, 379–383.

Ghanbari-Siahkali, A., Mitra, S., Kingshott, P., Almdal, K., Bloch, C. & Rehmeier, H. K. (2005) Investigation of the hydrothermal stability of cross-linked liquid silicone rubber (LSR). *Polymer Degradation and Stability*, **90**, 471–480.

Goldberg, A. J., Craig, R. G. & Filisko, F. E. (1978) Polyurethane elastomers as maxillofacial prosthetic materials. *Journal of Dental Research*, **57**, 563–569.

Goldfarb, C. A. & Stern, P. J. (2003) Metacarpophalangeal joint arthroplasty in rheumatoid arthritis – a long-term assessment. *Journal of Bone and Joint Surgery–American Volume*, **85**, 1869–1878.

Golomb, G., Barashi, A., Wagner, D. & Nachmias, O. (1993) *In vitro* and *in vivo* models for the study of the relationship between hydrophilicity and calcification of polymeric and collageneous biomaterials. *Clinical Materials*, **13**, 61–69.

Greil, O., Kleinschmidt, T., Weiss, W., Wolf, O., Heider, P., Schaffner, S., Gianotti, M., Schmid, T., Liepsch, D. & Berger, H. (2005) Flow velocities after carotid artery stenting: impact of stent design. A fluid dynamics study in a carotid artery model with laser doppler anemometry. *Cardiovascular and Interventional Radiology*, **28**, 66.

Griesser, H. J. (1991) Degradation of polyurethanes in biomedical applications: a review. *Polymer Degradation and Stability*, **33**, 329–354.

Gümüs, N. (2009) Capsular calcification may be an important factor for the failure of breast implant. *Journal of Plastic, Reconstructive & Aesthetic Surgery*, **62**, e606–e608.

Gunatillake, P. A., Martin, D. J., Meijs, G. F., Mccarthy, S. J. & Adhikari, R. (2003) Designing biostable polyurethane elastomers for biomedical implants. *Australian Journal of Chemistry*, **56**, 545–557.

Gunatillake, P. A., Meijs, G. F., Mccarthy, S. J. & Adhikari, R. (2000) Poly(dimethylsiloxane)/poly(hexamethylene oxide) mixed macrodiol based polyurethane elastomers. I. Synthesis and properties. *Journal of Applied Polymer Science*, **76**, 2026–2040.

Hemmerich, K. J. (1998) Accelerated aging. General aging theory and simplified protocol for accelerated aging of medical devices. *Medical Plastics and Biomaterials*, 16–23.

Hergenrother, R. W., Wabers, H. D. & Cooper, S. L. (1993) Effect of hard segment chemistry and strain on the stability of polyurethanes: *In vivo* biostability. *Biomaterials*, **14**, 449–458.

Hernandez, R., Weksler, J., Padsalgikar, A. & Runt, J. (2008) *In vitro* oxidation of high polydimethylsiloxane content biomedical polyurethanes: Correlation with the microstructure. *Journal of Biomedical Materials Research Part A*, **87A**, 546–556.

Hukins, D. W. L., Hickey, D. S. & Kennedy, A. P. (1983) Catheter encrustation by struvite. *British Journal of Urology*, **55**, 304–305.

Hukins, D. W. L., Mahomed, A. & Kukureka, S. N. (2008) Accelerated aging for testing polymeric biomaterials and medical devices. *Medical Engineering and Physics*, **30**, 1270–1274.

Kanyanta, V. & Ivankovic, A. (2010) Mechanical characterisation of polyurethane elastomer for biomedical applications. *Journal of the Mechanical Behavior of Biomedical Materials*, **3**, 51–62.

Kay, A. G., Jeffs, J. V. & Scott, J. T. (1978) Experience with silastic prostheses in the rheumatoid hand. A 5-year follow-up. *Annals of the Rheumatic Diseases*, **37**, 255–258.

Kennan, J. J., Peters, Y. A., Swarthout, D. E., Owen, M. J., Namkanisorn, A. & Chaudhury, M. K. (1997) Effect of saline exposure on the surface and bulk properties of medical grade silicone elastomers. *Journal of Biomedical Materials Research*, **36**, 487–497.

Khan, I., Smith, N., Jones, E., Finch, D. S. & Cameron, R. E. (2005a) Analysis and evaluation of a biomedical polycarbonate urethane tested in an *in vitro* study and an ovine arthroplasty model. Part I: Materials selection and evaluation. *Biomaterials*, **26**, 621–631.

Khan, I., Smith, N., Jones, E., Finch, D. S. & Cameron, R. E. (2005b) Analysis and evaluation of a biomedical polycarbonate urethane tested in an *in vitro* study and an ovine arthroplasty model. Part II: *In vivo* investigation. *Biomaterials*, **26**, 633–643.

Kirschenbaum, D., Schneider, L. H., Adams, D. C. & Cody, R. P. (1993) Arthroplasty of the metacarpophalangeal joints with use of silicone-rubber implants in patients who have rheumatoid arthritis. Long-term results. *Journal of Bone and Joint Surgery–American Volume*, **75**, 3–12.

Konkle, G. M., Selfridge, R. R. & Servais, P. C. (1947) Behavior of silastic on aging. *Industrial and Engineering Chemistry*, **39**, 1410–1413.

Lazennec, J. Y., Madi, A., Rousseau, M. A., Roger, B. & Saillant, G. (2006) Evaluation of the 96/4 PLDLLA polymer resorbable lumbar interbody cage in a long term animal model. *European Spine Journal*, **15**, 1545–1553.

Leslie, L. J., Jenkins, M. J., Shepherd, D. E. T. & Kukureka, S. N. (2008) The effect of the environment on the mechanical properties of medical grade silicones. *Journal of Biomedical Materials Research Part B: Applied Biomaterials*, **86B**, 460–465.

Mackay, T. G., Wheatley, D. J., Bernacca, G. M., Fisher, A. C. & Hindle, C. S. (1996) New polyurethane heart valve prosthesis: design, manufacture and evaluation. *Biomaterials*, **17**, 1857–1863.

Madhavan Nampoothiri, K., Nair, N. R. & John, R. P. (2010) An overview of the recent developments in polylactide (PLA) research. *Bioresource Technology*, **101**, 8493–8501.

Mahomed, A., Hukins, D. W. L., Kukureka, S. N. & Shepherd, D. E. T. (2010a) Effect of accelerated aging on the viscoelastic properties of ElastEon™: a polyurethane with soft poly(dimethylsiloxane) and poly(hexamethylene oxide) segments. *Materials Science and Engineering C*, **30**, 1298–1303.

Mahomed, A., Hukins, D. W. L., Kukureka, S. N. & Shepherd, D. E. T. (2010b) Viscoelastic properties of elastomers for small joint replacements. *IFBME Proceedings*, vol. 23, eds. Lim, C.T., & Goh, J.C.H., pp. 1191–1194.

Martin, D. J., Warren, L. A. P., Gunatillake, P. A., McCarthy, S. J., Meijs, G. F. & Schindhelm, K. (2000) Polydimethylsiloxane/polyether-mixed macrodiol-based polyurethane elastomers: biostability. *Biomaterials*, **21**, 1021–1029.

Metzner, A., Iino, K., Steinseifer, U., Uebing, A., De Buhr, W., Cremer, J. & Lutter, G. (2010) Percutaneous pulmonary polyurethane valved stent implantation. *Journal of Thoracic and Cardiovascular Surgery*, **139**, 748–752.

Middleton, J. C. & Tipton, A. J. (2000) Synthetic biodegradable polymers as orthopedic devices. *Biomaterials*, **21**, 2335–2346.

Naidu, S. H. (2007) Oxidation of silicone elastomer finger joints. *Journal of Hand Surgery–American Volume*, **32**, 190–193.

Naidu, S. H., Graham, J. & Laird, C. (1997) Pre- and postimplantation dynamic mechanical properties of silastic HP-100 finger joints. *Journal of Hand Surgery–American Volume*, **22**, 299–301.

Park, K. I. & Xanthos, M. (2009) A study on the degradation of polylactic acid in the presence of phosphonium ionic liquids. *Polymer Degradation and Stability*, **94**, 834–844.

Patel, M. & Skinner, A. R. (2001) Thermal ageing studies on room-temperature vulcanised polysiloxane rubbers. *Polymer Degradation and Stability*, **73**, 399–402.

Peng, Y. J., Kau, Y. C., Wen, C. W., Liu, K. S. & Liu, S. J. (2010) Solvent-free biodegradable scleral plugs providing sustained release of vancomycin, amikacin, and dexamethasone – an *in vivo* study. *Journal of Biomedical Materials Research Part A*, **94A**, 426–432.

Peters, W., Pritzker, K., Smith, D., Fornasier, V., Holmyard, D., Lugowski, S., Kamel, M. & Visram, F. (1998) Capsular calcification associated with silicone breast implants: incidence, determinants, and characterization. *Annals of Plastic Surgery*, **41**, 348–360.

Peters, W. & Smith, D. (1995) Calcification of breast implant capsules – incidence, diagnosis, and contributing factors. *Annals of Plastic Surgery*, **34**, 8–11.

Peters, W., Smith, D., Lugowski, S., Pritzker, K. & Holmyard, D. (2001) Calcification properties of saline-filled breast implants. *Plastic and Reconstructive Surgery*, **107**, 356–363.

Saber-Sheikh, K., Clarke, R. L. & Braden, M. (1999) Viscoelastic properties of some soft lining materials. II Ageing characteristics. *Biomaterials*, **20**, 2055–2062.

Santerre, J. P., Labow, R. S., Duguay, D. G., Erfle, D. & Adams, G. A. (1994) Biodegradation evaluation of polyether and polyester-urethanes with oxidative and hydrolytic enzymes. *Journal of Biomedical Materials Research*, **28**, 1187–1199.

Sato, M., Xi, T., Nakamura, A., Kawasaki, Y., Umemura, T., Tsuda, M. & Kurokawa, Y. (1995) Degradation of polyetherurethane by subcutaneous implantation into rats. II. Changes of contact angles, infrared spectra, and nuclear magnetic resonance spectra. *Journal of Biomedical Materials Research*, **29**, 1201–1213.

Schubert, M. A., Wiggins, M. J., Anderson, J. M. & Hiltner, A. (1997) Role of oxygen in biodegradation of poly(etherurethane urea) elastomers. *Journal of Biomedical Materials Research*, **34**, 519–530.

Schubert, M. A., Wiggins, M. J., Schaefer, M. P., Hiltner, A. & Anderson, J. M. (1995) Oxidative biodegradation mechanisms of biaxially strained poly(etherurethane urea) elastomers. *Journal of Biomedical Materials Research*, **29**, 337–347.

Shepherd, D. E. T. & Johnstone, A. J. (2005) A new design concept for wrist arthroplasty. *Proceedings of the Institution of Mechanical Engineers Part H: Journal of Engineering in Medicine*, **219**, 43–52.

Siggelkow, W., Faridi, A., Spiritus, K., Klinge, U., Rath, W. & Klosterhalfen, B. (2003) Histological analysis of silicone breast implant capsules and correlation with capsular contracture. *Biomaterials*, **24**, 1101–1109.

Simmons, A., Hyvarinen, J., Odell, R. A., Martin, D. J., Gunatillake, P. A., Noble, K. R. & Poole-Warren, L. A. (2004) Long-term *in vivo* biostability of poly(dimethylsiloxane)/poly(hexamethylene oxide) mixed macrodiol-based polyurethane elastomers. *Biomaterials*, **25**, 4887–4900.

Simmons, A., Hyvarinen, J. & Poole-Warren, L. (2006) The effect of sterilisation on a poly(dimethylsiloxane)/poly(hexamethylene oxide) mixed macrodiol-based polyurethane elastomer. *Biomaterials*, **27**, 4484–4497.

Simmons, A., Padsalgikar, A. D., Ferris, L. M. & Poole-Warren, L. A. (2008) Biostability and biological performance of a PDMS-based polyurethane for controlled drug release. *Biomaterials*, **29**, 2987–2995.

Smetana, M. & Vencalkova, S. (2003) Use of a silicone metatarsophalangeal joint endoprosthesis in hallux rigidus over a 15-year period. *Acta Chirurgiae Orthopaedicae et Traumatologiae Cechoslovaca*, **70**, 177–181.

Soldani, G., Losi, P., Bernabei, M., Burchielli, S., Chiappino, D., Kull, S., Briganti, E. & Spiller, D. (2010) Long term performance of small-diameter vascular grafts made of a poly(ether)urethane-polydimethylsiloxane semi-interpenetrating polymeric network. *Biomaterials*, **31**, 2592–2605.

Stokes, K., Mcvenes, R. & Anderson, J. M. (1995) Polyurethane elastomer biostability. *Journal of Biomaterials Applications*, **9**, 321–354.

Stokes, K., Urbanski, P. & Upton, J. (1990) The *in vivo* auto-oxidation of polyether polyurethane by metal ions. *Journal of Biomaterials Science Polymer Edition*, **1**, 207–230.

Swanson, A. B. (1972) Flexible implant arthroplasty for arthritic finger joints – rationale, technique, and results of treatment. *Journal of Bone and Joint Surgery-American Volume*, **A54**, 435–544.

Swanson, A. B., Meester, W. D., Swanson, G. D., Rangaswamy, L. & Schut, G. E. D. (1973) Durability of silicone implants – an *in vivo* study. *Orthopaedic Clinics of North America*, **4**, 1097–1112.

Swanson, A. B., Swanson, G. D. & Ishikawa, H. (1997) Use of grommets for flexible implant resection arthroplasty of the metacarpophalangeal joint. *Clinical Orthopaedics and Related Research*, **342**, 22–33.

Swanson, J. W. & Lebeau, J. E. (1974) The effect of implantation on physical properties of silicone rubber. *Journal of Biomedical Materials Research*, **8**, 357–367.

Talja, M., Korpela, A. & Jarvi, K. (1990) Comparison of urethral reaction to full silicone, hydrogen-coated and siliconized latex catheters. *British Journal of Urology*, **66**, 652–657.

Tanzi, M. C., Mantovani, D., Petrini, P., Guidoin, R. & Laroche, G. (1997) Chemical stability of polyether urethanes versus polycarbonate urethanes. *Journal of Biomedical Materials Research*, **36**, 550–559.

Trail, I. A., Martin, J. A., Nuttall, D. & Stanley, J. K. (2004) Seventeen-year survivorship analysis of silastic metacarpophalangeal joint replacement. *Journal of Bone and Joint Surgery–British Volume*, **86B**, 1002–1006.

Van De Velde, K. & Kiekens, P. (2002) Biopolymers: overview of several properties and consequences on their applications. *Polymer Testing*, **21**, 433–442.

Verdu, J., Colin, X., Fayolle, B. & Audouin, L. (2007) Methodology of lifetime prediction in polymer aging. *Journal of Testing and Evaluation*, **35**, 1–8.

Viljanen, J., Kinnunen, J., Bondestam, S., Majola, A., Rokkanen, P. & Törmälä, P. (1995) Bone changes after experimental osteotomies fixed with absorbable self-reinforced poly-L-lactide screws or metallic screws studied by plain radiographs, quantitative computed tomography and magnetic resonance imaging. *Biomaterials*, **16**, 1353–1358.

Wagner, W. C., Kawano, F., Dootz, E. R. & Koran, A. (1995) Dynamic viscoelastic properties of processed soft denture liners. Part 2. Effect of aging. *Journal of Prosthetic Dentistry*, **74**, 299–304.

Wheatley, D. J., Raco, L., Bernacca, G. M., Sim, I., Belcher, P. R. & Boyd, J. S. (2000) Polyurethane: material for the next generation of heart valve prostheses? *European Journal of Cardio-Thoracic Surgery*, **17**, 440–448.

Wilson, H. J. & Tomlin, H. R. (1969) Soft lining materials: some relevant properties and their determination. *Journal of Prosthetic Dentistry*, **21**, 244–250.

Wilson, R. L. & Carlblom, E. R. (1989) The rheumatoid metacarpophalangeal joint. *Hand Clinics*, **5**, 223–237.

Wu, L., Weisberg, D. M., Runt, J., Felder, G., Snyder, A. J. & Rosenberg, G. (1999) An investigation of the *in vivo* stability of poly(ether urethaneurea) blood sacs. *Journal of Biomedical Materials Research*, **44**, 371–380.

Wu, Y., Sellitti, C., Anderson, J. M., Hiltner, A., Lodoen, G. A. & Payet, C. R. (1992) An FTIR-ATR investigation of *in vivo* poly(ether urethane) degradation. *Journal of Applied Polymer Science*, **46**, 201–211.

Xi, T., Sato, M., Nakamura, A., Kawasaki, Y., Umemura, T., Tsuda, M. & Kurokawa, Y. (1994) Degradation of polyetherurethane by subcutaneous implantation into rats. I. Molecular weight change and surface morphology. *Journal of Biomedical Materials Research*, **28**, 483–490.

Yu, R., Koran, A., 3rd & Craig, R. G. (1980) Physical properties of maxillofacial elastomers under conditions of accelerated aging. *Journal of Dental Research*, **59**, 1041–1047.

Zhang, Z., King, M. W., Marois, Y., Marois, M. & Guidoin, R. (1994) *In vivo* performance of the polyesterurethane Vascugraft prosthesis implanted as a thoracoabdominal bypass in dogs: an exploratory study. *Biomaterials*, **15**, 1099–1112.

Zhao, Q., Agger, M. P., Fitzpatrick, M., Anderson, J. M., Hiltner, A., Stokes, K. & Urbanski, P. (1990) Cellular interactions with biomaterials: *in vivo* cracking of pre-stressed Pellethane 2363–80a. *Journal of Biomedical Materials Research*, **24**, 621–637.

Zhao, Q., Topham, N., Anderson, J. M., Hiltner, A., Lodoen, G. & Payet, C. R. (1991) Foreign-body giant cells and polyurethane biostability: *In vivo* correlation of cell adhesion and surface cracking. *Journal of Biomedical Materials Research*, **25**, 177–183.

Zhu, A. P., Diao, H. X., Rong, Q. P. & Cai, A. Y. (2010) Preparation and properties of polylactide–silica nanocomposites. *Journal of Applied Polymer Science*, **116**, 2866–2873.

9
The failure of synthetic polymeric medical devices

P. R. LEWIS, The Open University, UK

Abstract: Several case studies are used to show how failed medical devices are analysed for their failure modes and linked to witness evidence to show how accidents occurred. The analytical tools needed to investigate failures of medical products is reviewed briefly, with microscopy, spectroscopy and thermal analysis among the most important tools available for polymers. Other useful methods include mechanical testing, stress analysis, and gel permeation chromatography for molecular weight. Microscopic techniques include visual inspection, optical microscopy and scanning electron microscopy or environmental scanning electron microscopy. Fractures are often the starting point in any study, analysis of the fracture surface and surrounding features frequently allowing the failure mode to be identified uniquely. However, any single result must be corroborated with independent evidence, especially in cases which result in litigation. Improvements in medical product design must involve forensic study of failures, which implies preservation and conservation of the evidence, and an objective approach to independent analysis.

Key words: catheters, polymers, brittle cracking, failure, sutures, breast implants.

Note: This chapter is a revised and updated version of Chapters 1 'Introduction', 2 'Examination and analysis of failed components' and 3 'Polymer medical devices' by P. R. Lewis, originally published in *Forensic polymer engineering: why polymer products fail in service,* P. R. Lewis and C. Gagg, Woodhead Publishing Limited, 2010, ISBN: 978-1-84569-185-1.

9.1 Introduction

If one were to examine areas of great advance in the use of new materials, medical devices would surely be among the first to be noticed. One reason why synthetic polymers are now so widely used is their similarity to the proteins from which our bodies are built. They have similar mechanical properties, and so are flexible in response to body stresses. Some polymers are inert and unreactive to body fluids, and all can be designed into products of some complexity with great ease. The body environment is highly reactive because it is in a continual state of producing energy for body functions (such as muscle movement), with many complex chemical pathways both in the fluids (such as blood) and tissues (such as muscle and bone). Enzymes, or biochemical catalysts, target specific molecules in changing their structure, whether degrading them to simpler units, or changing their make-up. However, there are some relatively simple environments where the body breaks up the molecular constituents of food into much simpler units, and uses a strongly acidic environment to achieve that end. Thus, starch is effectively degraded to glucose monomer units by acidic hydrolysis in the stomach, the glucose then becoming a vital energy source for muscles. Implants must be able to resist such attack in other aggressive environments in the body, temporary implants such as catheters for short periods, and permanent implants such as hip joints for many years. On the other hand, degradation can be exploited in the case of sutures for stitching wounds, where the stitches disappear over a timescale matching the healing process.

In general, many common polymers show good biocompatibility, but care is needed to ensure their high purity owing to the problem of leaching of possible toxic additives which are usually added to commercial plastics to lengthen their lifetime. Additives such as antioxidants cannot be used for fear that they will contaminate the body. That then raises problems of enhanced sensitivity to degradation, especially thermal degradation during moulding for example. Ultraviolet (UV) absorbing additives present the same problem of leaching, toxicity and the chance of degradation before use. As if those problems were not difficult in themselves, there is another problem: sterilization. All devices to be used within the body must be totally sterile, so that no bacterial or viral contamination of the patient is possible. Equipment feed lines to patients must likewise be sterile, especially in the inner surfaces which make contact with fluids such as serum, blood, infusions of drugs or liquid nutrition.

There are several processes currently in use for sterilization: heat, ethylene oxide gas and gamma radiation. Each represents a different way of killing bacteria or viruses lurking on products, but exposure times and dose rates must be judged carefully to eliminate any possibility of affecting the polymer or polymers involved. Heat sterilization, for example, must be matched to the thermal behaviour of the polymer, not exceeding the glass transition temperature T_g, and never the melting point of the material T_m. Ethylene oxide is less aggressive, but cannot be used with polymers where there is any possibility of chemical reaction with the repeat unit. Gamma radiation is a highly energetic form of radiation, which can initiate degradation in sensitive chain molecules. Experiments before supplying new devices normally show what doses are effective only against extraneous bacterial contamination. Whatever form of sterilization is used, contamination from foreign matter of any kind is to be avoided with devices for medical use. This implies 'clean room' conditions of manufacture, with well sealed moulding shops, positive pressure of the internal (filtered) atmosphere to prevent ingress of dust, and a very high level of cleanliness. The feedstock polymer is usually a specific grade developed for a particular product, with traces of metal catalysts (or any other remnants of polymerization which might be harmful) removed because they pose a potential leaching risk. The moulding conditions must be chosen so as not to expose the hot melt to excessive temperatures when degradation starts to occur. Such traces might be difficult if not impossible to see by eye alone, remaining hidden unless special checks are made of product quality.

Most regulatory bodies, such as the Federal Drugs Administration (FDA) in the USA and the Medicines and Healthcare Products Regulatory Agency (MHRA) in the UK, insist on a programme of tests to ensure that a new product or device does not prove damaging to patients. The testing usually includes toxicity tests, integrity tests (such as for mechanical strength under expected loading conditions in the body) and *in vivo* tests as a final check on compatibility with the body. This might include tests using animals, the first balloon catheters being tested in this way, for example. Testing must be rigorous and demanding so as to assure the integrity of the final product. In reality, this is not always the case, as some of the following examples show very clearly. There is always the chance of unexpected damage, not caught by the rigorous quality testing demanded of medical products.

9.2 Forensic methods

Investigation should normally follow any serious failure of a medical product, starting with the remains of the product but also including a record of the circumstances of the failure. The way in which it failed often provides clues as to why the product broke, or otherwise did not fulfill its intended function. Comparison with intact or new products of identical design is a vital part of the process of assessing the failure modes concerned. When a product breaks into two or more parts, examination of the fracture can show how the cracks grew at the critical time, and here the fracture surface is an important piece of evidence.

Every product failure demands individual treatment, which usually starts with simple visual examination, careful measurement of its dimensions and determination of its condition compared with an equivalent intact component. Comparison is a simple way of checking if the parts really are identical and, if not, the reason for divergence. Many products are now identifiable from logos, date stamps and manufacturing codes either printed or embossed on the product outer surface. If the material is unknown, or degradation is suspected, it must be analyzed for the constituent parts: the matrix polymer, filler and any minor additives (such as UV absorbent). The analysis should aim to be non-destructive, but, if necessary, sampling needs to be away from critical features such as fracture surfaces. Although direct comparison with unaffected product or component is ideal, this is not always possible. Visual inspection aims to identify the following product features as a minimum:

- overall dimensions;
- distortion in dimensions;
- fit with matching parts;
- surface quality;
- traces of wear; and
- identity marks.

The search for key details does not stop at the fracture surface, however. Cracks which have not grown to completion are one objective of the search. Such subcritical cracks provide evidence of the way the component has been loaded in service, and might show why failure has occurred in the first place.

9.2.1 Microscopy

Optical microscopy of the fragments is essential, although it is often surprising how much information can be revealed by visual inspection with an eyeglass. Optical microscopy of reflected light is the easier to use, allowing manipulation of the sample under a wide variety of lighting conditions. Fibreoptic sources are particularly good for shadowing oblique surfaces so that fine details become visible through high contrast. Transmission is possible through transparent polymers such as silicone rubber, while birefringent polymers such as polycarbonate can show how the sample was made. Scanning electron microscopy (SEM) is the more powerful inspection method because the resolution is much higher and it gives a good three-dimensional view of surfaces. It also has the added advantage of providing elemental composition of the sample by analyzing the emitted X-rays from the polymer by electron irradiation.

9.2.2 Material analysis

Material analysis follows if any chemical change in the polymer used in the device or implant is suspected and it is often adopted to identify or confirm the polymer in question. Such methods include differential scanning calorimetry DSC and spectroscopy, of which the most important is Fourier transform infra-red (FTIR) spectroscopy. Calorimetry provides data on the thermal properties of the polymer such as the melting point T_m, the glass transition temperature T_g, and the presence of additives. It is important to compare the sample with known standards. Figure 9.1 shows the melting points of various types of polyethylene (PE), allowing characterization of unknown samples. Spectroscopy depends on detecting absorption of a

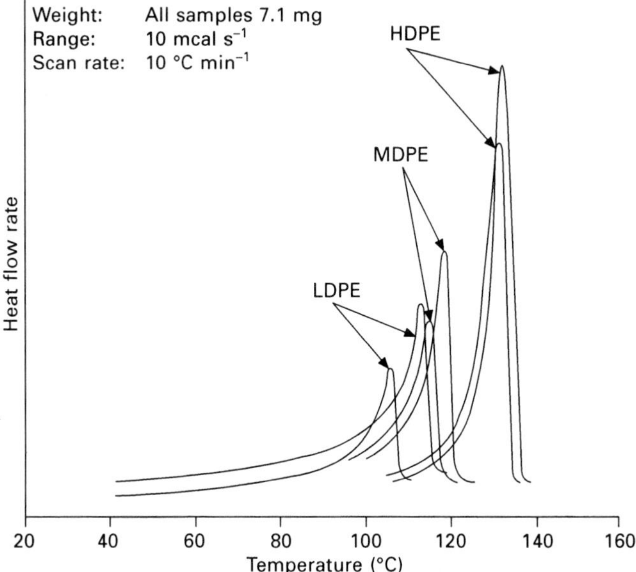

9.1 Comparison of melting points of low-, medium- and high-density polyethylenes (LDPE, MDPE and HDPE, respectively).

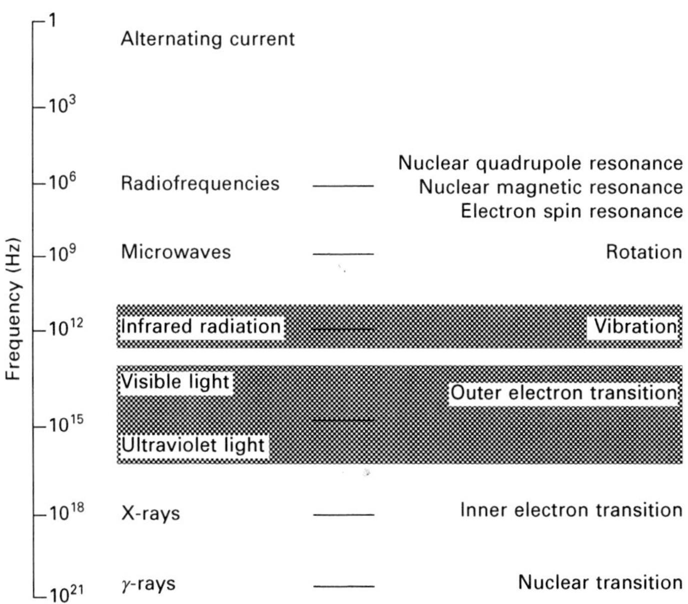

9.2 Electromagnetic spectrum and interactions with materials.

specific wavelength of electromagnetic radiation to characterize unknown compounds, and several types are used depending on the wavelengths (Fig. 9.2). FTIR detects functional groups within the polymer chain, and usually allows identification of the polymer used in the product when compared with standard spectra. Any evidence of degradation such as oxidation and hydrolysis, or contamination is detectable at specific wavelengths.

Mechanical testing is also often of use in determining the strength of samples compared with new products. There are many other tools specific to polymers which find more limited usage, as Table 9.1 indicates, although molecular weight determination is important because it is critical for the strength of the polymer and hence that of the product. Of the methods used, gel permeation chromatography (GPC) is the most useful because samples

Table 9.1 Analysis of polymer structure

Level of structure	Analytical technique	Information gained
1 Chemical composition and structure	Elemental analysis C,H,O,N; Group analysis e.g. OH, CO_2H; Infrared (IR) spectroscopy; UV spectroscopy; NMR; pyrolysis gas chromatography (PGC)	Type (and proportion) of repeating unit(s)
2 Molecular dimensions degrees of polymerization and molecular mass	Viscometry	An average molecular mass (viscosity average)
	Osmometry	An average molecular mass (number average)
	Light scattering measurements	Molecular dimensions and an average molecular mass (weight average)
	Gel permeation chromatography (GPC)	Molecular mass distribution
3 Type of molecular aggregation	Thermal analytical techniques: differential thermal analysis (DTA); differential scanning calorimetry (DSC); differential mechanical thermal analysis (DMTA)	Crystalline and amorphous phases; glass transition temperatures, crystalline melting points; levels of crystallinity: viscoelastic behaviour
	Electron microscopy	Fracture surfaces, orientation phase composition, crystalline state
	Optical microscopy	
	Scanning electron microscopy (SEM)	
	Birefringence	

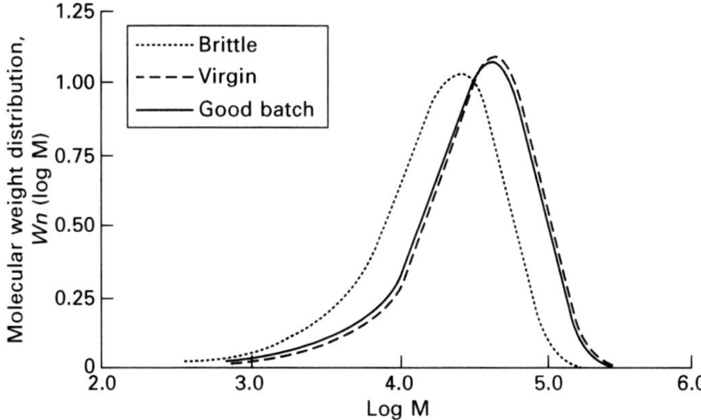

9.3 GPC molecular weight distribution showing effect of lower distribution.

can be analyzed rapidly and provide the molecular weight distribution (Fig. 9.3). The effect of lowering the molecular weight can often induce brittleness in ductile polymers, and so encourage premature cracking. The physical evidence of failure must in all cases be matched against witness and documentary evidence, as well as any standards which may apply. Only in that way can a credible sequence of events be established. Finding the root causes of failure can then lead to improvements in product design. Such methods are described in more detail in *Forensic polymer engineering* (P. R. Lewis and C. Gagg, Woodhead, 2010). The present chapter is based on Chapters 1, 2 and 3 of that book.

9.3 Catheter failure

Catheters are such a common item in hospital practice that they are usually taken for granted by all who use them. They are the plumbing tubes for infusing patients with drugs in intensive care, but if they break, damage to the patient can follow, or worse. Such products are easy to manufacture by extrusion, where hot molten polymer is pushed by a screw through a narrow circular die. The bore is created by an internal cylinder (or torpedo) within the die so that the difference between them forms the wall of the tube. Catheters of varying stiffness can be formed by varying wall thickness, but also by varying the material of construction.

9.3.1 Thermoplastic elastomers for catheters

Thermoplastic elastomers (TPEs) are a relatively new class of polymer which offer a wide range of stiffness because their microstructure can be controlled during polymerization. They are often block copolymers, made by reacting two or more different monomers together in such a way as to provide two or more different types of chain within the same molecule. Because different polymers are usually incompatible with one another, so-called domains are formed of one of the polymers. In the first of its type to be made in the 1960s, styrene–butadiene–styrene (SBS) copolymers form regular arrays of domains, which can be globular if styrene is the minor constituent (Fig. 9.4). Such domains act as a kind of physical crosslink because they anchor the flexible and elastomeric polybutadiene chains, the physical properties being much superior to polybutadiene (PB) alone. Creep is much reduced, so that shaped products retain their integrity. The stiffness of the material is similar to that of PB alone, but if the styrene content is increased, the modulus increases in step.[1] A different type of TPE is made from polyester and polyglycol (polyether) chains.[2] The stiffness is, in general, greater than the elastomeric part alone at high polyester content, thanks to the presence of crystalline domains (Fig. 9.5) rather than amorphous globules, as is the case with SBS materials. Other TPEs, which have all the advantages of thermoplastics, but a greater range of stiffness, include many varieties of polyolefin, such as ethylene propylene copolymers, where physical crosslinking is achieved by crystallization of small stereoregular blocks of one or the other component.[1] And there are also block copolymers of nylon and rubbery segments. Such a commercial material is Pebax (made by Elf Atochem), the trade name for a range of nylon TPEs. Like the polyester TPEs, they offer advantages for catheters owing to the great range of wall stiffness, giving doctors greater

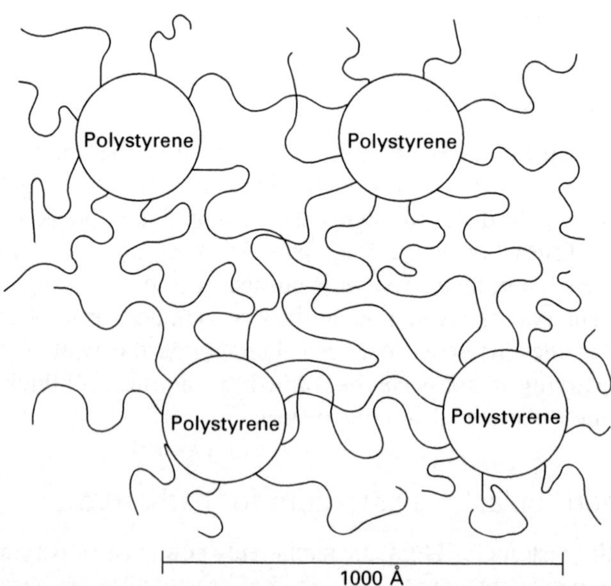

9.4 Microstructure of amorphous styrene–butadiene block copolymer.

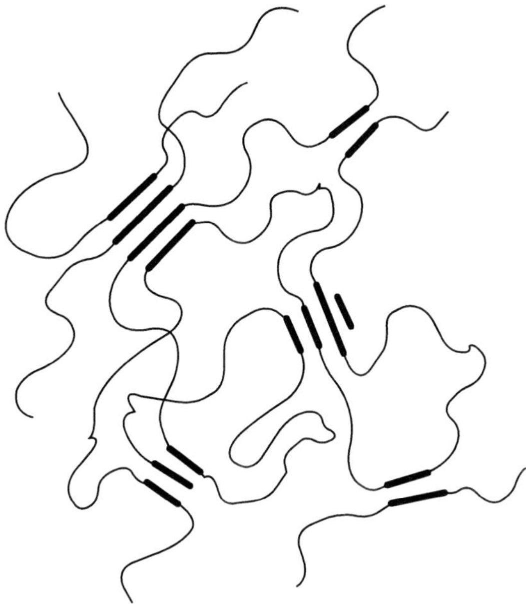

9.5 Microstructure of block copolyester with crystalline domains.

manipulative control of intravenous (IV) catheters designed for insertion into the body.

9.3.2 Accident during childbirth

One application found for Pebax was in catheters for infusing an epidural anaesthetic into pregnant women during labour. The anaesthetic may be requested to ease the lower abdomen pain when giving birth. The thin (1 mm outside diameter) catheter (1 m long) is sealed at one end, and three small holes are created by a hot wire in the adjacent side for transmitting the drug directly into the spinal fluid of the patient (Fig. 9.6). The distal or distant end of the catheter is threaded through a hollow steel needle (a so-called Tuohy needle) which punctures the spine (Fig. 9.7). It emerges into the fluid core of the backbone, and the drug can then be drip-fed safely into the patient. After birth, the Tuohy needle is withdrawn, carrying the catheter with it.

However, a problem occurred in 1990 when a Mrs K was giving birth to her first child. Following safe delivery of the baby boy, when the needle was withdrawn the catheter tip was found to be absent. Inspection of the remaining catheter showed that the tip had broken away across the proximal (or nearest) infusion hole and remained in the patient's spinal fluid. Any operation to extract the small piece of plastic was out of the question, because surgical

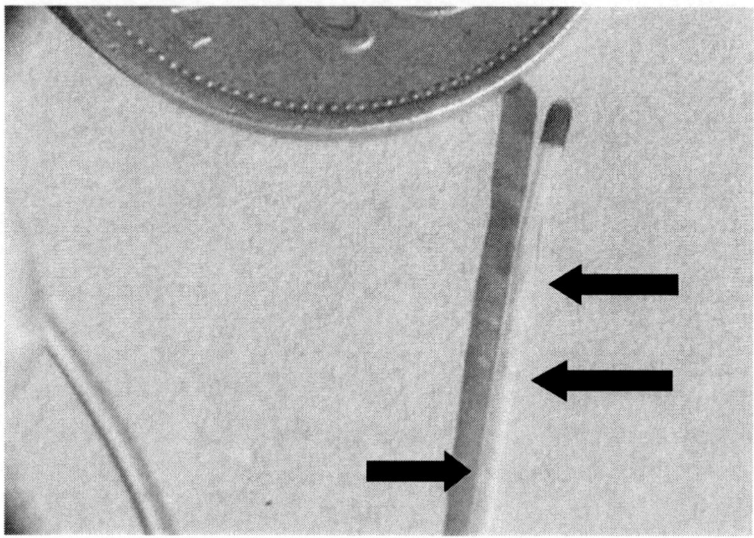

9.6 Tip of thermoplastic nylon catheter showing bleed holes and plastic deformation above distal bleed hole.

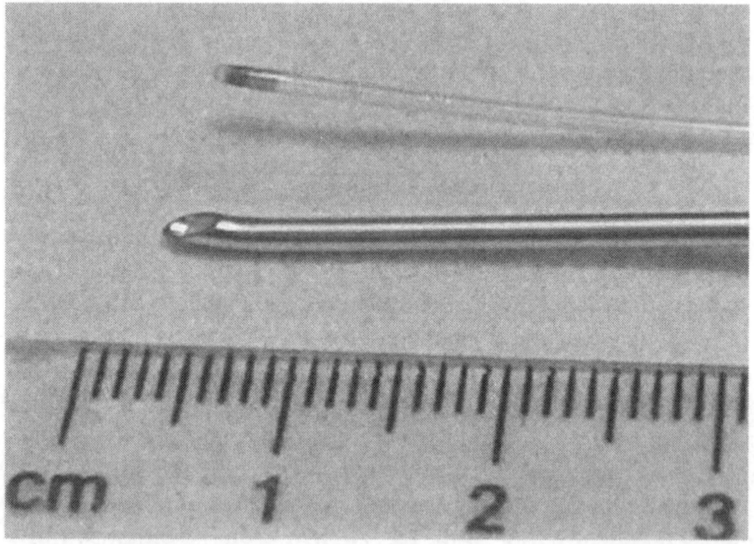

9.7 Tuohy needle used for epidural anaesthetic with catheter at top.

intervention might cause greater damage than justified. The tip was sterile and apparently presented no further risk to Mrs K. However, she thought otherwise, and brought an action against the hospital, and the makers of the catheter. In preparing expert reports, the failed catheter was clearly key evidence for the case, one way or the other. When first examined, the long length of remaining catheter proved to have been held in storage pinned to black card, and the proximal end through which the epidural fed showed signs of brittleness. Nurses had remembered having problems attaching the proximal end to the drip, and had to tape the parts together. There were brittle cracks present here, and at several other places along its length. In addition, there appeared to be a slight yellowish tinge to the failed catheter.

The expert acting for Mrs K examined the failed end of this length in a solicitor's office with a hand lens, not an ideal way of assessing the evidence. He thought he could see traces of score marks running across the failed end, perhaps created by the catheter being withdrawn over the sharp end of the Tuohy needle. This should not have happened, because there are strict guidelines given to hospital staff that the Tuohy needle should be taken out first, and then the catheter withdrawn through the needle. In his opinion, the staff had been negligent by withdrawing the catheter first, and thus damaging the end.

9.3.3 Microscopic analysis of fractured catheter end

The dispute entered a new phase when experts were appointed to act for the hospital and manufacturer. A joint meeting agreed that high-resolution microscopy of the fractured catheter could help resolve the main issues, whether to confirm or negate the score marks claimed by the claimant's expert. This was one of the first uses of environmental scanning electron microscopy (ESEM); the distal catheter end is shown in Fig. 9.8. Although

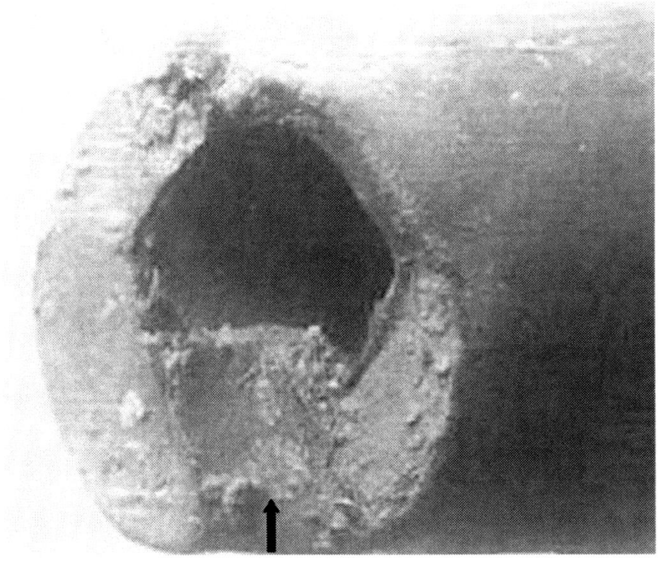

9.8 Fractured end of catheter showing bleed hole in section.

covered with dust from the solicitor's office, there appeared to be no trace of the score marks claimed by the claimant's expert. Another new catheter had been deliberately damaged by withdrawal through the Tuohy needle, and its surface (Fig. 9.9) was quite different to the failed sample. It does show score marks from tiny defects in the sharp edge of the needle blade, and cut debris at the edge. So how had the catheter actually failed? Another part of the proximal end was also examined, and its failure surface examined using conventional SEM (made conducting by a thin gold film). It exhibited a brittle glassy fracture over most of its end surface and a longitudinal crack, confirming what the nurses had said (Fig. 9.10). Most interesting, however, was the presence of a ductile tear (at left in the picture) of very similar type to that shown in the failed tip.

My interpretation of the features shown by the distal end (Fig. 9.11) indicated that the part had fractured in a mainly brittle, but also partly ductile way. There were two large flat zones next to the infusion hole with a thinned and torn part at the furthest extremity of the surface. There was no trace of the cut marks at all. Far from indicting the hospital staff, the evidence at both the distal and proximal ends showed a brittle catheter. Such a device should remain tough and ductile in response to loads, so how could it have become brittle?

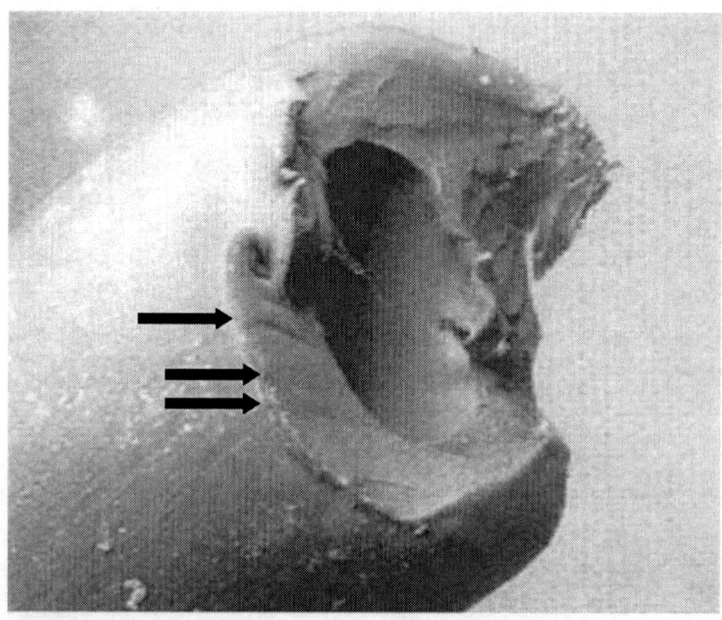

9.9 New catheter pulled back through Tuohy needle.

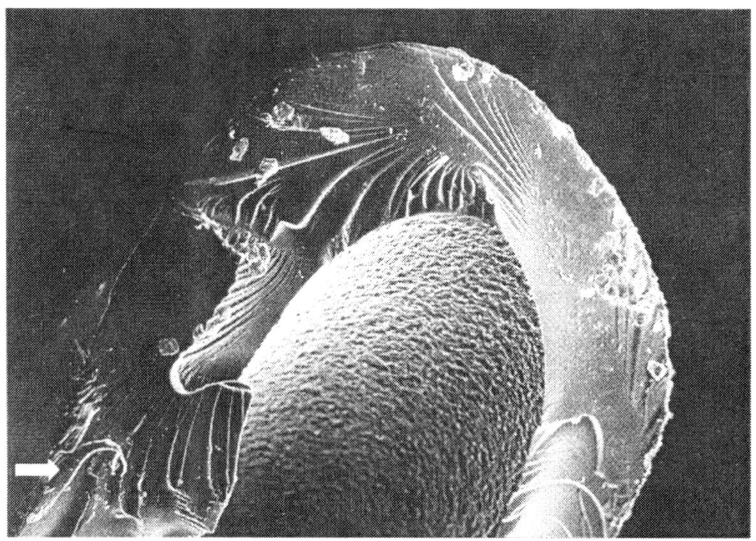

9.10 Brittle fracture in proximal end of failed catheter with ductile tear lower at left.

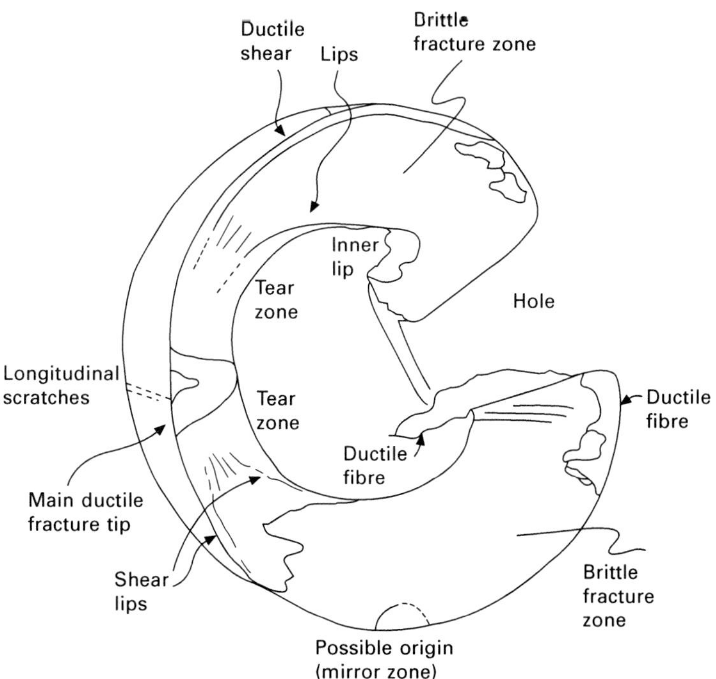

9.11 Fracture surface map of broken distal catheter end.

9.3.4 Material and mechanical testing

There was now some basis for tests to check the material quality of the polymer. It would be a multifold attack: first tensile testing of the remaining length of catheter, and second by infra-red spectroscopy near the brittle part of the tubing. Density tests showed little difference between the new and failed catheters, and DSC showed a single melting point (T_m) at about 170 °C in the failed sample, consistent with a separate and intact polyamide phase. However, there was a large difference in the heat of fusion (ΔH_f), a measure of the degree of crystallinity, as measured by the area under each peak of the new and failed catheters (Fig. 9.12). The upper curve of a new catheter showed a much smaller melting peak than that of the failed catheter, and the melting points and heats of fusion were significantly different:

standard new catheter, T_m = 184 °C, ΔH_f = 33 J g^{-1}; and

failed catheter, T_m = 171 °C, ΔH_f = 45 J g^{-1}.

The results were confirmed independently by the other experts, but what did they indicate? One possibility is that polyether chains had degraded in length, so fewer nylon blocks were held by polyether chains and, therefore, free to crystallize, thus increasing the heat of fusion. The small drop in T_m might indicate a loss of nylon block chain length too, because polymer melting points decrease with decreasing chain length.

The length of catheter provided several samples for straining to failure

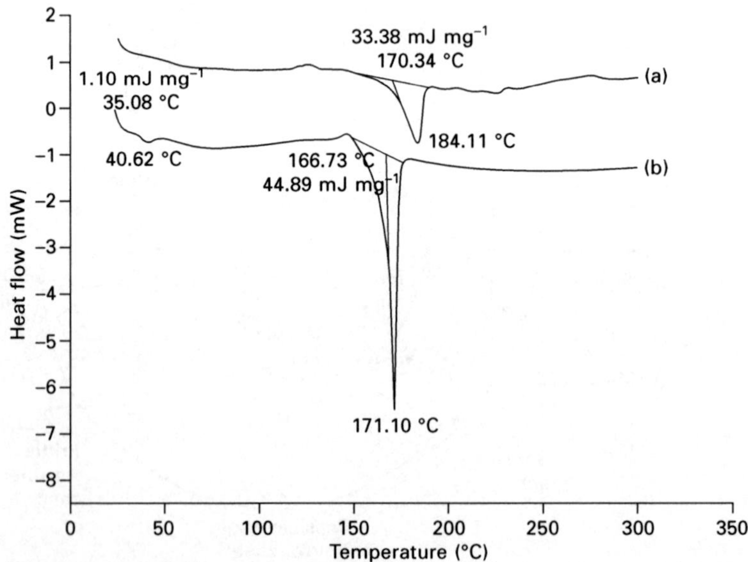

9.12 DSC curves: (a) new, (b) failed.

in simple tension, the results showing the used catheter to be much weaker than a new catheter tube. Samples from the proximal end were too brittle to withstand bending around the grips of the tensometer, but the distal end samples were tested successfully. The results on two such lengths of catheter were as follows:

mean tensile strength, 8 N; and

mean extension to break, 15%.

These results could be compared with five results obtained on a new catheter:

mean tensile strength, 28.2 N

mean extension to break, 650%

The new polymer thus exhibited a tensile strength well over three times the strength of the failed catheter, with no evidence of yield at all in any of the used tube samples tested.

Conventional infra-red spectroscopy yielded very little, with the spectra from both new and failed samples being effectively identical, a common result for polymers which may be in the early stages of degradation. However, the expert for the manufacturer chose a new method to analyze a very small piece from the failed catheter. It was FTIR microscopy, a newly developed technique which involves passing an infra-red microbeam over a chosen area of the sample in an optical microscope. The spectra are shown in Fig. 9.13 for both the failed and a new catheter. Although the spectra look similar, there are in fact subtle but significant differences, as noted by the arrows. Slight shoulders on bigger peaks indicate traces of compounds not present in new polymer, and their position pointed towards low molecular weight esters produced by photo-oxidation (possibly UV attack), as was supported by an independent survey carried out by Gauvin *et al.* in the 1980s.[3] Although the FTIR experiment was carried out by the expert acting for the manufacturer, the tensile tests were carried out in the presence of all the experts, so could not be disputed later when the case went to trial. Some NMR results were obtained for catheter material, indicating that the polymer comprised polyglycol and polyamide 12 chains of structure:

polytetramethylene glycol (PTMEG), $-[CH_2CH_2CH_2CH_2O]_n-$

and polyamide 12 (nylon 12), $-[(CH_2)_{11}-NH-CO]_n-$

The melting point of about 170 °C was consistent with the commercial brochure technical data supplied by the manufacturer Atochem.[4] However, it was surprising that a wholly aliphatic polymer should be sensitive to UV degradation, simply because the only chromophore in the repeat unit is the carbonyl group in the peptide bond (–CO–NH–). On the other hand, Gauvin

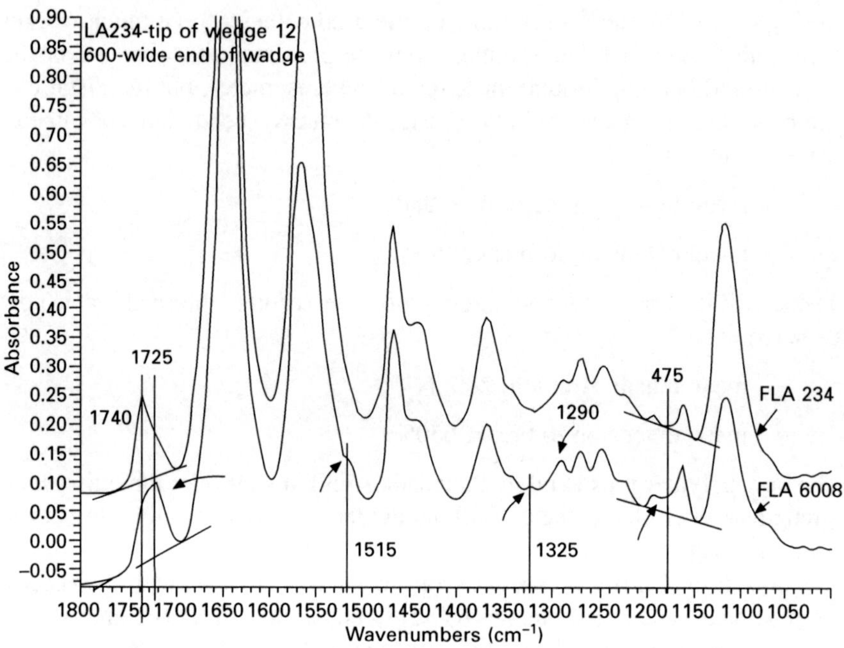

9.13 FTIR spectra of good (FLA 234) and failed (FLA 600B) catheter with anomalies arrowed.

et al.[3] found that photo-oxidation did occur, mainly within the polyether parts of the molecule. Alternatively, or in addition, the polymer may have been exposed to excessively high temperatures during moulding. Hydrolysis is less likely because the nylon blocks appeared unaffected in the failed catheter. Although GPC would have revealed the extent of chain breakdown, results were not obtained in time before the dispute was resolved.

9.3.5 Degradation theory

The sum total of all the tests (DSC, tensile and FTIR) now pointed to chain degradation of the catheter, but at what stage? There was no evidence that it had been carelessly exposed at the hospital to direct sunlight and, in any case, ordinary window glass screens out the most harmful part of the UV spectrum in sunlight. It was more likely that degradation had started earlier in its history. More information emerged from the manufacturer, enabling a flow diagram of the probable sequence of events in its life to be constructed (Fig. 9.14). There was no evidence that any other catheters made from the two batches, FLA 234 and FLA 235, had degraded in a similar way. Moreover, quality tests at several stages had not detected any problem, so how could it have happened? The fact that the brittle areas were isolated even on the

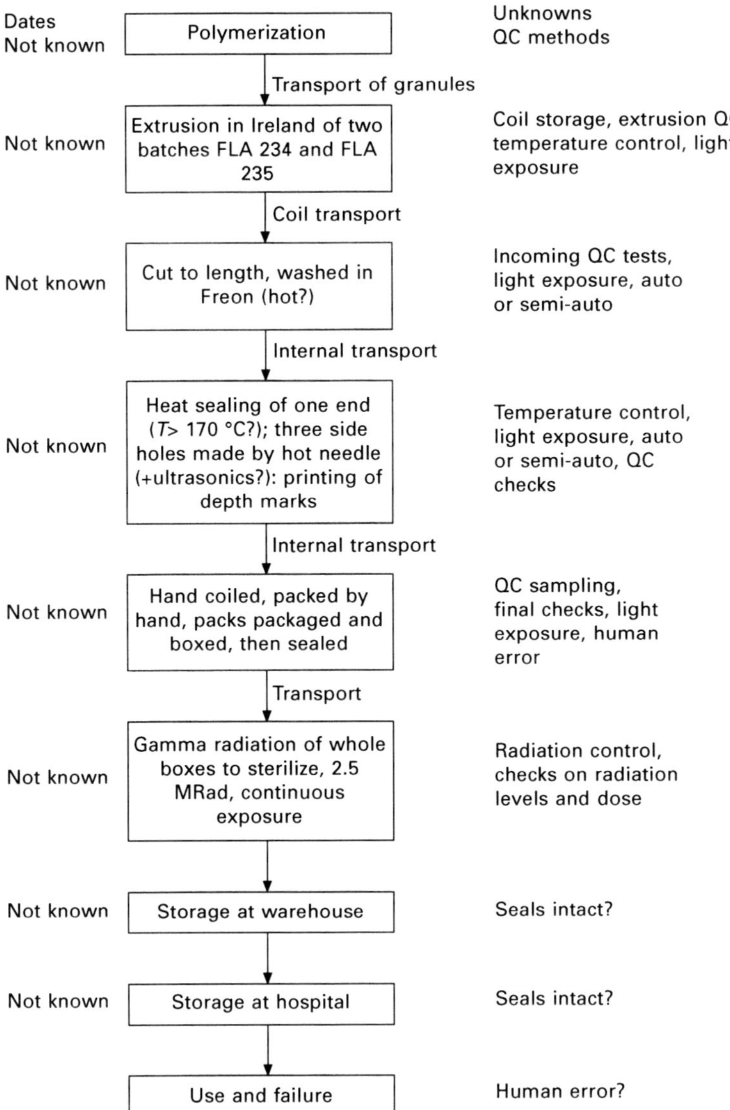

9.14 Flow sequence of catheter manufacture.

one metre length of the failed tubing produced one possible explanation. Extruded tube would have been stored in coils, and it is possible that the failed catheter was made from a length of tubing on the outside of the coil, where it might have been exposed to direct sunlight. Perhaps it occurred just after extrusion or at some stage in transport. A brief exposure to sunlight might have been enough to start the degradation in a small way, but the degradation was then accelerated by gamma sterilization at a further stage in its manufacture (Fig. 9.14). No antioxidant or UV absorber would have been used owing to the problem of leaching, so leaving the polymer unprotected. High moulding temperatures could also have enhanced the onset of UV degradation. An alternative possibility could involve environmental stress cracking (ESC) or stress corrosion cracking (SCC), but no data is currently available on the fluids which are known to crack the material. It is assumed that the manufacturer would have tested the polymer against known medical fluids to check its resistance, but there is always a chance that a new fluid cracking agent contacted the catheter after its removal from its protective packaging just before use.

9.3.6 Conclusion

The action proceeded towards a trial in the High Court, although all the evidence showed that a manufacturing defect was the most likely cause of the accident:

- The nurses discovered the proximal end to be brittle after it had been inserted.
- Calorimetry showed a big increase in heat of fusion, and a lowered T_m compared with a new catheter.
- FTIR microscopy showed traces of degradation products.
- The failed catheter showed low tensile strength in tests.

There was still substantial disagreement between the experts, despite a rather acrimonious meeting held between them. However, some new evidence emerged after the meeting, and just before the trial was due to commence. There was an unexplained feature of the damage to the catheter tip. What load could have caused the fracture to have occurred? After all, there should be no load at all if the catheter is enclosed by a hollow steel needle, and the end is simply resting in the spinal fluid. The answer came from a sample of a used catheter from a recent successful birth by epidural. The tip was intact, but was distorted at the tip: the consultant reported that it had been compressed by the adjacent vertebrae, and been deformed by the compressive load (Fig. 9.6). There was no sign of brittle cracking. This fact helped resolve the dispute, and the case was settled just before the trial was scheduled to start. The claimant received damages from the manufacturer, and the hospital was exonerated. The brittleness at the proximal end had only been discovered after the tip had been inserted into the spinal fluid, and the birth could not be suspended until a new catheter had been fitted.

A literature search failed to find any other reported examples of Pebax catheters failing by brittle cracking, informal evidence for cracking of other catheters came during the 2001 ANTEC conference in the USA, when a short paper of this case study was read in the Failures Analysis and Prevention section.[5] One delegate mentioned that he had had a similar intermittent problem with HDPE catheter tubing, also probably caused by UV exposure. Great care in manufacture of medical-grade polymers for catheters is clearly needed. The case study described in this section was published in full more recently.[6]

9.4 Balloon catheters and angioplasty

A life-saving operation which emerged during the 1980s is angioplasty, where a collapsed thermoplastic balloon is inserted into the artery of a heart patient (Fig. 9.15). Typically, the patient is suffering from blocked arteries, where fatty deposits accumulate on the walls of a blood vessel (artherosclerosis), restricting the blood supply and, when fragments break away, causing strokes or heart attacks. The balloon is carried on a flexible probe, a hollow tube carrying a guidewire for manipulating the device when being threaded through the artery to a blockage or restriction on the artery wall. The passage of the probe is followed using an X-ray body scanner or similar device, and when the balloon-carrying tip reaches the affected part, it is slowly inflated to 6–8 bar so as to crush the restriction and so improve blood supply. A further development of the device involves threading a hollow stent over the balloon. It is normally a perforated metal cage and is designed to expand permanently when the balloon is inflated. At its maximum extent it is in close contact with the artery wall, and should remain there when the

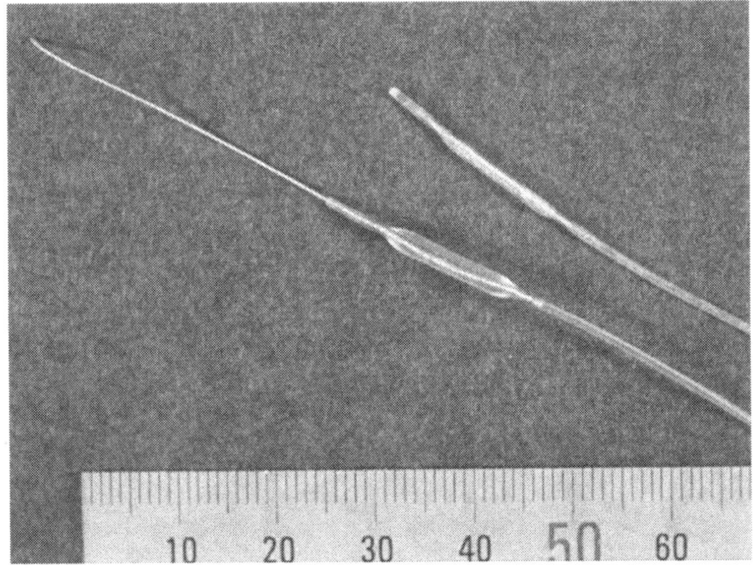

9.15 Balloon catheter and guidewire for angioplasty operation.

balloon is deflated and withdrawn at the end of the procedure. The stent remains in place because the metal has been deformed plastically. It supports the artery wall, where weakness may have developed over time because of the build-up of fatty deposits (plaque). The technique was first developed by Gruntzig working in Switzerland,[7] and further developed using the stent (Fig. 9.16) by Drs Palmaz and Schatz, surgeons working in Texas[8,9] The stent technique is now widespread, with many different designs available, and it is estimated that over 1 million such operations are carried out every year. It can eliminate the need for open-heart surgery, with all the risks involved. It is minimally invasive, involving insertion of the catheter through a small incision in the groin of the patient (with just the use of a local anaesthetic) to the spot where it is needed (Fig. 9.17). It has a high success rate, and is literally a life saver.

There were two major medical problems encountered with the method when first used: the deposits could grow back again (restenosis), requiring yet more intervention, and, secondly, if the fatty deposits are old they are frequently hard and calcified so that it is difficult to compress the deposit and more drastic methods must be used. Several other mechanical problems have also been encountered. Balloon catheters can be made from a variety of polymers, including polyvinyl chloride (PVC) (first used by Gruntzig), amorphous polyethylene terephthate (PET), PE and copolymers, but although tough and reliable balloon materials, they can fail under internal pressure from intrinsic defects or defects formed during the procedure. Failure is more likely when a stent covers the balloon, because of a hard metal structure being in close proximity to a softer material. Although sharp parts are obviously avoided, they can arise if failure of the stent occurs.[9] An elaborate kit is

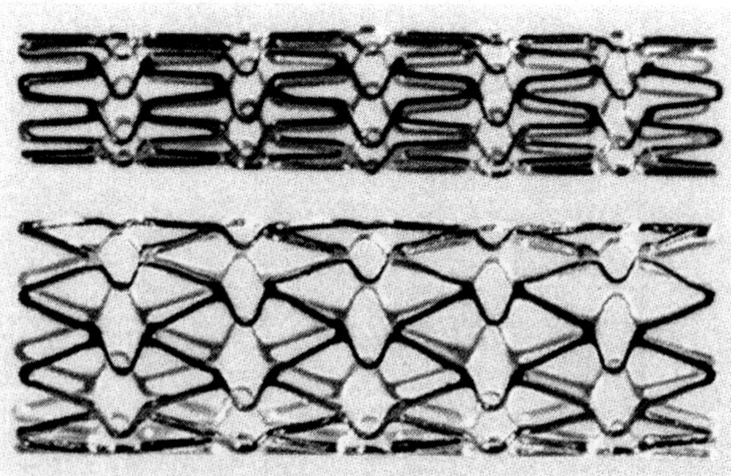

9.16 Compact and expanded metal stents.

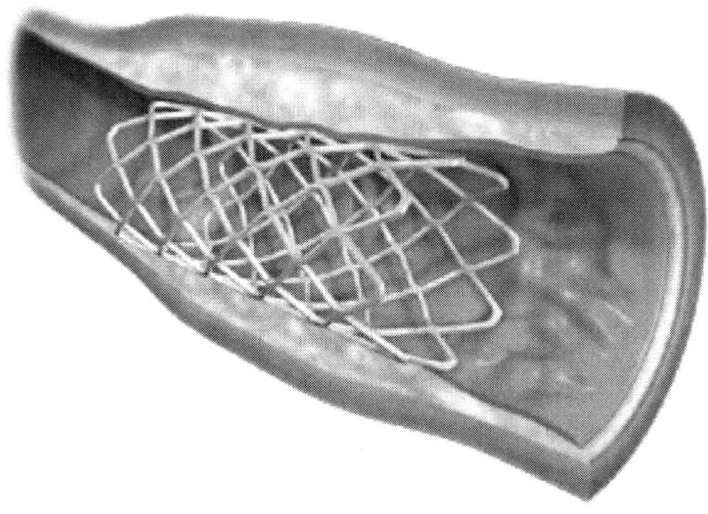

9.17 Expanded stent in artery acting to widen the channel.

needed to fish the broken parts from the artery. Use of balloon catheters and stents has been extended to the many other passages within the body, following the widespread development of endoscopy to explore the body. For example, special stents are available for supporting the lower aorta where aneurysm can develop with weak artery walls. An alert warning was issued by the MHRA in 2009 for one design of abdominal aortic aneurysm (AAA) endovascular graft, owing to problems with the trigger wire used to deploy the stent.[10] It seems clear that such operations will become more common as the technology develops, reducing the need for major invasive surgery.

9.5 Breast implants

There is a large range of implants available to surgeons for replacing diseased tissue which needs to be removed. Many employ silicone polymer for its inertness in the body and low modulus compatible with those of body tissues. One such device is the breast tissue expander. The balloon device is designed to be implanted after mastectomy under the chest muscles, and gradually filled with saline solution via a bulb connected to the balloon. When the process is complete, the device is removed and replaced with a permanent breast implant. Silicone elastomer is reinforced by PET (at the rear of the balloon), with a silicone catheter connecting the balloon to the bulb implanted just under the skin above. The major problem with silicone rubber, however, is its very poor mechanical properties, especially in fatigue.

9.5.1 Failure of tissue expander

The consequences of failure of implants are always serious for patients, involving trauma and loss of saline into their bodies. Just this happened to one woman one night several weeks after fitment of the device following mastectomy. The device had been filled at regular intervals and was apparently at or near capacity. The patient had already experienced the psychological shock of discovery of cancer, and loss of her breast, so the sudden loss of her shape was severe. On visiting her consultant, the device was extracted under anaesthetic and found to have fractured where the catheter joined the bag (Fig. 9.18). The bag was then made available for independent examination.

A check made using FTIR showed there to be no problem apparent with the polymer, all absorption peaks observed corresponding with the known spectrum for polysiloxane. However, the bag was supplied in a contaminated state with sodium chloride crystals visible on the inner surface in addition to congealed blood. There were relatively few absorption peaks owing to the thickness of the sample (c. 100 μm). However, in order to preserve the device intact, it was necessary to fold the membrane for insertion into the sample chamber of the spectrometer. The bending stress at the fold created a tear, showing the poor strength of the material when subjected to relatively low loads.

Optical microscopy showed that the original fracture extended across the catheter where it joined the bag, and showed how the fracture extended between two shoulders from the bag extension, one above and the other below the crack surface (Fig. 9.19). The survey confirmed the lack of clear features on the fracture surface itself although a cusp was found at one edge

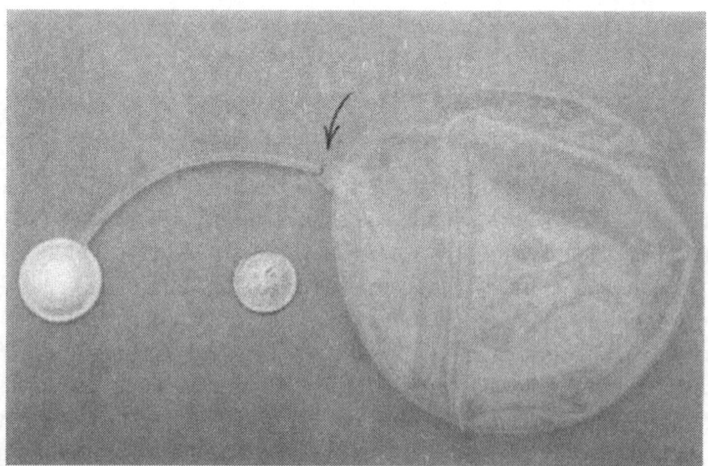

9.18 Fractured breast tissue expander in silicone rubber with crack between catheter and bag.

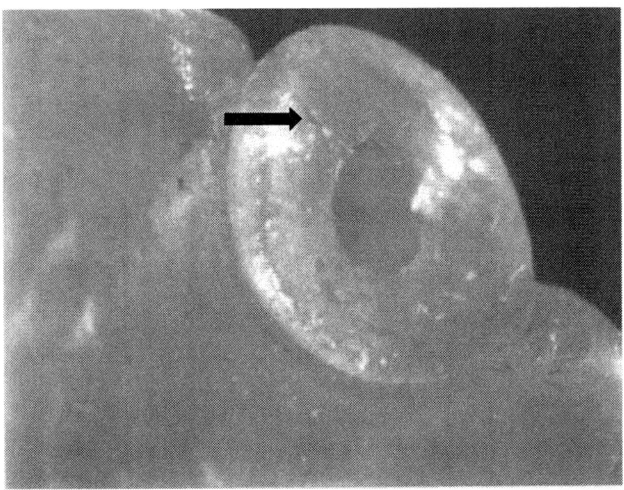

9.19 Oblique view of fracture surface in catheter showing cusp using optical microscopy.

representing the junction of two brittle cracks emanating from a common single origin on one side of the surface (the cusp at left in Fig. 9.19, with possible origin at right near the shoulder).

ESEM was needed to search for possible defects not detected in the optical microscope. An oblique shot confirmed the fracture to be relatively featureless (Fig. 9.20). There was no evidence of fatigue striations on the surface, therefore slow intermittent failure across the catheter could be excluded. The zone near the join with the bag showed many defects, and indeed some can be just seen at a deep cleft on the right (G) where the bag joins the tube. There appeared to be microcracks present here, which might explain how failure occurred. A more extensive survey revealed more cracks wherever the catheter met the bag, suggesting that either severe stress had created the cracks, or that these zones were inherently weak (Fig. 9.21).

A set of three cracks were seen in the neck near the origin (Fig. 9.22) but were not oriented to initiate a critical crack across the catheter. Just below was the remnant of a larger crack oriented at right angles to the first set, and this was very close to the main critical crack, suggesting that it initiated the final failure (Fig. 9.23). The many subcritical cracks present in the sample suggested the load of the whole bag was concentrated at the interface between the bag and catheter, and probably further raised at the sharp corner (Fig. 9.24). The interface might be regarded as the weakest zone for other reasons: it is where the catheter is adhesively bonded to the bag, so if the adhesive, itself a silicone polymer, had been poorly cured, then problems could follow.

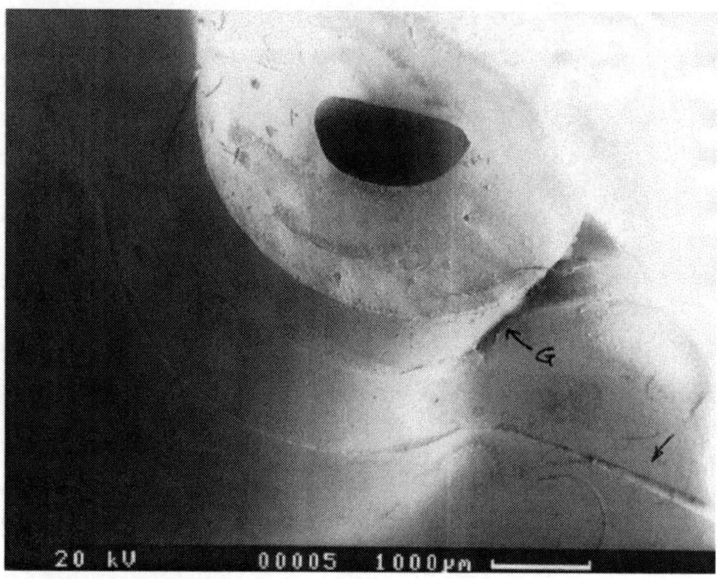

9.20 Oblique view of fracture in ESEM with crack at G.

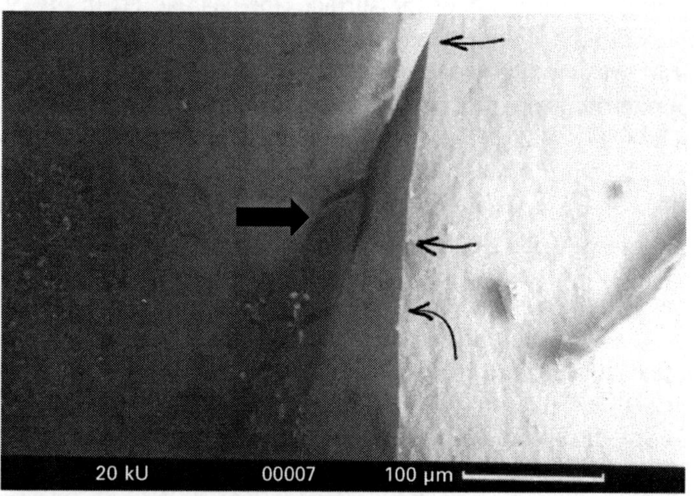

9.21 Close-up showing cracks at interface of bag and catheter.

9.5.2 Loading pattern

Thus microscopy provided good evidence that the device failed through poor manufacture. However, the history of the device was rather more complicated than at first thought. The sequence of infusions of saline solution is important in explaining why the device failed. The notes of the patient's

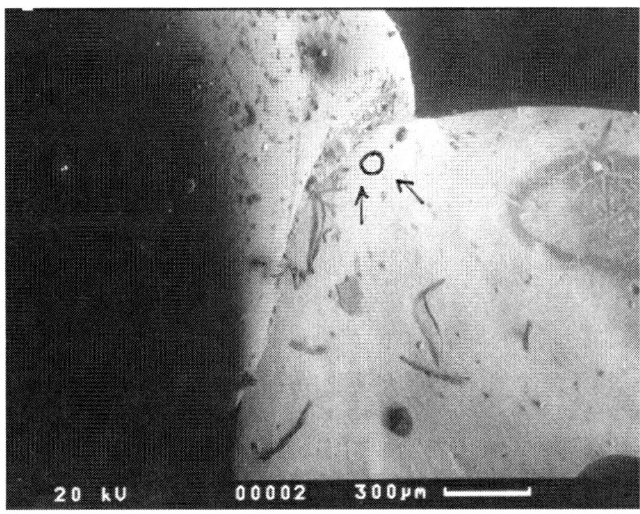

9.22 View of origin of main fracture showing crack origin, O.

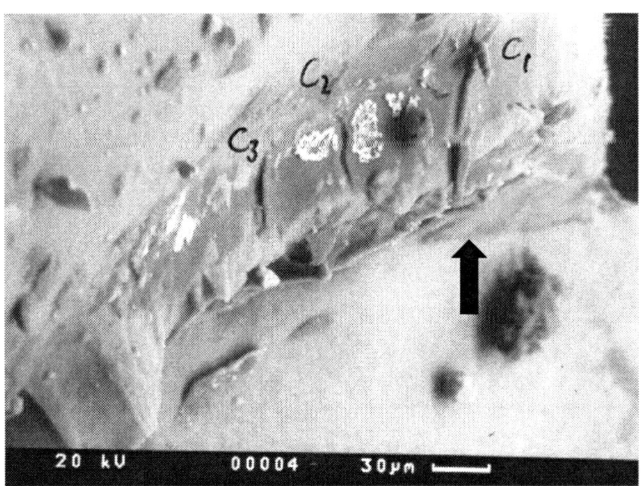

9.23 Close-up of origin showing brittle cracks, C_1 to C_3.

consultant showed a steady increase in volume of solution added to the nominal capacity of the bag of 550 ml (Table 9.2). The bag had been fitted by the consultant with 250 ml already present in the bag, and was followed by a further increment of 50 ml on August 22nd. A 100 ml portion was added on September 5th, giving a total of 400 ml added to that point. Then on September 19th, a volume of 170 ml was added, exceeding the nominal capacity by 20 ml. It was after this third addition, that the patient, Mrs H became disturbed because her chest did not appear to have grown. However,

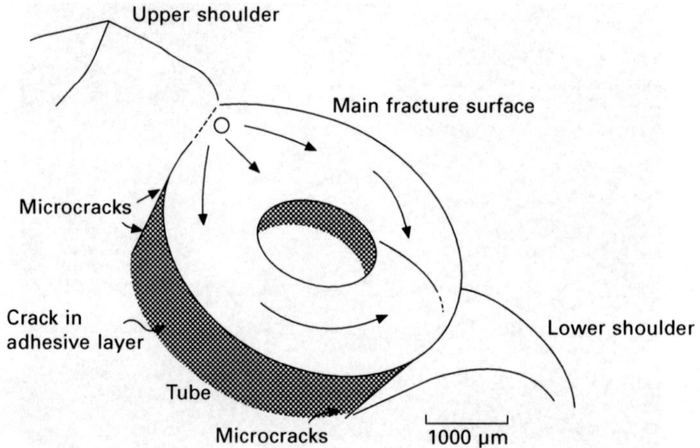

9.24 Fracture surface map of catheter showing crack growth from origin.

Table 9.2 Consultant's record of fills of breast expander

Date of fill	Volume of saline added (ml)	Comments
Aug 8	250	Operation with 550 ml capacity bag inserted by surgeon
Aug 22	50	
Sept 5	100	Total 400 ml added
Sept 19	170	Total 570 ml added
Oct 3	100	
Oct 10	150	Total 650 ml [*sic*] added (expander is probably leaking)
Post-Oct 17	–	Patient experiences total loss of fluid from bag

she did not inform her consultant. Further additions were made in October of 100 and 150 ml, and the consultant (presumably observing no increase in bag size) commented that the 'expander is probably leaking'.

Some time after October 17th, Mrs H experienced total loss of volume, and on visiting the surgery, the device was found on exploration to have fractured (Table 9.2). A check on the various additions was made by examining the elastomeric seal in the bulb. There were six puncture marks in total, confirming the testimony of the consultant (giving due allowance for a single mis-hit by the hypodermic needle). The rubber seal is designed to retract after puncture so as to retain the contents, although it is unlikely that any leakage occurred here simply because the saline drips down into the bag at a lower level. No defects could be found in the dome, in any case.

The final total of 650 ml shown in the consultant's notes was wrong. Her records showed that a total of no less than 820 ml of saline had been added by then, well beyond the capacity of the bag.

9.5.3 Conclusion

If the action had come to trial, there is no question that the uncertainty over the total solution added to the expander would have led defendant lawyers to attack the credibility of the consultant. A close relationship had grown up between the claimant and the consultant, and the former decided not to pursue the action for fear of indictment of the consultant. Such circumstances are not uncommon in medical litigation, where existing trauma can be deepened by open discussion of the case in public, because most courts are open for public attendance.

The case against the manufacturers, Mentor of California, was thus never tested openly, and no disclosure made of previous problems with the device, or evidence about tissue expander design and manufacture. It is possible to suggest the device may have been defective for the following reasons:

- the catheter possessed too small a diameter for the expected load of the full bag;
- the critical zone where it met the bag was poorly made, with stress raisers present at the deep corners; and
- the adhesive silicone used to bond bag and catheter was probably overcured, causing embrittlement.

It is not known what quality checks were in place with the device, or what tests had been performed before introduction to the market. The facts suggest weaknesses in product design and manufacture,[11] a conclusion supported by evidence from the largest market for medical devices, the USA.

9.5.4 Other cases

Litigation in the USA has been very extensive for a long period following the introduction of breast implants there in the 1980s. The situation was the subject of a class action and Dow Corning declared for bankruptcy, with many millions of dollars being awarded in compensation, mainly for failures and leaking permanent implants. There were also claims for damage caused by leakage of liquid silicone polymer gel used to fill those implants. Whatever the merit of those claims, there is no doubt that many of the implants fractured in the body, and the devices (like the one featured here) had been under-designed for their role. In the final event (May 2000), the Federal authorities (the FDA) only authorized two manufacturers (Mentor Corporation and Inamed Corporation) to make these devices, and under strict

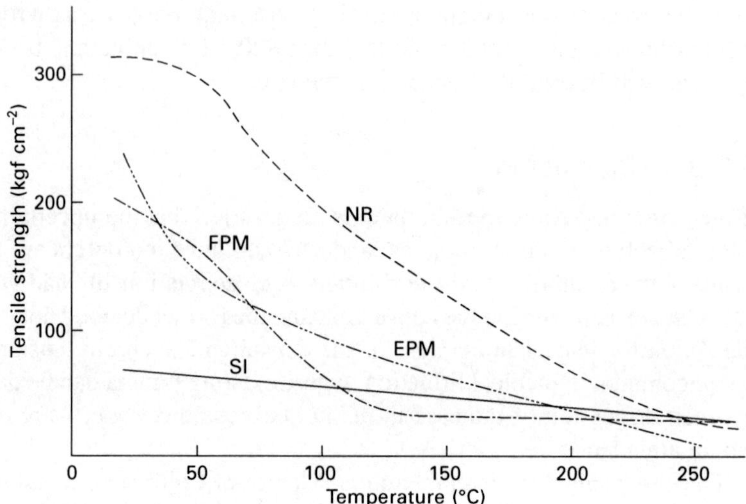

9.25 Tensile strength of various elastomers, showing silicone (SI) to be the weaker at most temperatures than natural rubber (NR), ethylene–propylene rubber (EPM), and fluoropropylene rubber (FPM).

government control.[12] They now use saline liquid as the infill rather than silicone gel. The design and manufacture of these devices has apparently improved, and other countries which also use them (such as the UK) will benefit from the tough attitude of the US authorities.[13,14] That is, however, of little help to users of the PIP implants imported from France, where high rupture rates have been experienced, and where criminal prosecution of the manufacturers is underway in 2012.

It is not difficult to see why the design of silicone implants is so important. Fig. 9.25 shows the nature of the problem.[15] The tensile strength of silicone elastomer (Si) is very low at 25 °C and certainly much lower than ethylene propylene rubber (EPM) or natural rubber (NR). The tensile strength drops very slowly with a rise in temperature (unlike the much steeper drops for other rubbers), but this is no consolation for users of the material at body temperatures (c. 40 °C). The material is also very weak in repeated loading, and fatigues easily at low applied loads; therefore, where body movement is normal and expected, product design must be conservative. It means eliminating or ameliorating stress concentrations (such as the deep corners where the bag meets the catheter, Fig. 9.20), using thick sections of material and ensuring adhesives are cured correctly.

9.6 Intraocular lenses

Many attempts have been made to strengthen silicone rubber using a wide variety of different fillers, but a solution is still awaited. In other implants, such as intraocular lenses (IOLs), silicone is an excellent choice for the replacement lens (Fig. 9.26). They replaced the original PMMA lenses developed in the UK for RAF pilots who had been injured during the Battle of Britain. Unreinforced silicone lenses are optically clear and replace a diseased lens, where cataracts have reduced if not eliminated vision in the eye affected.[16] The silicone lens is rolled up and injected through a small slit in the outer eye covering; it then unrolls and fills the cavity. The device is only lightly stressed throughout injection, and almost unstressed when in the eye, so the chance of mechanical failure is very low. However, problems can arise in delivering the lens to the eye via the polypropylene injector in its rolled-up state (Fig. 9.27 and 9.28). Low friction in the tube is critical and this is achieved by adding calcium stearate to the polymer

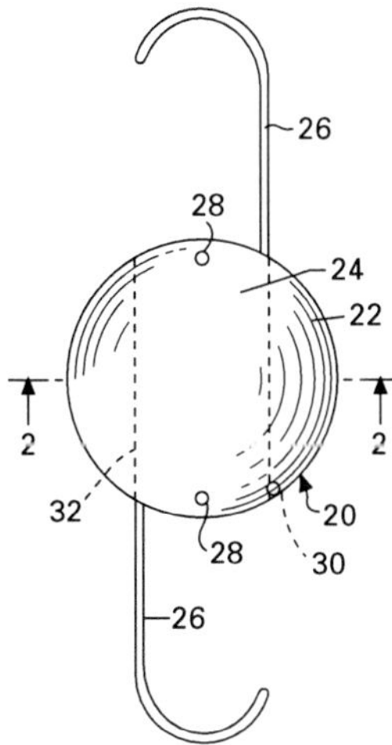

9.26 Design of flexible intraocular lens (US patent 4,717,906; 1988).

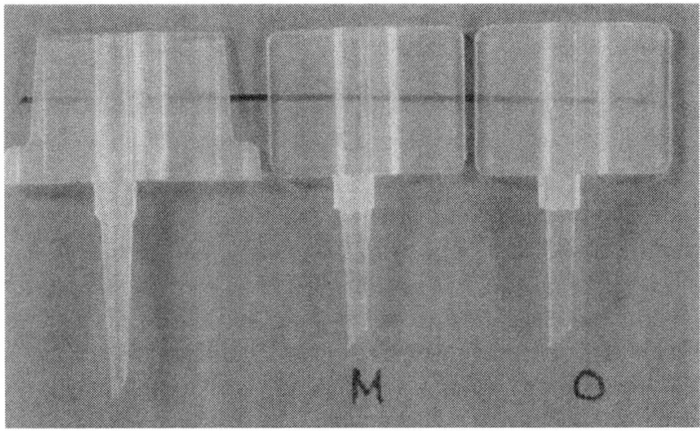

9.27 Plastic injectors for inserting the IOL into the eye.

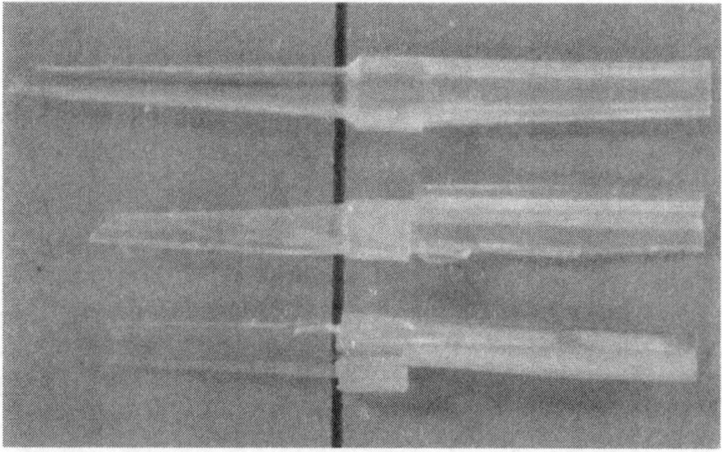

9.28 Thin and flexible wall on injector tubes.

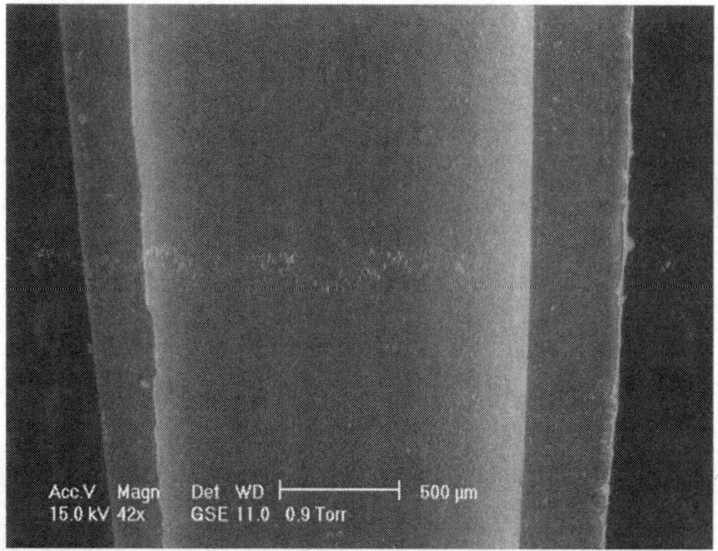

9.29 ESEM of injector inner surface with smooth stearate film.

before moulding, the idea being that it migrates to the surface and provides a low friction monolayer (Fig. 9.29 and 9.30). We were able to advise a company developing a new injection system to alter moulding conditions, because early models failed to deliver the lens effectively. The additive had not formed a uniform layer on the surface of the injector (Fig. 9.31), and so the lens became stuck in the injector. Providing a longer dwell time in the injection moulding tool eventually solved the problem by giving the lubricant time to migrate to the surface.

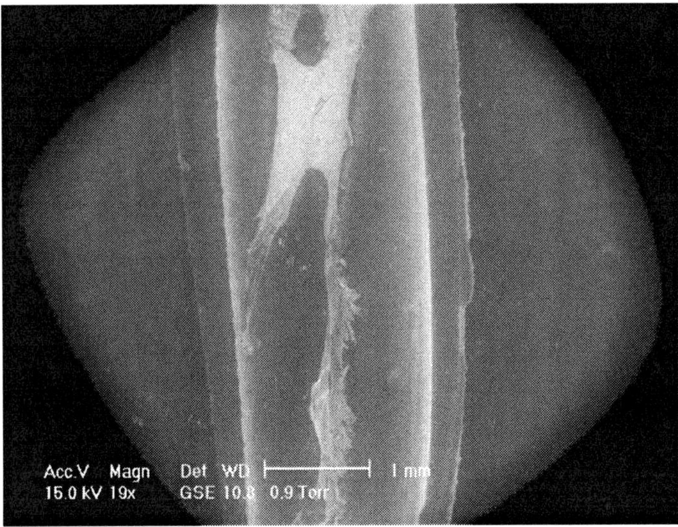

9.30 Break-up of stearate film after injection.

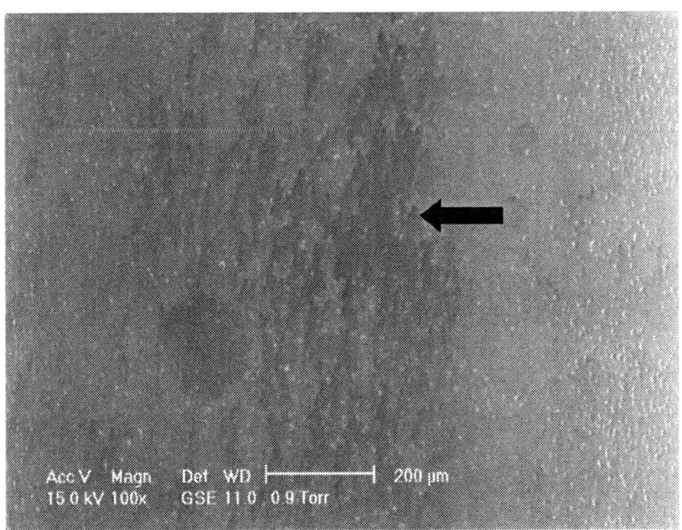

9.31 Faulty stearate film with gaps in section.

9.7 Failure of Foley catheters

However, crosslinked silicone rubber is used so widely in catheters that other problems are more common than one might expect. For example, Foley catheters are used for urinary drainage in patients and, if the tube breaks, serious problems can follow for the patient (Fig. 9.32). The catheter is more

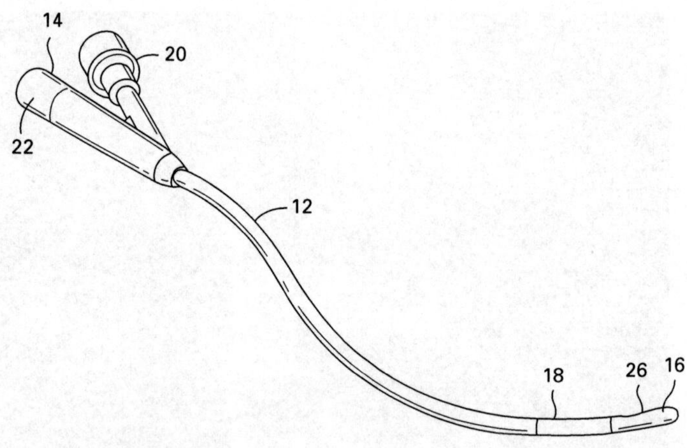

9.32 Structure of Foley catheter (US patent 6,602,243; 2003).

complex than normal because it has two channels within the tube, the larger being the drainage channel, the smaller being a channel for water pumped externally via a hypodermic needle to a side seal (20 in the figure) to inflate a bladder (18) near the tip (16). Urine is bled off from the large hole (26) in the side of the catheter behind the tip. After threading through the urethra to the bladder, the balloon is expanded by pumping water until the bulb near the end is large enough to prevent the tube slipping away.

Catheters must withstand often substantial stresses, from the weight of urine when the collection bag is full, as well as from movement of the user, and these stresses induce fatigue. The catheter can break near the tip, in which case the end must be extracted surgically.[17] Just this happened to a patient, Miss C, in 2007, and she experienced great discomfort and pain, not to mention distress without the device before a new catheter was implanted. The failed parts were returned, and she gave them to her pharmacist for examination, but they were discarded or lost, and so the cause of failure was never determined. However, the replacement catheter she was sent showed failure of almost exactly the same kind, and she sued the manufacturer as a result. The presence of a clean radial fracture (Fig. 9.33) without any applied stress implied a manufacturing defect in the material, vulcanized silicone rubber.

Although optical microscopy was used initially, the transparency of the polymer made ESEM obligatory and also provided higher resolution images. The transverse fracture showed a clear origin (Fig. 9.34), and a cusp marking the meeting point of the cracks opposite was clearly visible (Fig. 9.35). Detailed inspection showed the presence of numerous defects, including numerous voids revealed by the passage of the crack (Fig. 9.36).

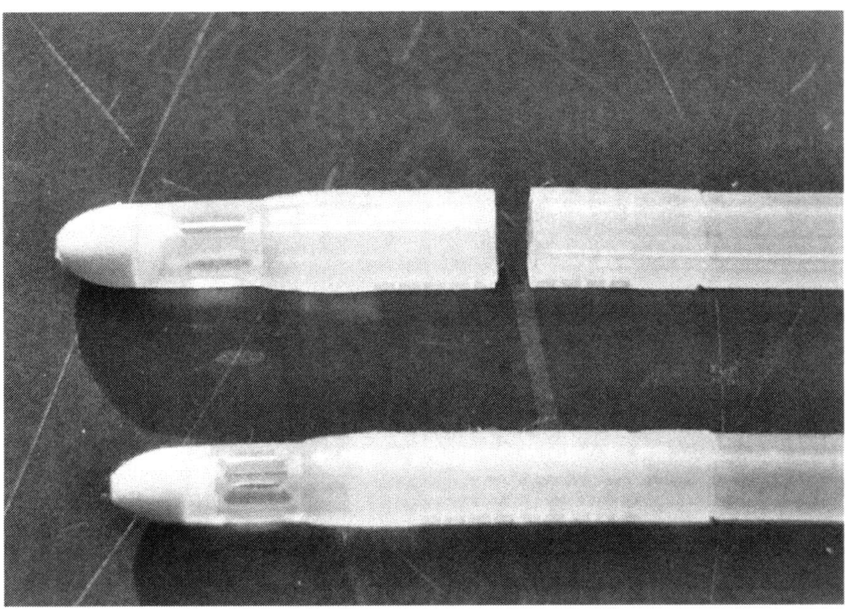

9.33 Fracture in the balloon section of the Foley catheter.

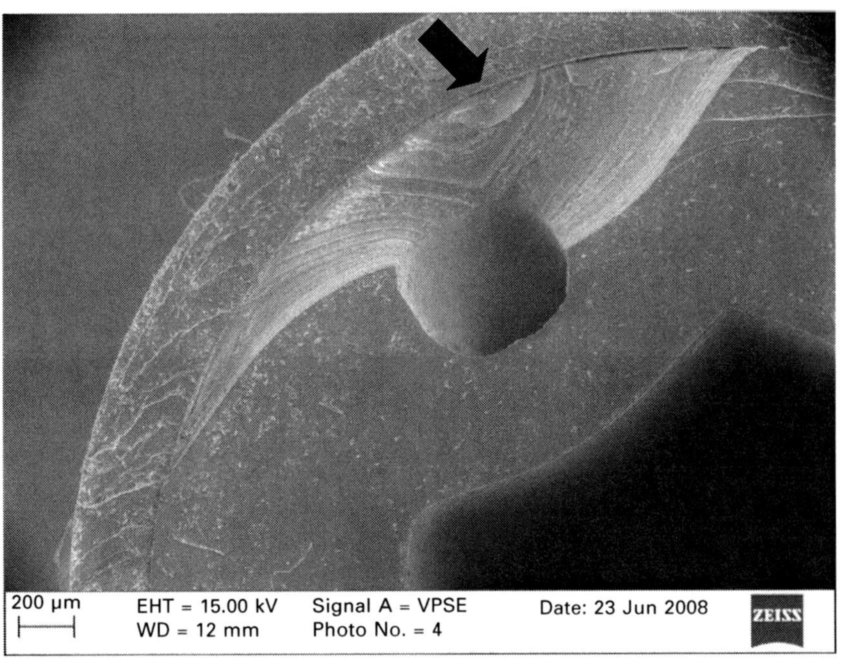

9.34 Brittle fracture in ESEM showing the origin (arrow).

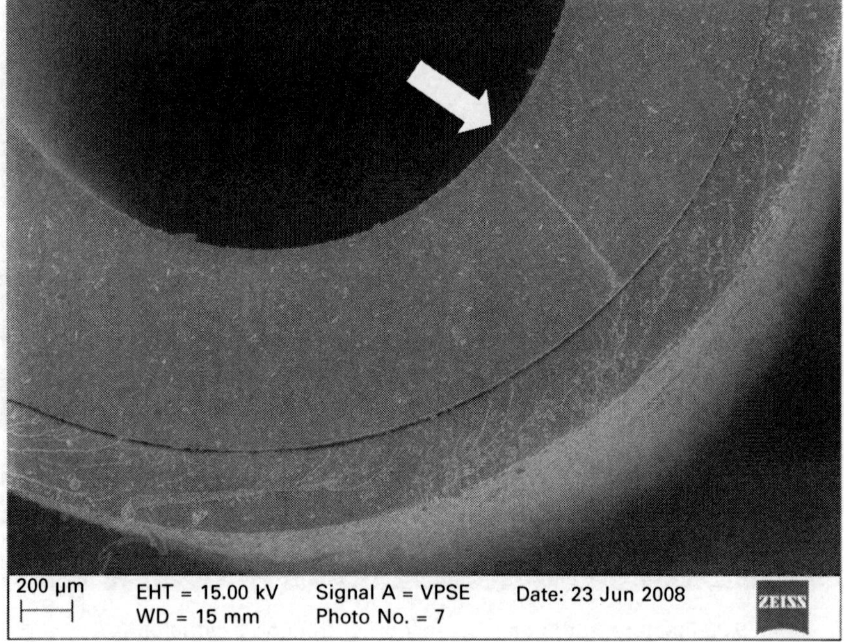

9.35 Cusp in opposite fracture surface showing meeting of cracks (arrow).

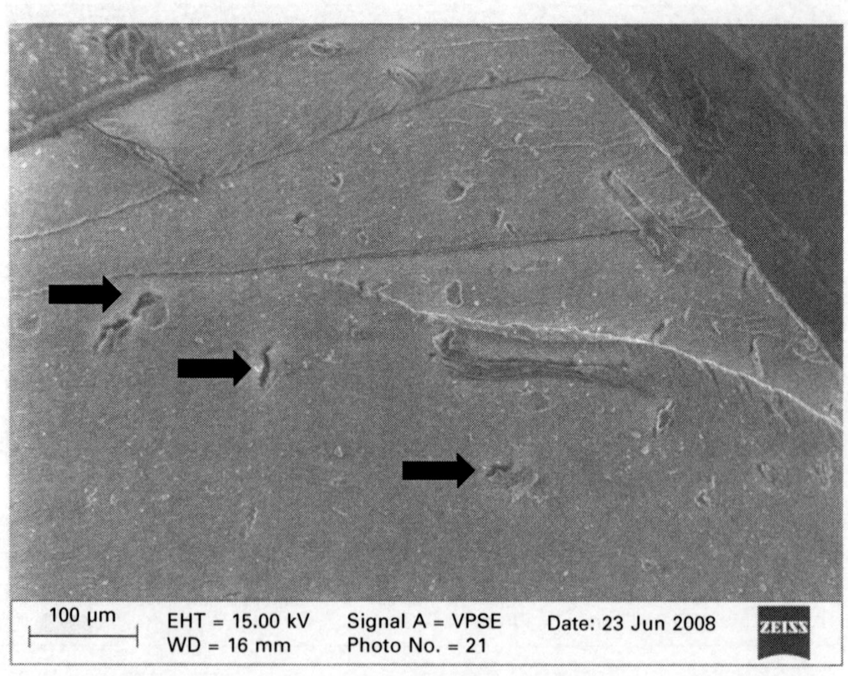

9.36 Voids revealed by crack growth in fracture surface (arrows).

In addition, the broken halves did not match up, indicating that the bleed hole had been lost in a separate fragment which had fallen away, and been lost entirely. That the fractures had been initiated at the bleed hole seemed to be confirmed when another intact catheter was inspected. It showed that fragments had been lost from the sides of the hole, leaving a rough and jagged appearance (Fig. 9.37). This was confirmed when a new catheter obtained independently was examined: it had a round and smooth bleed hole (Fig. 9.38).

The defective catheters had been poorly manufactured, and the data supplied by the manufacturers (based in the Far East) proved to be of no assistance in tracing the origin of the faulty batch of devices. There are several dangers during manufacture, including overcure, when too high a density of crosslinks are present. Other parts may be undercured and the purity of the raw material must also be carefully controlled to prevent inclusions. If the distribution of crosslinks varies across the walls of the device then asymmetric stresses are set up when loaded, and these encourage crack growth. It is likely that the main tube was extruded (given that it is of constant section), and that the other parts were either hot moulded onto the tube or attached by silicone adhesives. A selection of finished devices are normally selected for detailed inspection and testing, but for several defective catheters to penetrate the security is unusual, and indicative of a serious lapse in quality control.

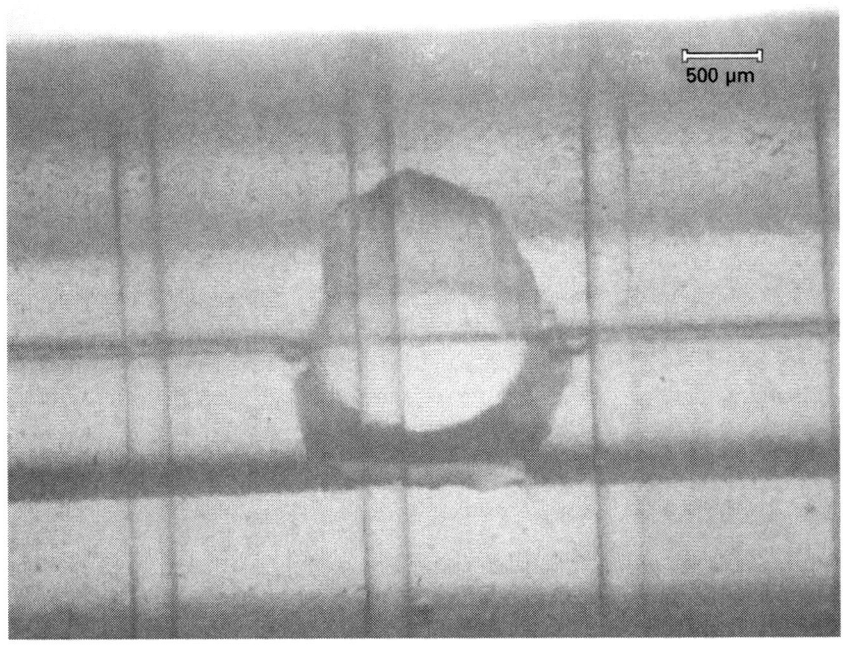

9.37 Irregular bleed hole in new intact catheter.

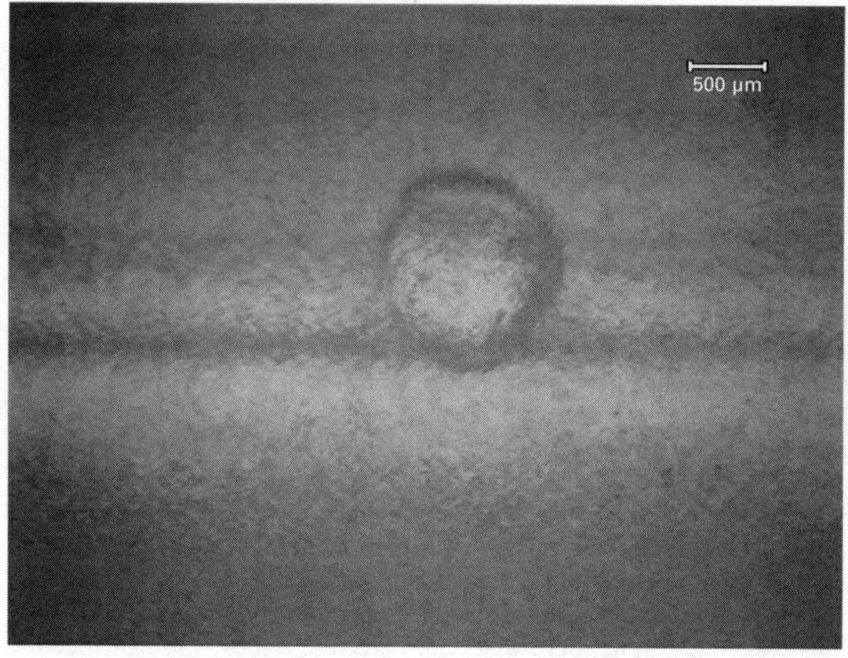

9.38 Regular bleed hole in new catheter.

Miss C eventually received damages from the makers in the Far East in 2010 as compensation for the distress and pain she had experienced as a result of a poor batch of catheters. Contrary to the findings of a previous study,[17] it is clear that such failures are not at all uncommon, as a review from 1993 of five failed catheters indicated.[18] Other materials used include polyurethane and natural rubber, and these too have suffered failures, judging by the more than 18 adverse incident reports on the FDA Maude database from US hospitals, from about 2000 to the most recent report from March 2011. Several alerts have also been issued by the MHRA in the period up to 2008/9. Such problems highlight the importance of quality control of manufacture, and close control of the polymers used in forming such products.

9.8 Sutures

Catgut is a traditional monofilament used to stitch wounds together, but there are now many alternative fibrous materials available. Another natural product, braided silk fibre can also be used, and individual doctors make a choice appropriate for each particular type of wound. Stitches that dissolve in body fluids to produce harmless products have been known for many years, the polymers of interest producing non-toxic monomers or starting units. One of the most widely used absorbable suture materials is polyglactin 910, a polysaccharide (commonly sold under the trade name Vicryl). The material is a copolyester of lactic acid and glycolic acid, both of which are harmless products easily excreted by the body:

glycolic acid repeat unit: $–[OCH_2CO]–$

lactic acid repeat unit: $–[OCH(CH_3)CO]–$

The lactic acid content is about 10% in Vicryl, the repeat units being randomly distributed among blocks of glycolic acid. The crystallinity is lower than pure glycolic acid, but amorphous zones are needed to enhance breakdown by absorbing body fluids. It is hydrolyzed by body fluids at a rate similar to that of wound healing, thus disappearing when it has finished holding tissues together, and the tissues are by then self-supporting.

9.8.1 Suture failure causing wound opening

Absorbable sutures are ideal for internal wounds, such as those made after childbirth, but things may not always go to plan. A Mrs P was recovering after successful delivery of a baby boy, using an emergency Caesarean section. The following morning, she began to bleed heavily and was transferred to the labour suite and underwent corrective surgery. However, she suffered continuing problems with the outer wound, which was oozing a pink sticky fluid. The conventional stitches were removed, but about 10 min later, she stood up, and the wound opened. She was horrified to see her intestines spilling out, an incident witnessed by her shocked partner at the bedside. She subsequently brought an action against the hospital and makers of the Vicryl sutures used to stitch her uterus.

The medical records showed that following delivery of the baby, her uterus was stitched in two layers with Vicryl, and externally with Prolene (polypropylene). She lost a considerable amount of blood during recovery, about 1.44 litre (including that lost at delivery). An ultrasound scan showed her uterus distended with blood clots, about 1 litre being removed under general anaesthetic via her cervix. A clinical note made the next day stated that the 'uterus had well contracted'. Her outer dressing was changed owing to oozing of fluid, but appeared to have diminished the next day. Later that same day, the external Prolene sutures were found to be 'digging into her skin', so were cut and taped with paper sutures. The following day the wound was clean with only slight oozing, and the paper sutures removed. The attending midwife said that the wound was clean and dry, and the outer Prolene stitches removed 'easily'. The notes then record wound dehiscence (opening), and she was transferred quickly to theatre where the wound was restitched by another doctor not involved in the original stitching. He made the observation that 'all the layers of the wound closure were still present, but the sheath suture had snapped in the middle'.

The statement claimed that the Vicryl suture had not broken at the knots, and the knots had not slipped. But the failed suture had been discarded after the operation, making investigation of the evidence impossible, a not uncommon problem in medical negligence cases.

9.8.2 Analysis of a new suture

Although the failed suture had been unfortunately lost, equivalent new sutures were made available for inspection. One of the lengths was strained to break on a tensometer, by tying a granny knot to form a loop and then stringing the loop over round supports on the machine. The results of two tests gave tensile breaking loads of 70 and 58 N for failure strains of 74% (in free fibre) and 96% (at knot), respectively. There is clearly substantial variation in strength, depending on the knot, which could be attributed to slippage and perhaps knot orientation as well. Knots are well known stress concentrators in ropes and cords, and this also applies to knots in braided fibre. At the high rate of test, the broken ends showed melting of individual fibres to form blobs of solidified molten polymer (Fig. 9.39). On the other hand, the failure loads of about 7 and 5.8 kg are high compared with expected loads in soft tissue.

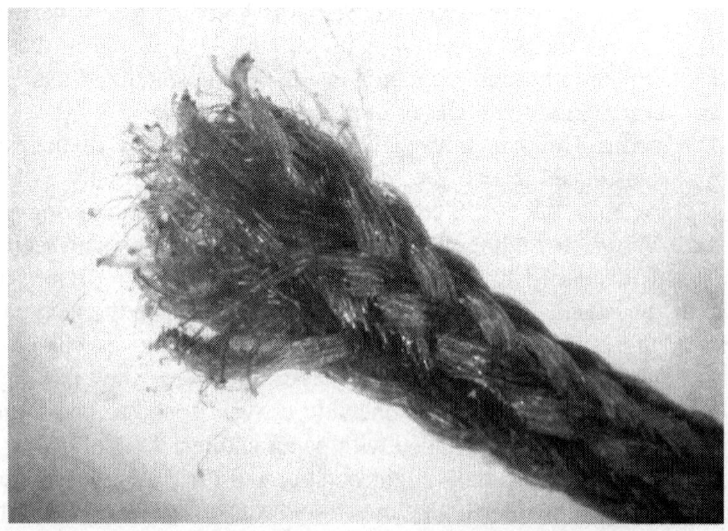

9.39 Fractured test end of Vicryl suture showing fibre melt at tips.

The thermal properties of the polymer showed a main melting point of about 200 °C, with subsidiary peaks at 180, 126 and 73 °C. It is known that the suture was coated with another polyglactide of different composition, probably exhibited by a large peak at 180 °C while the smaller peaks represented lubricants such as calcium stearate. Finally, the fibre proved soluble (several hours immersion) in strong caustic soda of pH 14, showing that alkaline conditions were needed for hydrolysis. Some body fluids are slightly alkaline, so enhancing degradation.

9.8.3 Possible causes of failure

It was therefore necessary to examine how the suture failed at such a critical moment. The company Ethicon publishes guidelines on their Vicryl suture on their website, www.ethicon360.com, stating that the sutures retain 75% of their original tensile strength after 2 weeks implantation in rats, and 50% at three weeks. Because the sutures failed the day after they were emplaced, it was thus unlikely that they failed by dissolution in her body. However, the doctor who restitched the wound said that the Vicryl suture had fractured in the middle. Unfortunately the suture was discarded, so no forensic examination could be made of the remains, and his assertion could not be tested.

It is unusual for cords to break centrally, fractures tending to occur at knots or other attachment points, as experiment had shown. Alternatively, the stitch could simply have not been tied correctly in the first place using approved knots and placements in the soft tissues to be joined together. Evidence from the staff involved in the original stitching was contradictory, but it was known that very junior staff had been involved when the patient was stitched.

9.8.4 Outcome

The legal action did not proceed in the absence of clear evidence of either medical negligence or a defective suture, and the patient could not be compensated for her distress. It is unfortunate that the physical evidence of failure in many medical cases is frequently lost or discarded, perhaps because the items are disposable anyway. However, it may leave patients uncompensated, and product manufacturers uncertain of the state of their product. If the design and manufacture of products is to be improved, then analysis of failures is vital to determining the cause or causes of the specific problem in question. That task is impossible if the failed products are no longer available for examination. Even a photograph of a failed product is better than no product at all, for much can be learnt from good photographs of failures, especially now when even a mobile phone can be used to record evidence.

9.9 Conclusions

There are many problems in tackling failures of medical devices. They include:

- a reluctance to retain and store failed samples returned by hospitals to manufacturers;
- failure to retain failed products by hospitals;
- the poor quality of reports analyzing samples (poor photography, or no photography at all); and
- the tendency to blame users without investigating the problem in depth.

Such difficulties are not normally encountered in other areas of engineering failure (although of course not unknown), but tend to recur in case after case of failed medical products. Breast implants have been lost by hospitals and even, in one case, by the Medical Devices Agency (MDA), the forerunner of the MHRA. A failed Foley catheter was discarded by a pharmacist, but the replacements were also faulty, so the investigation could proceed. However, a failed suture disappeared completely at the hospital, leaving the victim unable to prove negligence. In short, there seems to be little general awareness among both product designers and some medical staff of the importance of failure analysis in improving product quality, especially for safety-critical products like catheters and ancillary equipment. It is also certainly true that most medical staff are aware of their importance, and do often retain samples and report about the circumstances of failure. However, frequently those samples are sent away to the manufacturer and then discarded, without photographs or other information on the failed device(s).

Reports of medical device failure are numerous because responsible staff are aware of the safety critical nature of many of the products used to assist patients. Doctors and consultants do report and describe the failures encountered in their practice, both in technical and professional journals, and often about individual pieces of equipment. They are an invaluable aid for investigators researching specific designs, as are the adverse incident reports from the FDA Maude website and more recently, a similar website run by the MDHA.

However, not all relevant details are published as might be hoped, such as the materials of construction or the loads to which they have been exposed. But the stresses experienced by implants such as breast expanders or external devices such as catheters are often difficult to estimate with any degree of accuracy. The traditional engineering approach involves providing products with a high safety margin, using very conservative estimates of load so that the device should be capable of surviving normal loads without failure. Standards also provide a useful way of assuring medical staff that a medical product will resist normal handling and body stresses. However, standards authorities usually lag by several years, so that standards appear after failures have been widespread. The standard for breast implants for example, only appeared in 2000, several years after the first failures were experienced by patients.[19] The standard describes numerous tests to evaluate the mechanical strength of implants, which, if applied rigorously, should help to improve product performance. Fatigue behaviour remains uncertain, however, especially when body loads can vary so greatly from person to person, tending to be higher the younger the patient. The artificial hip joint is perhaps the most obvious implant which experiences millions of cycles during its lifetime, and where there have been severe problems caused by fatigue crack growth as well as excessive wear in the joint itself.[20] There have also been examples of premature fatigue fracture of artificial heart valves, most notably the Bjork–Shiley valve made from tantalum and carbon fibre composite. A design variant of a hitherto successful design failed suddenly and many patients died prematurely as a direct result. The problem was traced to faulty welds on some of the valves, emphasizing the importance of quality control during manufacture.[22]

9.10 Acknowledgements

The author would like to thank Gordon Imlach for scanning microscopy, DSC, and FTIR spectroscopic analyses, and Stan Hiller for optical microsocopy. He also thanks Dr Patrick A Lewis of the Institute of Neurology, UCL for assistance in the literature searches related to medical products, and his colleagues, Drs Colin Gagg and Sarah Hainsworth for useful discussions of some of the cases reported here.

9.11 References

1. Holden, G, Legge NR, Quirk, R and Schroeder, HE, *Thermoplastic elastomers*, 2nd edition, Hanser Publishers (1996).
2. Adams, RK, Hoeschle, GK and Witsiepe, WK, *Thermoplastic polyether ester elastomers*, in *Thermoplastic elastomers*, Holden, G, Legge NR, Quink R and Schroeder, 2nd edition, Hanser Publishers (1996).
3. Gauvin, P, Philippart, J-L and Lemaire, J, Photo-oxydation de polyether-block-polyamides, *Makromol Chem*, **186**, 1167–1180 (1985).
4. Elf Atochem technical brochures, available at http://www.pebax.com.
5. Lewis, PR, Premature failure of a thermoplastic epidural catheter, Society of Plastics Engineers, *ANTEC 2001*, Dallas, USA.
6. Lewis, PR and Gagg, C, *Failure of an Epidural Catheter*, *Eng Fail Anal*, **16**(6), 1805–1815 (2009).
7. Mueller R and Sanborn T, The History of Interventional Cardiology, *Am Heart J* **129**, 146–172 (1995).
8. Myler R and Stertzer, S, Coronary and peripheral angioplasty: historic perspective,

Textbook of Interventional Cardiology (2nd Ed.) Vol. 1. Topol, E. (Ed.) WB Saunders Co., Philadelphia (1993).

9. King, SB, Angioplasty from bench to bedside to bench, *Circulation*, **93**, 1621–1629 (1996).
10. MHRA, *Medical device alert*, MDA/2009/023.
11. Lynch, W, *Handbook of silicone rubber fabrication*, Van Nostrand Reinhold (1978).
12. FDA, *Study of rupture of silicone gel filled breast implants*, available at http://www.fda.gov.
13. Young, VL and Watson, ME, Breast implant research: where we have been, where we are, where we need to go, *Clin Plast Surg*, **28**(3) 451–483 (2001).
14. Brandon, HJ, Young, VL, Jenina, KL and Wolf, CJ, Variability in the properties of silicone gel breast implants, *Plast Reconstruct Surg*, **108**(3), 647–655 (2001).
15. Blow, CM (Ed), *Rubber technology and manufacture*, Newnes Butterworth, 135 (1971).
16. Holladay, JT, Ting, AC, Koester, CJ, Portney, V and Willis TR, Silicone intraocular lens resolution in air and in water, *J Catatact Refract Surg*, **14**, 657–659 (1988).
17. El-Sherif, AE, Taweela, N and Nagi AK, Complete fracture of urethral Foley's catheter: a rare complication, *J Royal Soc Med*, **84**, 563 (1991).
18. McKenzie, JM, Flahiff, CM and Nelson, CL, Retention and strength of silicone-rubber catheters: A report of five cases of retention and analysis of catheter strength, *J Bone Joint Surg Am*, **75**, 1505–1507 (1993).
19. British Standards, Non-active surgical implants – body contouring implants – specific requirements for mammary implants, BS EN 12180: 2000.
20. Lewis, PR, Reynolds, K and Gagg, C, *Forensic materials engineering*, CRC Press (2004).
21. Blackstone, EH, Could It Happen Again? The Björk-Shiley Convexo-Concave Heart Valve Story, *Circulation*, **111**, 2717–2719 (2005).

10 Manufacturing defects in polymeric medical devices

P. R. LEWIS, The Open University, UK

Abstract: Injection moulding, extrusion and other processes for manufacturing polymer components are discussed. Several case studies are presented where manufacture of polymer components is crucial to product performance, such as injection-moulded polycarbonate connectors in a catheter, cylinder guard fractures, sight tubes, a crutch failure, and ozone cracking of tubing and a condom.

Key words: medical devices, implants, manufacturing defects, anaesthetics, sight tube, condom, crutch.

Note: This chapter is a revised and updated version of Chapters 2 'Examination and analysis of failed components', 3 'Polymer medical devices' and 8 'Tools and ladders' by P. R. Lewis, originally published in *Forensic polymer engineering: why polymer products fail in service*, P. R. Lewis and C. Gagg, Woodhead Publishing Limited, 2010, ISBN: 978-1-84569-185-1.

10.1 Introduction

Medical equipment, such as the implants and other devices discussed in the previous chapter, has developed rapidly as medical treatment has advanced, and polymeric materials have played a large part in the progress in providing effective relief for patients suffering from all manner of illnesses. Their low densities make them ideal for prostheses for example, and the high strength of composite materials has led to many innovative designs in artificial limbs. Such materials can exploit the extraordinary properties of carbon fibre, which when combined with a strong matrix such as epoxy resin, gives products which resist fatigue or repeated loading to a much greater extent than conventional materials. However, their high cost both as raw materials and manufacturing prohibits their use in common medical equipment, where mass manufacture demands low unit costs. Thermoplastic polymers have been widely adopted for many different parts of medical equipment, but their design and manufacture demands very high quality constraints, an objective not always met in practice, as described in some of the cases discussed in this chapter.

The way products are made is important for the features that can arise from the particular way a polymer is shaped, and when those features turn into defects. Two kinds of manufacturing defect were discussed in the previous chapter, including faulty extrusion of the Foley catheter and faulty assembly of the breast implant (combined with under-design for strength). However, many other types of defect are known in moulded polymers.

10.2 Polymer moulding

Shaping of polymers occurs via several routes, in particular:

- injection moulding;
- extrusion;
- rotational moulding; and
- compression moulding.

Each process produces characteristic faults, most of which are detected by the machine operator. Many, however, are difficult to spot without access to microscopes or other methods, and result in defective products entering the market.

10.2.1 Injection moulding

Injection moulding involves injection of molten polymer into a shaped tool which can be separated at the end of the moulding cycle (Fig. 10.1). The tool has at least one gate where the polymer enters and, in some cases where the shape to be created is complex, several gates. Because the metal parts of the tool must be able to separate, there are several important design rules. Polymer products frequently need supporting ribs, so they must be aligned with the direction of withdrawal of the tool, for example. The cycle time is dominated by the cooling period (Fig. 10.2) caused by their low thermal

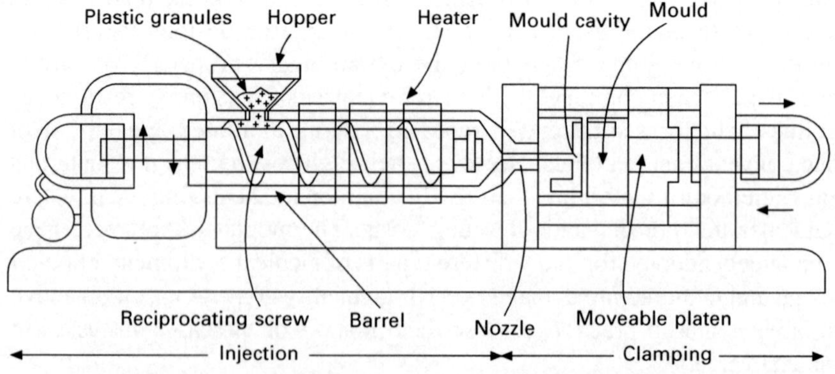

10.1 Section of injection moulding machine with mould at right.

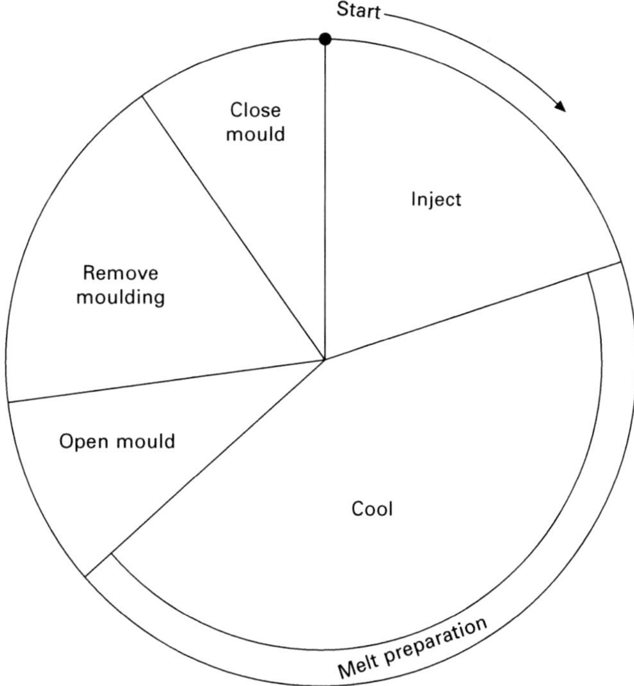

10.2 Injection moulding cycle with cooling the largest component.

conductivity. Many polymers must be cooled slowly so as to relieve internal strains and stresses that can result from quenching, otherwise, a seriously defective product can be created. Where holes are needed in a product, the flow of the melt has to divide, creating the problem of weld lines where they rejoin. Voids and sinks can act as stress concentrators if in the load path when the product is in service. Moulding features can include:

- frozen-in stress and strain;
- poor fusion at weld lines;
- voids in the centre of thick sections; and
- sink marks at the surface.

Other features may be created when the polymer granules are not dried correctly, leading to degradation at the high temperatures of moulding molten polymer. Because thermoplastic polymers have to be processed well above the glass transition temperature T_g or melting point T_m, the process temperature is usually well above the boiling point of water. Any traces of moisture therefore result in voids and surface 'splay marks'. Hydrolysis may occur, thus causing a reduction in the molecular weight. Whether a moulding feature becomes a defect depends on its location on the product, its further treatment and its final environment. Thus, a weld line in an unstressed part of the product may not cause failure. However, if it falls along a load path, it can act as a nucleus for a brittle crack.

The polymer melt viscosity is an important variable in the process because it effectively controls not just the way the process works, but the strength of the final product. The root variable is molecular weight M which controls both these properties; the greater the molecular weight of the polymer, the greater both the melt viscosity and the product mechanical strength. Molecular weight is a simple measure of chain length. The shear stress τ of a Newtonian fluid such as water is related to the shear rate γ and the viscosity η by the simple equation

$$\tau = \eta\gamma \qquad [10.1]$$

However, polymer melts are governed by a so-called rate law, where the shear stress is more sensitive to shear rate, or the rate at which the melt moves when sheared:

$$\tau = \eta(\gamma)^{n} \qquad [10.2]$$

or

$$\log\tau = \log\eta + n\log\gamma \qquad [10.3]$$

and

$$\log\eta = \log\tau - n\log\gamma \qquad [10.4]$$

with the exponent n being a negative value. In other words, the melt viscosity decreases with increasing shear rate, and such fluids are generally known as 'pseudoplastic' in nature, a specific example of a non-Newtonian liquid (Fig. 10.3). Thus, as the shear rate increases, the shear stress falls. Figure 10.3 shows how several different polymers react as shear rate rises, and there are considerable variations between them. Thus, acrylics such as poly(methyl methacrylate) (PMMA) and poly(vinyl chloride) (PVC) fall faster than more rigid chains such as those of polybutylene terephthalate (PBT) and polyethersulfone. The melt flow index (MFI) is an empirical measure of melt viscosity used by moulders, which is inversely related to molecular weight. The shear rates encountered in the pipes of moulding machines is typically above 10^3, so the melt viscosities used in moulding are those to the right of Fig. 10.3. There is a subtle implication that some polymers are more difficult to mould than others, those polymers with inflexible chains generally being more difficult than simple chains such as low-density polyethylene (LDPE). Greater care is needed for such polymers, which includes polysulfones and polycarbonates as well as PBT since the melt is more Newtonian than simpler polymers. Similar care is needed with composites such as short glass fibre (GF) reinforced materials such as GF nylon owing to the thickening effect of the short fibres present in the melt.

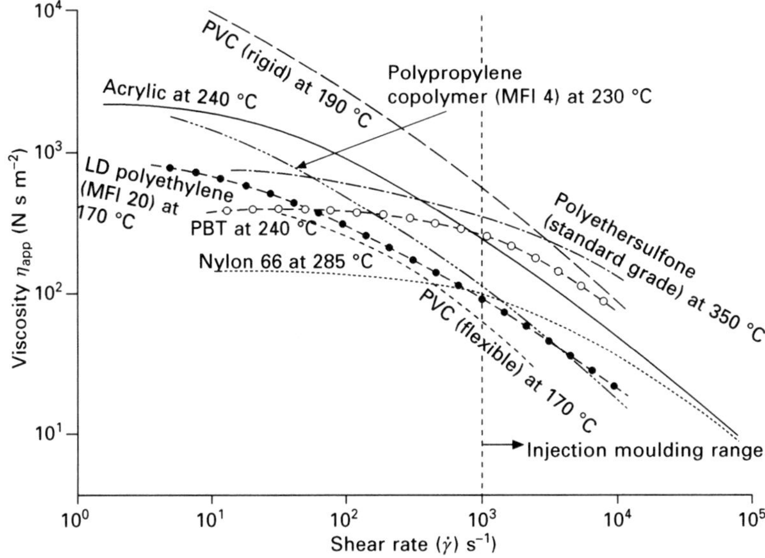

10.3 Effect of increasing shear rate on polymer melt viscosity.

The melt viscosity below entanglement is proportional to molecular weight:

$$\eta = k\mathrm{M_w} \quad [10.5]$$

However, when the chains start to entangle with one another, the melt viscosity rises very steeply according to a power law:

$$\eta = k\, M_w^{\,3.4} \quad [10.6]$$

The influence of the two equations is illustrated for some polymers by Fig. 10.4, where the molecular weight is now plotted in terms of the number of atoms in the backbone chain N_B. This is why injection moulding grades of polymers tend to be chosen near to the entanglement molecular weight in order to minimise melt viscosity. However, the tensile strength lies at the lower end of expectations, and is sensitive to any mechanism that cuts or degrades chains. It might only need a few single-chain scissions to lower the molecular weight locally to below entanglement, thus causing the tensile strength to drop dramatically and a brittle crack to be initiated.

Injection moulding is the most sophisticated moulding technique, and the tools are an expensive part of the process, their cost being determined by their complexity. Production runs must be long to justify their cost, and there are various ways of increasing the rate, by using multicavity tools for example.[1, 2]

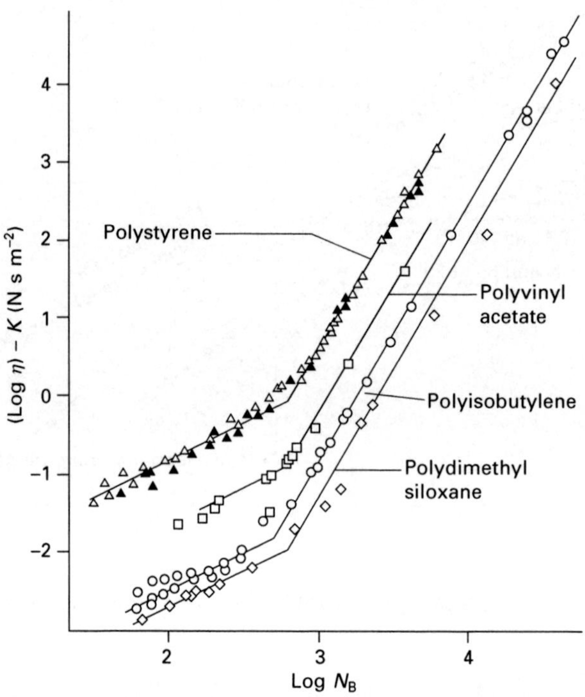

10.4 Effect of molecular weight or chain length on melt viscosity.

10.2.2 Extrusion

The process of injecting a stream of molten polymer through a die of constant section is known as extrusion, and it is generally simpler than injection moulding. Pipe, sheet and profiles are made using the method, but there are several features in the final product that can be deleterious. Perhaps the most important is the equivalent of weld lines, so-called 'spider lines', which are aligned along the axis of a pipe, for example. They are formed by the internal metal supports for the die head, where the melt divides before reforming. If the melt is too cold, then reformation is poor, so leaving lines along the extrudate. They can be seen clearly in the section of a pipe in Fig. 10.5.

Figure 10.5 also shows another problem encountered in all processes: poor mixing of ingredients, in this case carbon black in polyethylene. To achieve the best product strength, such fillers must be mixed to make a uniform material, combining both high dispersion and an even distribution of particles.

Owing to the simplicity of extrusion, polymers of higher molecular weight can be used, so extruded products tend to be stronger than moulded products. The problem of residual strain is also usually much reduced in extrudates.

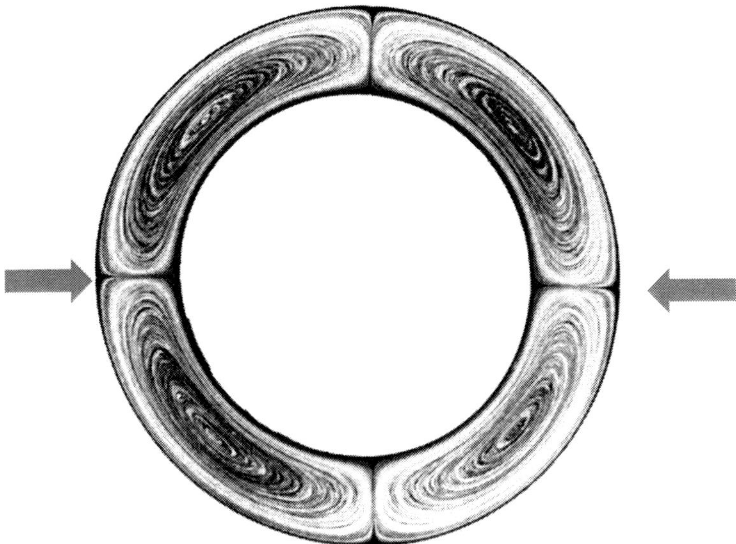

10.5 Section of poorly mixed extrudate with spider lines (two arrowed) from die head.

Thus, pipe is generally very strong, with failures tending to occur at welded joints.

10.2.3 Other moulding methods

Rotational moulding is a way of shaping products without two matching tools. Only an outer tool is used, and a weighed quantity of powder is added to the tool which is then rotated in an oven. The particles gradually melt and fuse to create a uniform wall, which can then be removed at the end of the cycle. Because high pressure is not used, higher tool temperatures are needed, thus raising the chance of thermal degradation. The inner surface can also be rough owing to incomplete particle fusion. Both oxidation and geometric irregularity can weaken this surface, making products weak to external impact loads.[3]

Compression moulding, a primitive form of injection moulding, is widely used for elastomers and some thermosets. However, it suffers from the primitive control of melt flow, although tools are simple and production rates high. The features that may become defects are similar to those of injection moulding. Perhaps the most sophisticated method is used in tyre building, where temperature control is crucial to achieving the best properties of the many different parts of the product.

For materials of extremely high molecular weight, which are impossible to mould or extrude, sintering is a possible forming route. The process involves use of high pressures to compress powder particles together into simple shapes in a closed mould. It is used for ultra-high molecular weight polyethylene (UHMWPE) used in hip joint sockets for example. Shaping by machining can then be used, although costs are high because each product must be shaped individually. UHMWPE has the advantage of a very high strength needed to resist hip loads owing to its high molecular weight of several millions.

10.2.4 Other manufacturing routes

Welding is an important secondary process used to bond components together to make a composite product. Thermal or fusion welding presents the problem of temperature control. Because high temperatures are needed, the problem of oxidation is ever present, and good control of the process is needed to achieve a reliable bond. Ultrasonic or radio frequency vibrations can also be used to weld two plastic surfaces in contact by means of the heat generated at the interface. However, care is needed to ensure that the two surfaces are always in direct contact so as to achieve a good bond and, as it is almost impossible for a weld to match the strength of the bulk polymer, welds are a key zone where failure can occur. Adhesives are also widely used to join separate parts. The manufacturing method, always an important part of product design, is of particular importance for medical products that have to resist a very wide range of stresses, abuse, and environments. In determining root cause of specific incidents, the manufacturing process must be considered alongside the physical design of the device as well as the documentary and witness evidence.

10.3 Catheter systems

Intravenous (IV) catheter lines find extensive use in intensive care and for drip feeds to many other groups of patients (the elderly, chronically sick and premature babies, for example). It is natural, therefore, that systems have been developed for allowing different drugs to be fed through the same tube, for other fluids to be supplied, such as serum and total parental nutrition (TPN), which is a synthetic equivalent of milk. Multiple supply implies use of junctions (Y-junctions for example), connections and ways of supplying drugs via hypodermic needles to prevent any possibility of contamination within the lines. There are many such medical plumbing systems available to medical staff in hospitals, and indeed for self-medication to chronically ill, but stable patients, who have been transferred home. Many systems were developed in the 1980s and 1990s, and they are still being actively developed further. Various materials have been used for the catheters of such systems, including crosslinked silicone rubber, for example, which is a very stable polymer, inert to most body and medical fluids, but of low strength. The catheter ends are supplied with connectors to enable infusion of drugs via hypodermic needle; such connectors typically comprise a rubber seal embedded in a plastic connector. The needle can be pushed through the seal and retracted, the rubber relaxing back and so providing a secure way of delivering a measured dose with no external contamination.

10.3.1 Connector failures

However, there have been problems with the quality of the thermoplastic fittings. The connectors at the ends of the catheter are often injection moulded from polycarbonate, and, in some instances, these have broken, either partly or completely. The hairline brittle cracks formed before separation of the components are very difficult for medical staff to spot in time, and can lead to bacterial contamination of the fluid supply to the patient. The problem was highlighted by investigators in the early 1990s when large numbers of such devices first started to appear on the market. Splits in hubs were often encountered, especially in connections known as 'luers' (from the first user of such devices), where a smooth conical end is pushed into a shaped female receptacle. The problem arises from the hoop stress applied by the pushing action tending to initiate cracks from defects on the edge of the joint or elsewhere (such as poorly formed gates, the point where plastic was injected into the tool of the moulding machine). In addition, any variation in fitment dimensions puts extra hoop stresses on the female part of the joint.[4]

Another device uses a screw fitting, where the male part is twisted into the female luer. However, there are several problems with this fitting too. Such fittings are covered by an ISO standard,[5] but there are still problems of fitment. The first problem is that screw fittings are insecure unless some means of locking the fitting can be made. This problem is well known to motor engineers, and various devices have been developed to stop joints unscrewing. The second problem is the fit between connectors from different suppliers in the absence of a common standard. Owing to small dimensional differences, the joint can unscrew quite readily, thus making the joint unsafe.

10.3.2 Premature cracking of connectors

The problem of premature cracking of connectors became critical when one design was introduced into the British market in the mid-1990s.[6] The connectors are designed to join lengths of catheter and are typically used in Hickman lines, which are usually made in silicone rubber (Fig. 10.6). Each device is made by welding two parts of the outer casing together to form the final shape (Fig. 10.7). The device is 25 mm long and 10 mm wide at its widest point. The casing conceals an inner working mechanism, which

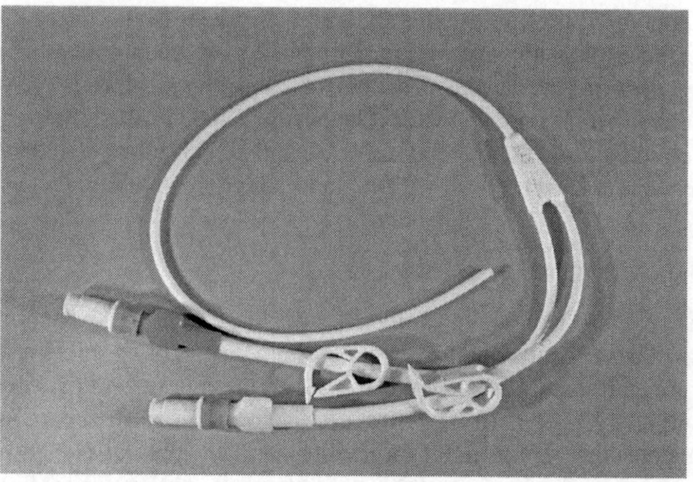

10.6 Hickman IV line fitted with coloured polycarbonate connectors.

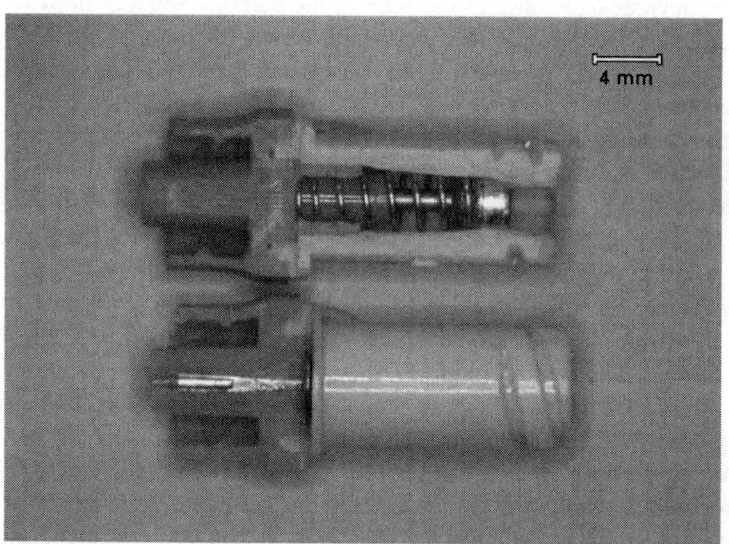

10.7 Section through connector to show internal structure.

consists of a stainless-steel helical spring behind a latex rubber seal. The stainless-steel tube within the spring runs along the centre line of the design and provides the pathway for the liquids used in the IV line (Fig. 10.7). The rubber seal has a resealable cut at its centre to allow luers to be inserted easily for a new line. Such a female luer also has an external screw thread for secure attachment of the connection. The other end of the device consists of a male luer which can be connected to the main line, and is also fitted with a screw thread.

The device was tested to standards current to the early 1990s,[5] and appeared to fulfil all requirements. The device offered a sealed unit so as to prevent contamination of the central feed line by pathogenic bacteria. The problem of infection in hospitals is well known, and hospital authorities have been tackling it by a variety of routes including cleaning and disinfection of working surfaces, improved staff hygiene and so on. The IV lines need extra special care because the lines offer direct entry to the body to pathogens, bypassing the normal defences of the body. Lines carrying nutritional fluids such as TPN are especially at risk because they offer nutrition to bacteria as well as the patient.

That the design was faulty emerged later,[6] during a court action brought by the mother of a premature baby born in a hospital in the south-west of England in 1995. The premature baby was fed intravenously via a Hickman line, but suffered infections in the early part of 1996 when the new connectors started to be used by that particular hospital. According to nurses, doctors and the mother herself, the connectors kept cracking, and would last no longer than a day. Sometimes brittle cracking was so bad that they had to be replaced even more frequently. On one occasion, when the baby was being transferred between hospitals by ambulance, the Hickman line snapped and the assembly was retained by the mother after surgical removal (Fig. 10.6). It was to play a central role in the subsequent proceedings. Both of the green polycarbonate shrouds on the connectors exhibited brittle cracks (Fig. 10.8). In June 1996, the baby contracted meningitis while cracked connectors were still in use, and he almost died. It later was found that the little boy

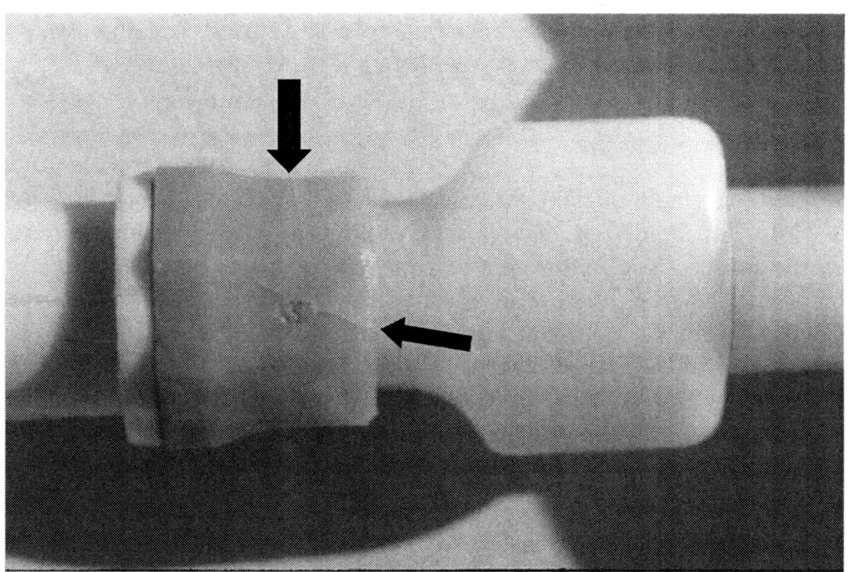

10.8 Cracked joint in coloured polycarbonate connector.

had suffered brain damage which medical experts assigned to the near fatal episode in June 1996. The mother then started proceedings in 2002, accusing the hospital of negligence in using such devices, and the manufacturer for supplying faulty products.

The surviving samples retained by the mother were examined using macrophotography, but were not subjected at that stage to the more revealing methods of optical or electron optical microscopy. The solicitor in charge of the case was very protective of the samples, and it later transpired that they were the only surviving examples of many similar failed connectors. The low magnification survey showed that brittle cracks were present at the gate of the green shroud, where molten polymer was injected during manufacture. The cracks were entirely brittle and extended over large parts of the outer shroud. No examination was made of the inner parts of the devices because that would have involved dissembly of the joint, involving extra stress on the samples.

Brittle cracks tend to occur at the gate because this is where frozen-in strain or chain orientation is greatest, making this a common problem with many polymers, and where polycarbonate is susceptible if moulded incorrectly. Early work conducted with mining products (especially miners' backpack batteries) showed that the polycarbonate battery cases cracked in a brittle fashion when exposed to organic solvents (methylene chloride and ethylene chloride) used during solvent welding of the product. It was concluded at an early stage in the investigation that the catheter connectors had been poorly moulded, although their birefringence could not be measured directly because they had been filled with pigment. Birefringence is a useful tool in examining transparent products for high levels of chain orientation, which is the root cause of the cracking problem.

10.3.3 Disclosure

Several years later, in 2006, the case advanced with the claimant asking for disclosure of the design, manufacture, testing and failure documents from the defendants. The failure reports from UK hospitals made particularly interesting reading. There were records from the first introduction of the device in 1994 of numerous and sometimes distressing complaints from many different hospitals of the problem of cracked connectors, and the then Medical Devices Agency (MDA) was asked to investigate. They passed the problem to the company who examined the reports. The first failure reports made by internal workers at the manufacturer were unimpressive:

- the reports lacked a systematic approach with only two photographs provided;
- the users were blamed for 'forcing' joints open with forceps; and
- no samples were preserved.

That broken products had indeed been sent for inspection was proved by photocopies of the letters of complaint, often with the broken device attached to the letter, and so photocopied as well. The many published reports on polycarbonate failures seemed to have been ignored, however. Because the users were blamed for the problem, no serious action was taken to either withdraw the faulty products from supply to hospitals, or to re-examine the design and manufacture of the connectors. Even when a new design using different polymer was introduced in early 1996, the older designs continued to be used by hospitals, including that where the premature baby was being treated.

10.3.4 Published reports of problems

In fact, there had been many warnings published in the technical press about the problems of using polycarbonate in luers and connectors similar to the type made in France and the subject of the investigation, and they were published before the French design was launched. Particular warnings were expressed in papers presented to the Failure Analysis Group of the (SPE) Society of Plastics Engineers at their annual ANTEC conferences. Stubstad was one of the first researchers to warn of the problems of premature cracking of polycarbonate luers in a paper at ANTEC 1992.[7] He reported that female luers were susceptible to lengthwise brittle cracking owing to the hoop stress imposed by the incoming male luer, especially if there were any dimensional differences between the two. However, the underlying problem could be cold moulding, where high chain orientation exists in the luer, thus encouraging brittle cracking.[8] Failures in clinical situations were also being reported in the medical literature, and were detailed in a review in *Neonatal Network* in 1992.[9] The method examined was extra corporeal membrane oxygenation (ECMO) where, of 445 accidents, 45% caused loss of blood and 55% involved cracked circuit components such as connectors. A specific accident involving polycarbonate was detailed in another study.[10] 'Bathing alcohol' was accidentally spilled onto a polycarbonate casing of an oxygenator, causing it to crack. The fluid was composed of 70% ethyl alcohol, 1.6% acetone and other organic fluids. The oxygenator was being used during a heart operation on an elderly man, and its malfunction was life-threatening. Many other studies of the 1990s reported cracked connectors, but failed to identify the polymer used in the devices. For example, a hub on an epidural catheter connector cracked and emergency methods were adopted.[11]

10.3.5 Joint expert examination

As the trial approached (set for May 2008), the experts engaged by each of the three parties to the action, organised a new examination of the connector remains. Optical microscopic inspection of the connectors was the first to be used; both the external shroud and the inner recesses of the two devices were examined by disassembly of the connectors. The results were dramatic because they revealed two key features which had not been seen in the original inspection:

1. many surfaces were contaminated by stains and particles, and
2. brittle cracks extended to the inner recess.

The traces of yellow stains over much of the exterior and some of the inner parts of both connectors implied that they originated during their period of use (Fig. 10.9). They were probably urine stains from the baby because the connectors would have been in close proximity to his body, probably lying on his skin. The particles trapped in the sharp facets at the remnant of the gate were probably traces of faeces and coagulated blood. The fracture surfaces of the cracks were also contaminated both with the yellow stain and by particulate matter, so that contamination and crack formation were probably contemporaneous.

Contamination extended to the inner recess of the connector attached to the red end of the Hickman line when the joint had been separated. More importantly, the tip of the male luer exhibited a brittle crack very close to the part of the device where the inner steel pipe ended (Fig. 10.10). This observation was unexpected because it had not been seen before (the joint was only dissembled once and the tip was not examined) but it showed that

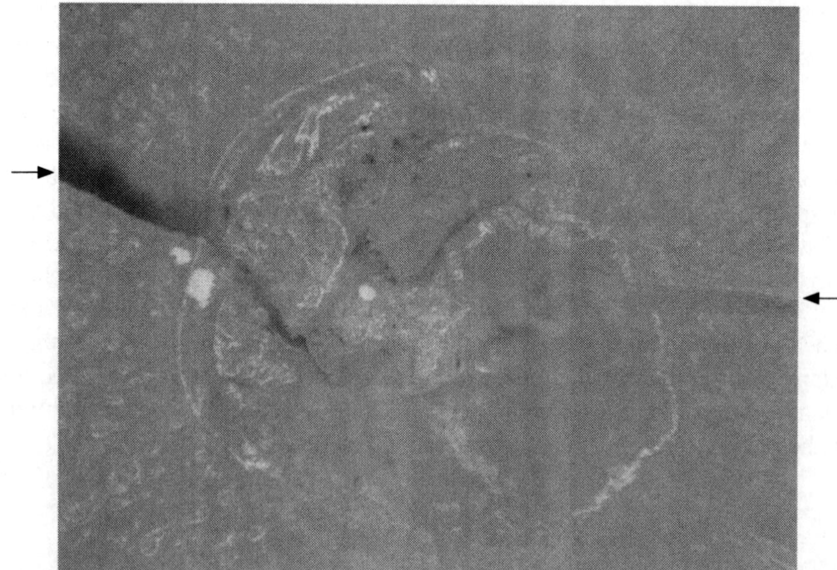

10.9 Optical micrograph of gate showing cracks and contamination.

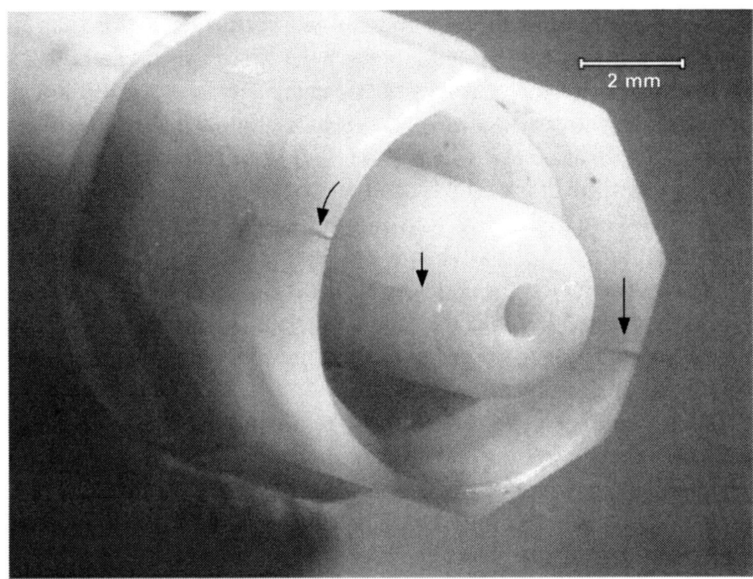

10.10 Connector end showing extensive cracking and contamination.

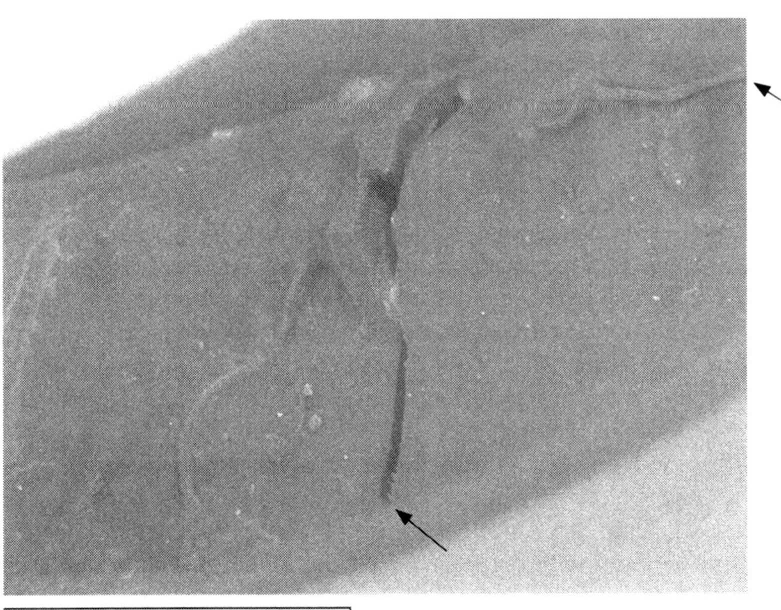

10.11 ESEM of inner crack in connector.

brittle cracking was much more extensive than had been appreciated. That conclusion was reinforced by the observation of brittle cracks in the base of the recess (Fig. 10.11). Clearly, the external cracks had penetrated the body of the connector and allowed contamination to enter the recess. The second male luer showed little contamination but there was a crack near the tip.

The quality of the seal was tested using air pressure and a test in water appeared to show no leaks of air (a test familiar to cyclists for a leaking inner tube). However, it was not at all clear whether such a test would have shown a hairline crack which had penetrated through to the bore of the tube at the tip owing to the slow rate of air movement through such a small crack (also familiar to cyclists when a tiny hole exists in the tube: a well known cause of slow punctures and very difficult to detect by the water test). If the cracks had extended into the side of the tip then there would have been a path for pathogens to enter the bore of the tube where contamination of the TPN feed or drug line was possible.

The three experts followed up by re-examining the same samples using environmental scanning electron microscopy (ESEM) shortly afterwards. The results confirmed the existence of large cracks at the base of the recess of the male luer (Fig. 10.11). The crack in the base was about 20 μm wide, and it was, therefore, easy for 0.2 μm diameter bacteria to penetrate. Although the experts did not find a crack at the tip of the male luer, the top of the steel inner pipe appeared misplaced in the polycarbonate moulding. No X-ray analysis was carried out at the time which might have revealed the nature of the contamination that was clearly seen by both optical and electron microscopy.

10.3.6 Injection moulding

Consideration of the bundles of documents disclosed by the manufacturer produced some moulding records, but they were not contemporary with the first design of the connector, and in fact dated to several years later when the company returned to use polycarbonate after using polyester. Those records showed that a tool temperature of 80 °C was being used, a temperature within allowable limits (according to technical brochures from the manufacturers, and our experience of the problem).

No further moulding details were forthcoming despite repeated requests, and it was said by the defendants that 'such moulding details would be recorded on "a scrap of paper"'. Even in the early 1990s, most injection moulding machines were fully computerised, and all setting conditions (such as melt pressures and temperatures and tool temperatures) were recorded automatically. The reason why it is important to record such details is very simple: when it comes to repeating a batch run, it is essential to use the setting conditions already established for that product.

It was thus likely that the original design had been cold moulded, producing high levels of chain orientation in the polycarbonate parts of the device.

10.3.7 Environmental stress cracking (ESC) or stress corrosion cracking (SCC)

Environmental stress cracking (ESC) or stress corrosion cracking (SCC) seemed the most likely cause of the brittle cracks seen in the retained samples, but no records had been kept by the hospital of what fluids the connectors had made contact during service. Polycarbonate is sensitive not just only to solvent cracking, such as those seen on battery cases, but to a range of other common liquids that are likely to be found in hospitals, as previous studies had shown.

It was very unlikely that the connectors came into contact with methylene chloride or ethylene chloride, but much more likely that cleaning fluids used on wards may have made contact. Such liquids as bleach (sodium hypochlorite) and strong detergents are used for disinfection, and contact with them could initiate brittle cracks. They do so by an SCC rather than ESC mechanism because the alkaline solution hydrolyses polycarbonate by attacking the carbonate group in the repeat unit. Indeed, methanolic KOH or NaOH degrade the material extremely rapidly back to monomer, a method for destructive removal of the polymer.[12] Other organic fluids, including acetone, organic alcohols and ethers, can act as ESC agents.[13–15]

However, it was known that TPN itself can attack polycarbonate, knowledge which was publicised before 1994/5 particularly in US studies,[7] and, therefore, the company should have been very wary of introducing the connectors without extensive testing in TPN. Stubstad, for example, in his 1992 study[8] had referred to the problem of cracking in "fat solutions", which includes TPN. Other liquids containing lipids and used for carrying drugs were also a problem, judging by the failure reports from UK hospitals in 1994/5. However, it was difficult to explain how a fluid in the bore could have caused such extensive external cracking in the retained connectors unless leakage had occurred elsewhere in the system. Unfortunately, the manufacturer had disposed of all failed connectors which had been sent back for inspection by many hospitals (and the MDA), so that there was no prospect of a more complete analysis of the problem.

It was also of some interest to observe from the numerous hospital failure reports that cracking was usually detected by nurses seeing fluid leaking from the devices, so in many cases of reported failures, cracking must have linked the bore with the external world. Even the external cracks visible on the retained connectors were not spotted either by the baby's mother or the solicitor dealing with the case when the action was first started, such is the small size of the device, and the difficulty of observing small hairline or even partly open cracks (Fig. 10.6).

Given the published failure reports, a survey of the Federal Food and Drugs Administration (FDA) website at www.fda.gov showed a number of reported failures of luer connectors made on the 'Maude' compilation. (The Medicines and Healthcare products Regulatory Agency (MHRA) also has a similar anonymous reporting database on their website at www.mhra.gov.uk.) The records (made anonymously by medical staff) showed failures of IV sets in 1991, many involving fracture or detachment of luers. Several reports mentioned failure of the French design although the records did not provide the detail needed to pinpoint the exact cause of fracture. FDA enforcement notices also showed that a number of recalls were made in the same period. The French company issued a recall of 60 000 infant feeding systems in France in 1994 because the 'end cap may become loose'. A larger recall of 60 million was made by another company in the same year owing to cracks produced by certain solutions in the female luer. Two further recalls were made in 1996 and 1998, the first being a recall of the subsidiary of the French company of 3068 neonatal catheters owing to cracking in the female luer lock, and a smaller similar recall made in 1998. Thus, recalls could be adopted by the manufacturer in question, although none appeared to have taken place in the UK.

10.3.8 Discussion

It was most likely that the brittle cracks seen on many connectors, and in some examples quoted by hospitals, leading to total disintegration, were caused either by ESC or by SCC, or by a combination of both failure modes. Although the cracks on the retained connectors had not apparently reached a critical state, they were very close to penetrating the inner bore of the feed tube (Fig. 10.10). They supported the mother's contention that connectors were cracking on a daily basis, needing regular replacement before they in turn had to be replaced.

The experts for the defendants resisted these conclusions, however. An important point which arose in discussions related to the ISO standard, which advised that the materials of construction of such devices should resist all fluids with which it could make contact within a hospital environment. The net result of several expert meetings produced a much more reasonable document just before trial, allowing the lawyers to proceed to a fair settlement without the need for what would have been a very expensive trial. There were up to 30 experts on all sides in the action, most of whom were medical experts rather than scientists or engineers. Substantial damages were paid to the mother of the disabled child.

10.4 Security cap for gas cylinders

There have been many innovative ways in which polymers have been used to create new designs fulfilling unexpected functions, such as the development of security guards for gas cylinders used in hospitals. The product was designed to be fitted around the tops of gas cylinders to protect the valve as well as show the user what gas was present in the cylinder by colour coding the plastic (Fig. 10.12).

A problem was discovered in 1988 by the manufacturer, an injection moulder in Leicester, who found that caps were cracking before ever being used on gas cylinders, even in storage at the moulders. The devices were made in talc-filled polypropylene in four colours and made with two flaps which are brought together in a secure joint around the top valve of the cylinder. The flaps are hinged at two points to allow rotation of the flaps (Fig. 10.12). The non-return parts of the joint can be seen at left in the figure. The cap is removed at the hospital by applying a hexagonal spanner to the front of the fitted device. Although disposed of after removal from a cylinder, the unattached caps must be able to resist dropping and handling loads before fitment.

10.4.1 Failures in storage

However, whole batches were found to be failing at the critical hinges when held in storage, and had to be returned to the moulders for scrapping. Indeed, the warehouse at the factory was full of rejected products, a sight

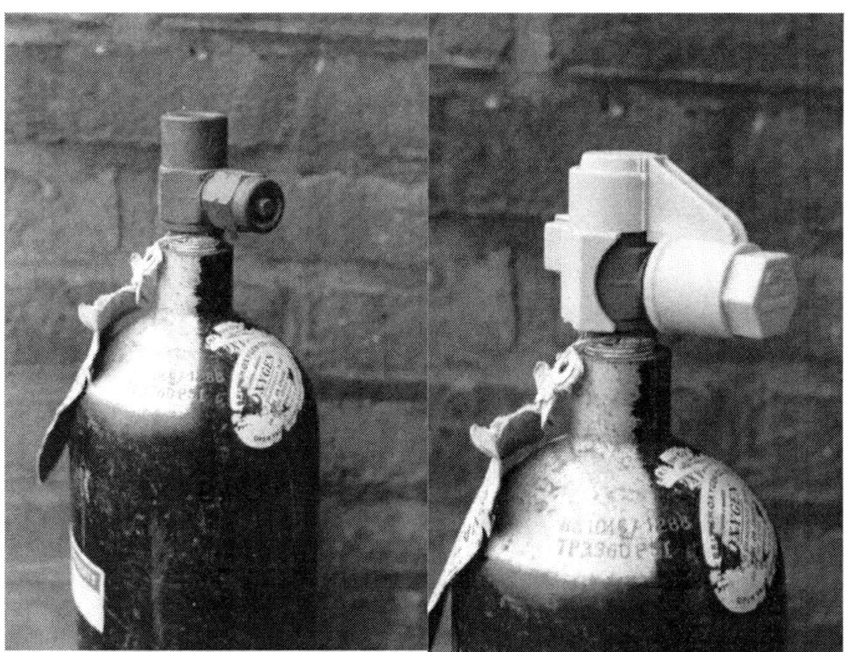

10.12 Safety guard for oxygen cylinder.

which horrified the moulders and led to a panic phone call to help resolve the crisis. A considerable amount of production had been lost by the time of consultation.

There were several possible causes, poor material being the one favoured by the moulders, perhaps not unsurprisingly, given the natural tendency to blame others before oneself. Samples of material were thus cut from a selection of good and failed mouldings to test the theory using Fourier transform infra-red (FTIR) spectroscopy and differential scanning calorimetry (DSC). However, no anomalies could be found at all using the methods, so poor material by degradation for example, could be excluded. The spectroscopy showed a polypropylene with a high ethylene content of about 10%, making the material both tough and very flexible. Attention turned to the way they were moulded, because this was now the likely source of the problem.

The device was moulded via no less than four gates: one at the centre of the hub of the cap (Fig. 10.13 shows the sprue remnant of this gate), two on each of the side flaps and one at the centre of the device diametrically opposite the first gate, as shown by the arrows in the photograph. There were a number of irregularities in the moulding parameters, especially the barrel temperatures of the moulding machine. The setting sheet used to determine the moulding conditions showed the temperature sequence along the barrel of the machine as 211, 212 and 219 °C, whereas the thermostat set temperatures were 236, 243 and 263 °C. These large discrepancies could change the product in unexpected ways since the temperatures were much higher than those originally specified.

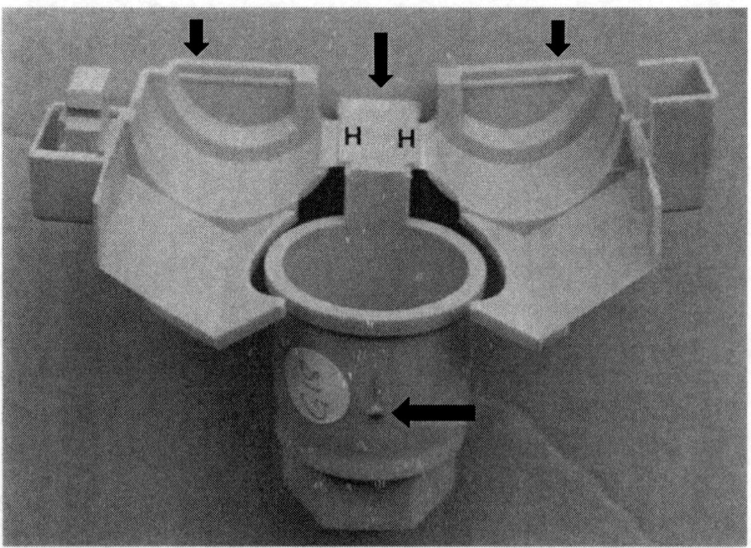

10.13 Security cap before fitment showing hinges (HH) and gates (arrows).

10.4.2 Inspection for defects

A large number of new devices were then examined for any defects, and were also tested by fitting on a cylinder head. A key observation came very quickly: the weakest parts were the hinges about which the flaps rotated to lock the device in place. They consisted of plastic only 0.5 mm thick and running the length of 20 mm along each side of the flaps at the base of the hub (Fig. 10.14). The two lengths of polymer had to be strong enough to resist handling and bending to form the hinge, but yet weak enough to give way when the cylinder was needed. It was noticed that many samples which failed prematurely exhibited weld lines at or on the hinge, the weld lines having formed by impingement of the three streams of molten polymer entering opposite the hub of the device. Failed samples invariably possessed such weld lines in the hinge rather than in the bulk polymer (Fig. 10.14) and those weld lines varied erratically from sample to sample.

Of sixteen samples tested, only five survived fitment to the oxygen cylinder (Fig. 10.12). The remainder showed splits or cracks in the hinges. A quantitative test was needed to test the strength of the guards, and close attention to moulding conditions was required.

10.4.3 Development of torque test

A simple objective test was required to mimic the needs of the end user and yet be easily applied in the factory. To develop the test, a mole wrench and

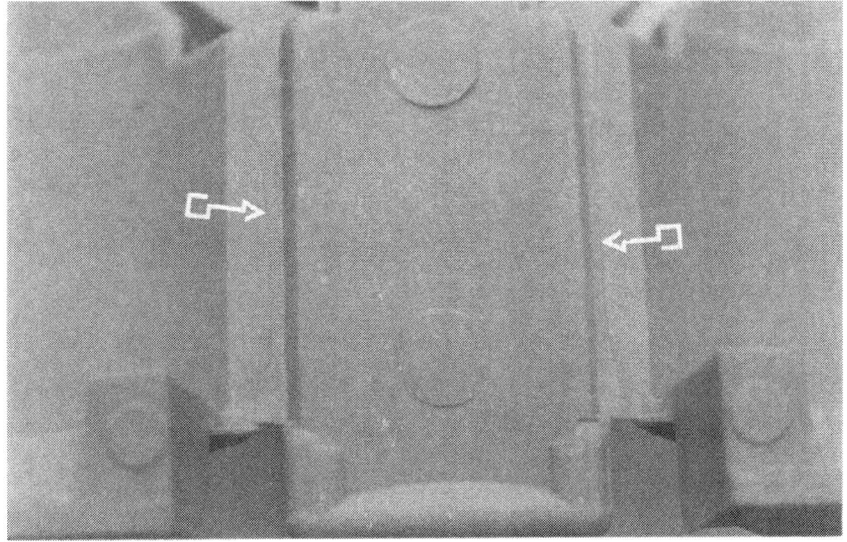

10.14 Weld lines in thin polymer hinges of cap guard (arrows).

spring balance were used under standard conditions to measure the torque strength of the fitted caps. The caps which showed hinge cracks or weld lines gave very low failure torques, ranging from 0 to a maximum of 8.3 N m, but the average result was only about 4 N m. By contrast the five intact caps gave an average of 8 N m with a maximum value of 19 N m (although these failed in the case rather than the hinge). There was a linear relation between the length of weld line in the hinges and their torque strength, confirming that weld lines were indeed the cause of the problem of premature failure.

Such a spread of results was quite unacceptable for the customer, who needed a reliable guard cap which would fail only when a spanner was used on the device. Moreover, the failure torque needed to be relatively high to necessitate use of a spanner. Ergonomic studies (Fig. 10.15) showed that when the hand gripped cylinders of various surface textures and diameter, there was a maximum torque that the hand could exert. The maximum was lower for women, and the obvious choice was that for males because it was greater.[16,17] Using the results shown in Fig. 10.15 and the diameter of the hub as 35 mm, then the maximum torque that can be exerted is about 0.8 kgf m or 8 N m for a knurled steel cylinder. Moulding conditions should be varied first, to move the weld lines away from the hinge, and second to give the hinges a torque strength of at least 8 N m. This would mean that the hub could not be removed by hand action, requiring a spanner to twist the guard free.

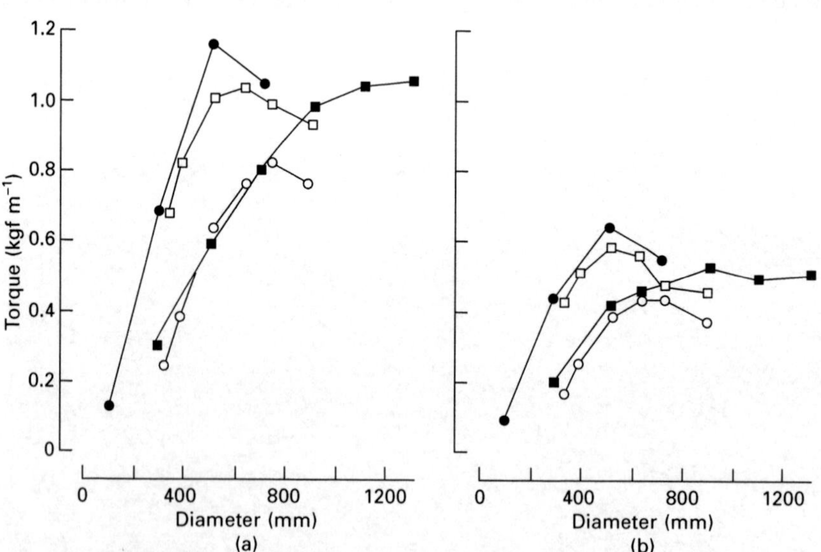

10.15 Torque as a function of handle diameter: (a) men; (b) women; ● knurled steel cylinders; ■ knurled discs; □ polished wooden cylinders; ○ polished wooden spheres.

10.4.4 Aftermath

Returning to the factory with the recommendation that moulding be stopped to reset the moulding machines, did indeed save the situation. The change in conditions moved the weld lines away from the hinges, and samples were again taken for testing. The strength of the new samples averaged 12 N m and was much more consistent. Far from being a material problem, the moulders should have taken greater care in monitoring their moulding conditions, and inspecting their products to eliminate the damaging weld lines. A systematic approach to troubleshooting the problem revealed the cause of the premature failures, led directly to remedial measures and a solution to a problem which had caused a great deal of concern as well as loss of production. Such action would strengthen the guards to such an extent that they would survive harsh handling during transport and any casual vandalism, so as to reassure the final user, the hospital technician, that the cylinder contents remained intact and tamper-free.

10.5 Breathing tube failures

The medical appliances market has developed greatly in recent years with the demand for ever better patient care both in hospital for acute cases, and at home for patients with chronic ailments. Respiratory illnesses are among the most common such ailments, and often require breathing apparatus for supplying the patient with humidified air or oxygen in a controllable way. The breathing equipment for such applications must be made to a very high standard, so that bacterial contamination of the bore is impossible. The case reported here concerns the quality of a large transparent sight tube developed for use in breathing apparatus, the material being injection moulded polysulfone.

The alleged defects related to the quality of finish of the tubes, rather than any structural or functional problems in use. The manufacturer of the breathing apparatus brought an action against the toolmaker, alleging that the tool for making the tubes was incapable of moulding sight tubes in polysulfone.

10.5.1 Development of sight tube

The breathing equipment was already in existence when the decision was made to develop a moulded sight tube. The tube sat at the top of a longer metal pipe, and enclosed a float giving visual indication of flow rate in the tube (Fig. 10.16). The float must not fall below the lower marker so as to ensure air or oxygen is being sent to the patient. The transparent tube was machined from acrylic resin (high molecular weight PMMA) to a high quality,

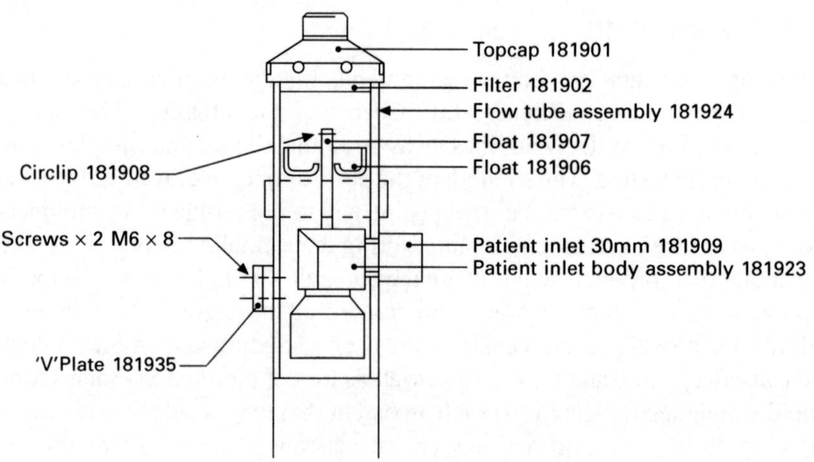

10.16 Section of breathing tube showing float assembly.

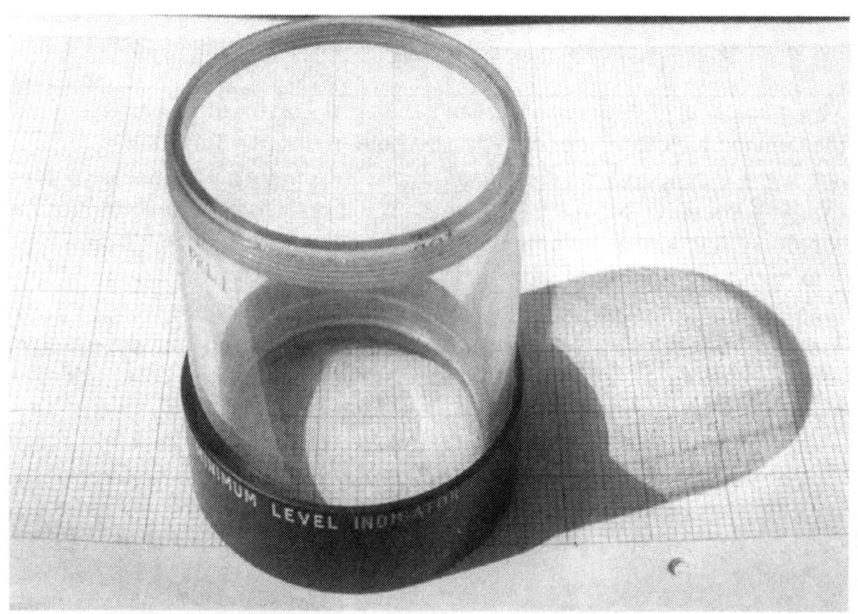

10.17 Original PMMA sight tube with regular wall (as shown by shadow).

but at correspondingly high cost (Fig. 10.17). Not only was the process very labour intensive (and thus expensive), but also required two parts being attached together. Injection moulding would offer economies of scale and parts consolidation, a common design objective when improving products.

A tool was commissioned and the first prototypes in acrylic proved encouraging (Fig. 10.18), although many moulding defects were present, such

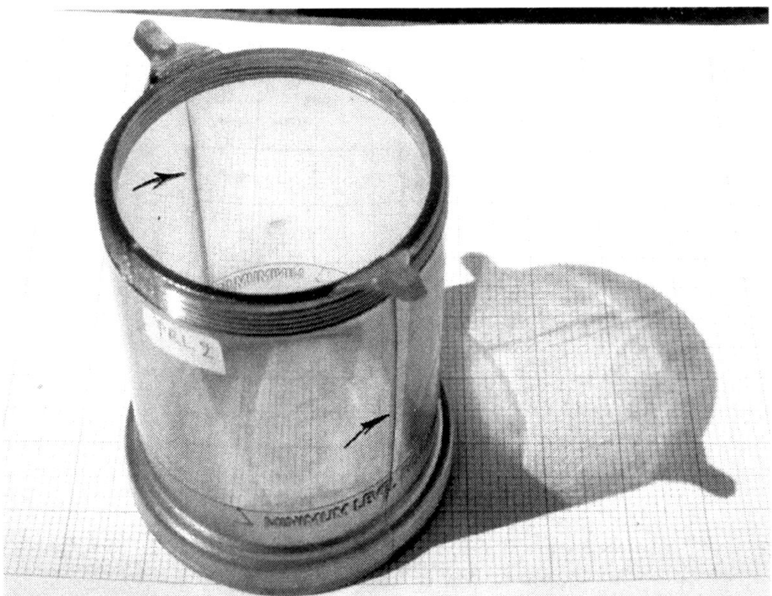

10.18 Prototype moulded sight tube in acrylic showing severe weld lines and flow marks (in shadow).

as severe weld lines (the vertical lines either side of the tube). The decision was made to use Udel polysulfone (made by Union Carbide), a strange decision given the high cost, and difficult moulding problems presented by this polymer. Apparently, it was felt that alternative transparent plastics such as polycarbonate (and acrylic itself) were too susceptible to ESC by attack from common fluids used regularly in hospitals, such as ether and alcohol. The manufacturer clearly envisaged high sales to justify the considerable capital investment needed for an injection moulding tool. Having commissioned the tool, several moulders were then engaged to manufacture the tubes.

10.5.2 Faulty tubes

Because the critical proof of the quality of a tool is in the moulding, the set of about 40 faulty sight tubes held by the plaintiff was central to the dispute. The tubes had been moulded by three different moulders. The tubes were examined for the defects alleged by the plaintiff, with very mixed results. It was clear that the moulders used by the plaintiff had experienced severe problems in moulding polysulfone, largely because of its high melt viscosity and Newtonian behaviour with increasing shear rate in the tool.[18]

Most common thermoplastics exhibit shear thinning, which means that the melt viscosity drops substantially in the runners of the tool, and thus makes moulding to shape much easier (Fig. 10.19). Thus, LDPE and polystyrene

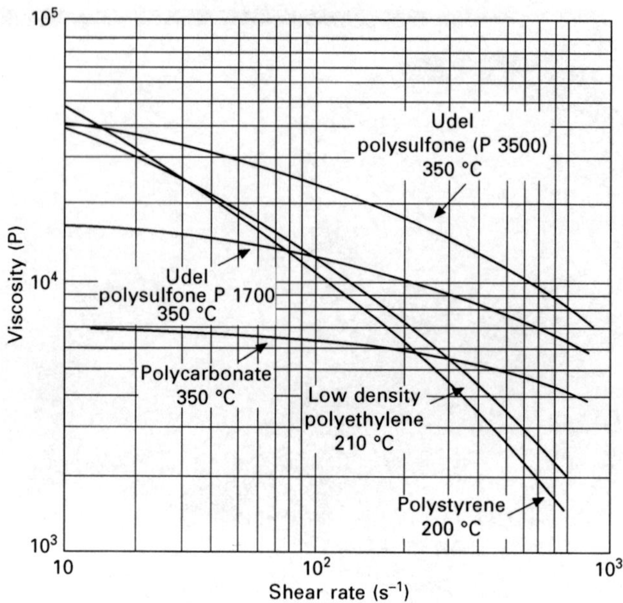

10.19 Melt viscosity of polysulfone and other polymers as a function of shear rate at various temperatures.

are usually much easier to mould than polycarbonate or polysulfone because their melt viscosity drops rapidly as the shear rate increases in the narrow runners into the tool cavity. In addition, the tools must be held at high temperature to minimise frozen-in strain in the final product. Accurate temperature control is needed because the melt viscosity is more sensitive to change in temperature than other polymers. The raw granules must be dried before moulding to eliminate surface defects such as splay or splash marks.

Such manufacturing constraints had not been considered by at least one of the moulders, who had needed to buy an oil circulation system to heat the tool so as to mould the polysulfone. Of the many defects seen in the 40 or so sample tubes, most if not all were moulding defects caused by poor material preparation, and cold tools, showing inexperience in moulding this material. Figure 10.20 for example, shows flow lines in the barrel of the tube caused by poor temperature control, the flow lines being visualised by their effect on the shadow cast on graph paper. The tube shown in Fig. 10.21 displays splash marks caused by inadequate drying of the granules, an effect usually appearing on exposed surfaces, and clearly unacceptable for a sight tube where optical clarity was essential. Sink marks in the barrel were relatively common owing to low pressures in the tool. Inclusions were seen in some samples (Fig. 10.22). Discolouration was also present in some

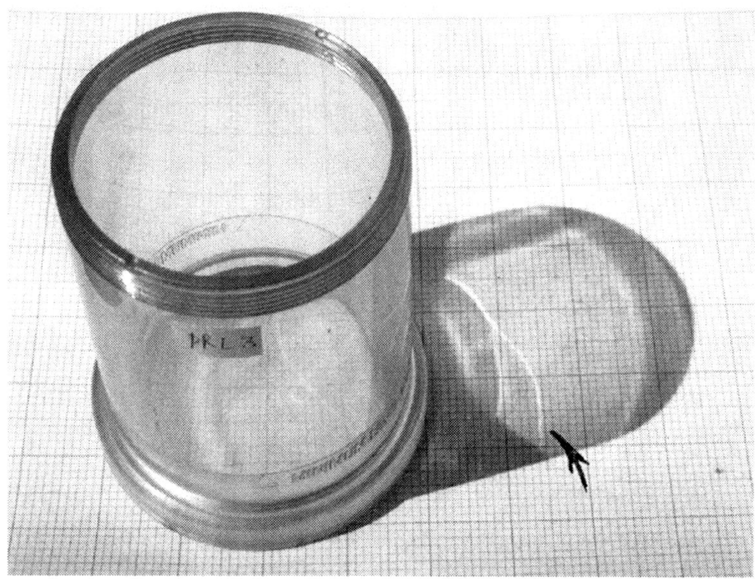

10.20 Flow lines in polysulfone moulding shown by shadow (arrow).

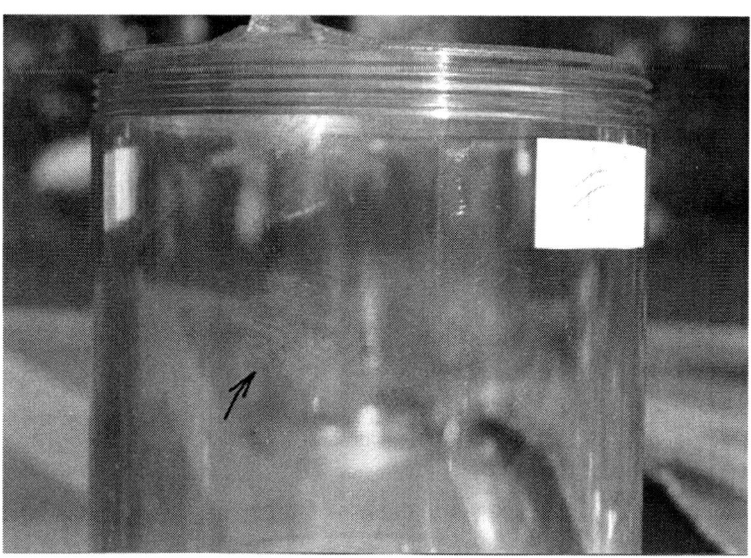

10.21 Flash marks caused by wet polymer granules (arrow).

samples (Fig. 10.23), showing a range of temperatures at which the melt and tool had been held.

Detailed inspection of the available tubes showed that all defects were attributable to moulding problems and could not be blamed on the tool.

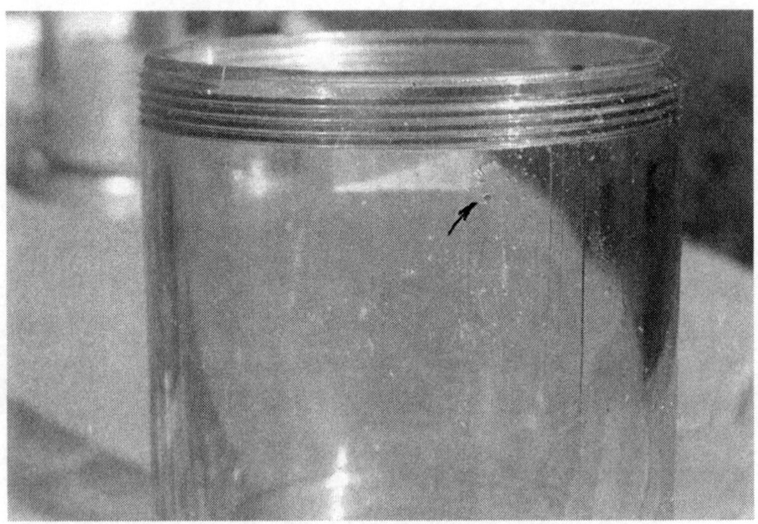

10.22 Inclusions in polysulfone tube moulding (arrow).

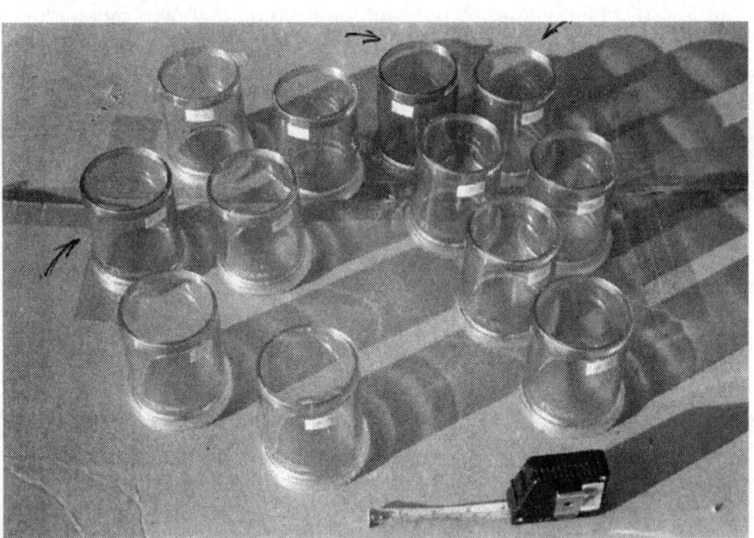

10.23 Colour variation in set of mouldings, darkest arrowed at top and left.

Furthermore, several samples showed score marks caused by the operator levering the moulding from the cavity. However, despite the overwhelming evidence of poor moulding practice, the plaintiff decided to proceed with the case. A meeting between the two opposing experts in the case failed to resolve any of the contentious issues concerning injection moulding.

10.5.3 Trial

The dispute came to trial in London in the mid-1990s. But the trial itself was to yield yet further revelations and some surpises. In the first place, the lawyer for the claimant had been briefed only at the last minute and had a poor grasp of the case essentials, so the opening speech had to be made by the defendant's barrister! Then it was the claimant's role to enter the witness stand and be questioned. The defendant's barrister was very well equipped to cross-examine and, as is usual in such trials, much depended on the documentary evidence that had accumulated over the several years during which the dispute had been ongoing.

There were reports from the moulders describing the problems of using the tool with polysulfone, but the judge noticed that the last sentence of the last page of one report appeared to be ungrammatical. One possible explanation (offered by the judge) could be that the report had been doctored by photocopying with part of the report deliberately obscured by plain paper, so that it would not be copied. Such manipulation of evidence could be taken as contempt of court, a serious charge if proven, and subject to severe penalties.

The judge ordered that the original be produced in open court. It was never produced because the case took yet another dramatic turn. It was clear from cross-examination on the stand that the claimant could not remember key features of the details of the dispute, and when he returned for further cross-examination on the third day of the trial, he broke down and accepted an offer from the defendant to settle the case. The defendant withdrew his counterclaim in return for the claimant withdrawing his claim. But there was a sting in the tail of the case: the plaintiff had to pay most of the costs of litigation, including the large costs accrued before the trial, bringing the case to trial and the two days of the trial itself. The total costs were in fact much greater than the original sum in dispute. So none of the voluminous technical evidence was ever heard in open court, although the judge had clearly read the salient reports in the action and, indeed, made many pertinent comments during the hearing.

10.5.4 Lessons learned

It was never clear why the manufacturer specified polysulfone for the sight tube. Although injection moulding would have lowered unit costs in the long term, it was still a risky venture and depended on achieving high sales of the apparatus. To specify polysulfone was even riskier, because the several injection moulders chosen were inexperienced in moulding the material. The tool was sufficient to mould the material, but the quality of the end product was mainly in the hands of the moulders and not the toolmaker. It was not a complicated product, having a simple shape. The only element of complexity lay in the screw threads at either end of the tube (requiring a rotating core), but this was not an insuperable problem in moulding. The polysulfone chosen was very expensive and also costly to injection mould correctly, especially by moulders with little or no prior experience of moulding the material.

10.6 A failed crutch

An elderly woman (Mrs S) suffered serious injury when one of the pair of crutches she was using to support herself suddenly broke at the junction of the aluminum handle and the main shaft. The woman was recovering from an operation to remove the lower part of one of her legs, and she fell onto her stump as she was moving through a doorway. The fall was severe and traumatic, especially so for a patient in convalescence. Each crutch (Fig. 10.24) consisted of an aluminum tube into which was fitted an aluminum telescopic leg, the telescopic action being utilised for height adjustment to suit the individual user's needs.[18] The top of the crutch was fitted with an arm rest, designed to rotate about a riveted hinge (Fig. 10.25). The hinge was mounted in a polypropylene plastic insert which fitted the top of the aluminium

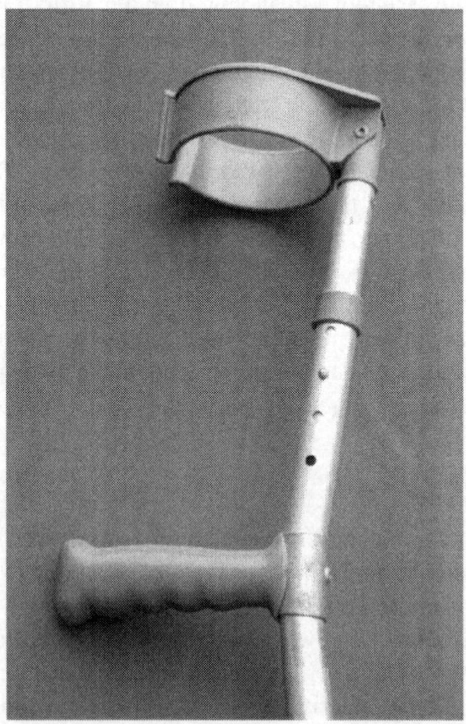

10.24 Adjustable crutch with handhold and arm support.

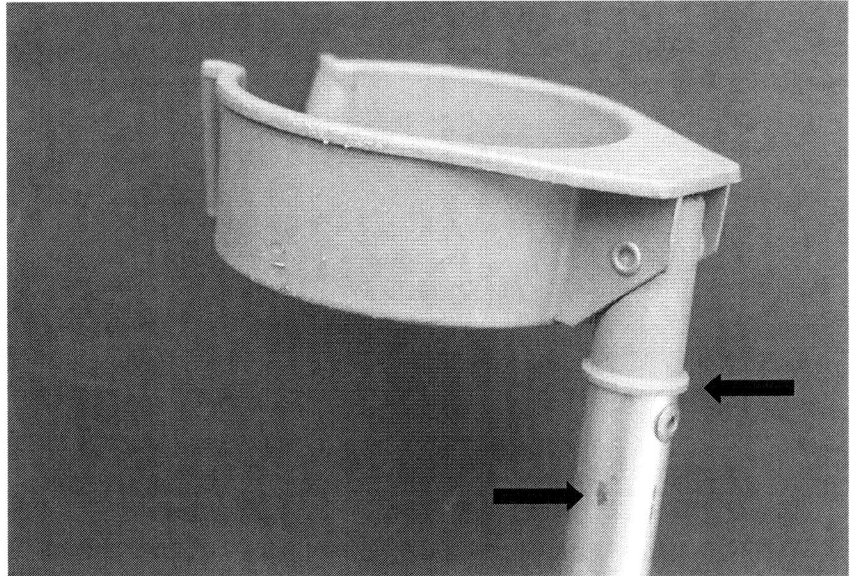

10.25 Intact arm rest showing rivets and wear mark (lower arrow). The device broke at the junction of the metal tube and plastic insert (right arrow).

leg, and penetrated the tube for some distance. The insert was designed with an outer lip or rim so as to rest against the top of the metal tube. Owing to its irregular shape, the insert had clearly been injection moulded.

10.6.1 Brittle fracture

The crutch in question had fractured near the junction of the two tubes, inside the plastic insert (Fig. 10.25) that connected them. The fracture surface itself was not very revealing, but did show completely brittle behaviour (Fig. 10.26), unusual behaviour for what is normally a highly ductile polymer. There were traces of jumps in the crack as it grew around the periphery of the circular insert. The origin probably lay on the outer side of the insert where the tensile stress would have been greatest when the crutch was used. The user's arm naturally exerts a load against the back of the arm rest, and thus caused the plastic insert to bend, with stress concentrated at the outer side opposite the lower rivet. The inner corner of the moulding resting against the top of the tube exhibited a sharp corner which also exacerbated the stress there, making that zone the weakest part of the design. Examination of the interior of the polymer tube under magnification revealed several subcritical cracks or crazes close to the edge of the fracture surface. The service loading had clearly exceeded the tensile strength of the plastic.

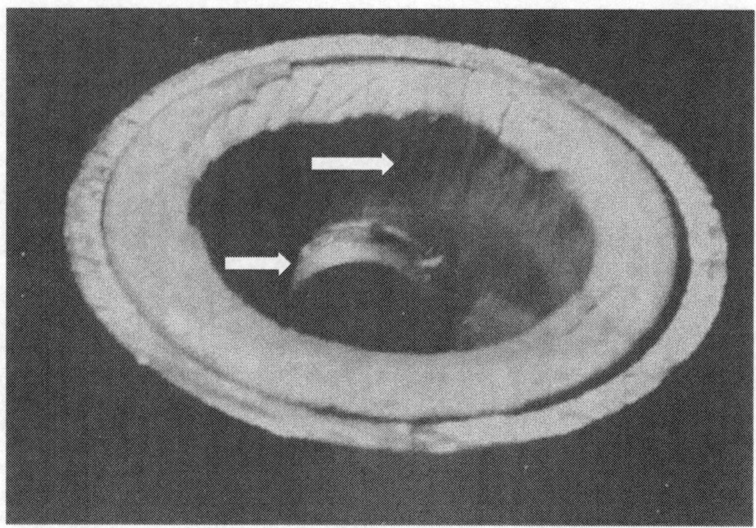

10.26 Brittle fracture surface of failed crutch showing rivet and flutes on inner surface.

Moreover, there were signs of defects on the plastic inside the metal tube, at a point below the subcritical cracks. They comprised a series of flutes (Fig. 10.26) and a curious wavy line on the inner surface (Fig. 10.27). This combination of features observed on the plastic insert indicated material degradation, because this part should have had a smooth blemish-free surface. Being an injection moulding, the surface had been in contact with the steel core. If the polymer had flowed, then the viscosity must have dropped to allow the material to flow when the product was removed from the tool, showing that the molecular weight was too low.

10.6.2 Wear pattern

The pair of crutches showed superficial scratches together with several zones of heavier wear. Those zones were identified as representing contact between the metal tubes at the head of the crutch (Figs 10.25 and 10.28). The wear pattern on the aluminum tube showed that the failed crutch had been used much more heavily, judging by the area affected, and it was consistent with the greater support needed for the user's amputated leg. The loads on the failed crutch would have been greater than those on the intact crutch, simply because the user had placed more of her weight there. This meant that the loads on the critical plastic insert were considerably greater than its equivalent on the intact crutch. But what mechanism had caused the polymer to become brittle and why had the viscosity of the polymer fallen so drastically?

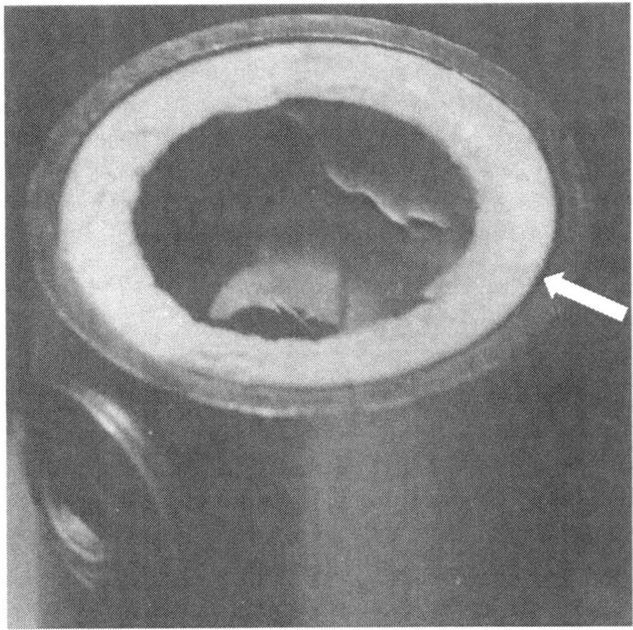

10.27 Broken crutch with external view of rivet showing misfit.

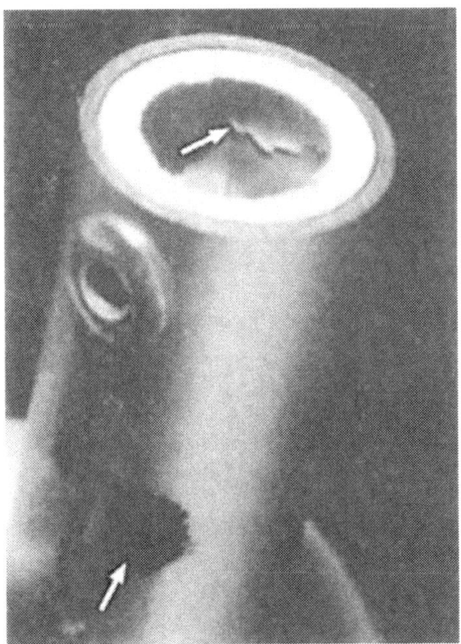

10.28 View of the top of the broken crutch showing large wear zone where the pin of the adjustment device had rubbed against the surface of the tube. The upper arrow shows the inner defect on the plastic moulding.

10.6.3 Infra-red spectroscopy

A thin film was made by scraping off the outer surface of the polymer insert and dissolving it in decalin solvent to create a thin (30 μm thick) film. The IR spectrum recorded on the thin film showed the polymer to be a polypropylene copolymer with ethylene, but it also showed an anomalous peak at 1735.7 cm^{-1} (Fig. 10.29). This is the characteristic position of the carbonyl group (C=O) produced by premature oxidation of the polymer:

$$-[CH_2–CH \cdot CH_3]- + O_2 \rightarrow -[CO -CH \cdot CH_3]- + H_2O$$

Further oxidation occurs at carbonyl group, eventually splitting the chain:

$$-[CO–CH \cdot CH_3]- + O_2 \rightarrow -CO_2H + HOCH \cdot CH_3-$$

The extent of oxidation was judged by comparing the height of the carbonyl peak with that from a standard sample, and it indicated a very high level of degradation, so explaining the deterioration in the tensile strength of the insert.

10.6.4 Conclusions

The cause of the premature fracture which injured Mrs S lay in a defective plastic insert at the arm rest of the crutch. The polymer used, polypropylene-

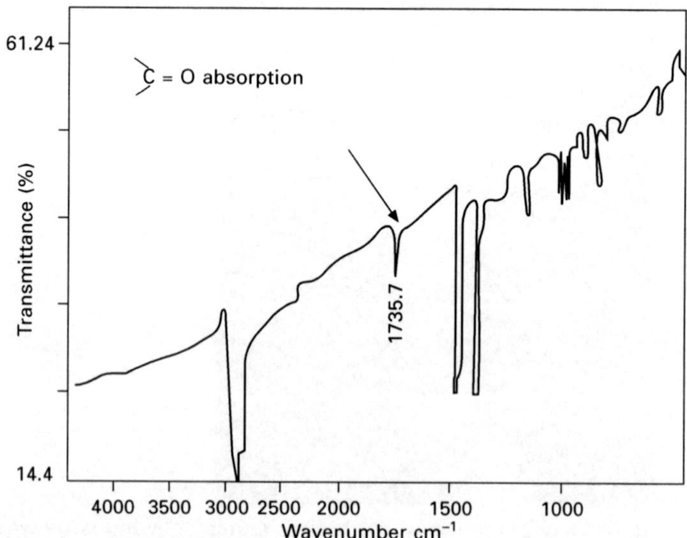

10.29 Infra-red spectrum of polypropylene from crutch insert showing oxidation peak.

co-ethylene, had degraded through oxidation during moulding, leading to chain breakage and a fall in tensile strength. There was no trace of fatigue striations in the fracture, so the crutch had failed suddenly by overload. The polymer degradation could have been brought about by recycling of polymer in the factory, each addition increasing the degraded content of material. Polypropylene is especially susceptible to oxidation and, unless protected (by an antioxidant, for example), it oxidises at the high temperatures used during injection moulding. Degraded polymer builds up continuously through moulding, weakening the resultant product. The problem should have been detected at an early stage in quality control, but evaded the normally strict controls operated by responsible moulders. The stringent demands of the relevant product standard BS 4988:1990 had not been observed, and resulted in injury to the user.[20] Mrs S received compensation for the trauma and injury after the manufacturer accepted the findings of our investigation.

The design of the crutch has proved very successful since inception, and many variants are currently available, but this should not detract from the fact that its structural integrity is paramount. As a safety-critical product, extra vigilance is needed to ensure that all component parts are made to the highest standards. It is not known whether other similar failures of the polymer inset occurred, but it is worth noting that failures of the metal leg have been reported by the MHRA in an alert issued in 2005.[21] Five similar leg failures were mentioned in the alert, and although serious injury did not occur, the alert asked that health managers be aware of the possible problem. All crutches in the affected batch were recalled by the manufacturer. The rivet holding the handle to the shaft was found to be loose in some crutches, leading to another alert in 2009.[22]

10.7 Cracked medical tubing

A problem was encountered when investigating cracking found in operating theatre gas tubing. The tubing had cracked radially where bending had occurred in the 10 mm diameter rubber tubing (Fig. 10.30). The tubing was composed of a natural rubber vulcanisate and the operating theatre had just been built. The technician who supplied the sample was puzzled by the problem because there appeared to be no obvious cause. However, the cracking was a visible manifestation of a long-known problem with many elastomeric components. A similar problem was found soon after in an acrylonitrile–butadiene rubber (NBR) fuel pipe brought in by insurers from a new car which had been destroyed in a fire (Fig. 10.31). In both cases, the cause of the cracking was attack by low levels of a powerful oxidising agent, ozone gas. Analysis of the cracking showed the extent and severity of the problem in the fuel pipe sample.

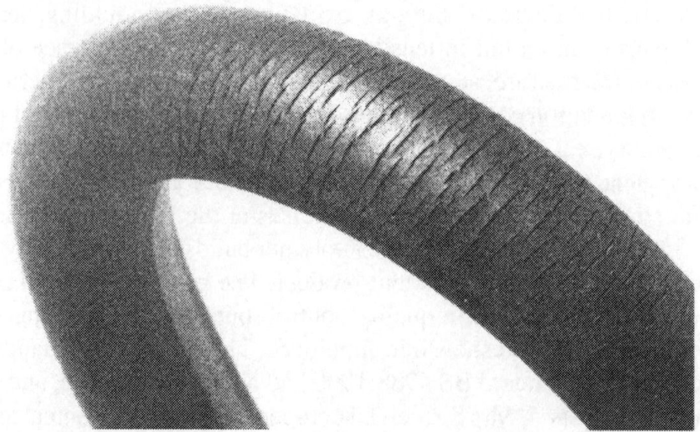

10.30 Radial ozone cracks in anaesthetic gas tubing.

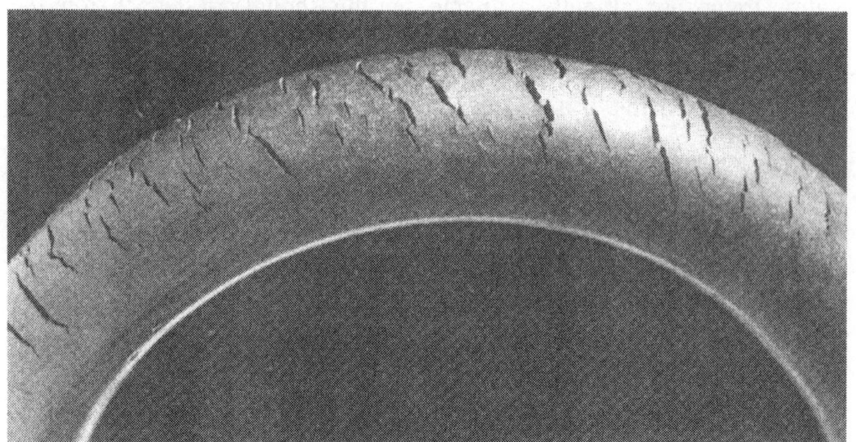

10.31 Ozone cracks at bend in fuel pipe.

10.7.1 Fuel pipe problem

The fuel pipe sample exhibited deep ozone cracks oriented at right angles to its length, in such a way as to suggest that the cracks had formed when the tube was bent to a low radius (as one might expect when in place in the engine compartment). The form of such cracks is shown schematically in Fig. 10.32. The main cracks were measured using a depth gauge (a stiff wire) and analysed, the distributions for crack depth and length, respectively, being shown in Figs 10.33 and 10.34. The worst cracks were about 2.5 mm deep, compared with tube dimensions ID of 5 mm and OD of 16 mm with a wall thickness of 4.5 mm. The worst cracks were thus over half way through the wall.

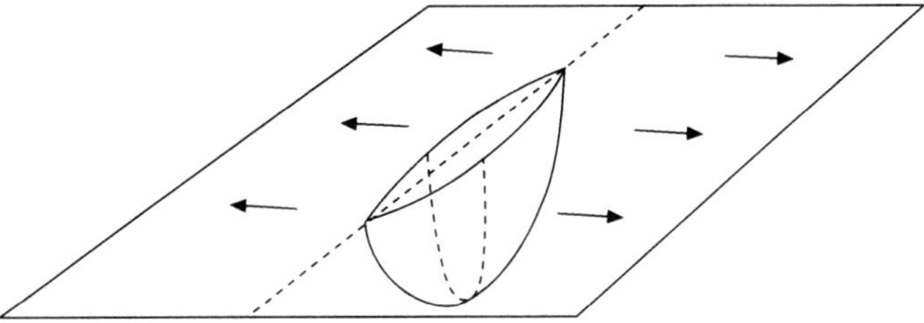

10.32 Single ozone crack oriented at right angles to tensile stress.

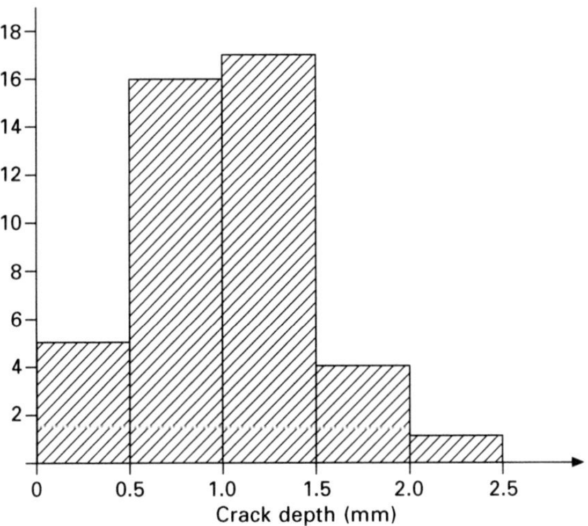

10.33 Histogram of ozone crack depth in fuel pipe.

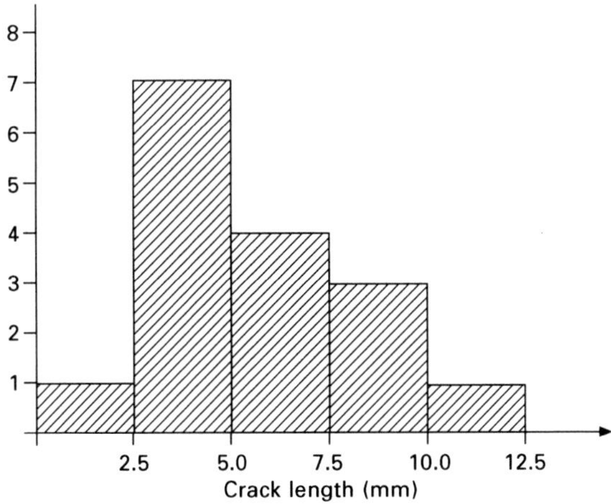

10.34 Histogram of crack length in fuel pipe.

The rubber was identified from simple swelling measurements, where cut sections of hose are dipped into several different organic solvents: the degree of swelling shows the type of elastomer present. Identification can be achieved somewhat more rapidly and more exactly using attenuated total reflectance (ATR) IR spectroscopy by pressing a free surface against a single germanium crystal and obtaining the absorption spectrum on an FTIR spectrometer. Because germanium is transparent to IR radiation, the beam strikes the surface of the polymer from within the crystal and is reflected back for analysis.

10.7.2 Presence of ozone

Ozone gas is produced near electrical circuits, especially where either sparking or silent discharge of current occurs. Rubbers with double bonds in their chains, natural rubber (NR), styrene–butadiene rubber (SBR) and NBR in particular are susceptible to cracking because the gas attacks the bonds and cleaves them very quickly. Only very low gas concentrations are needed (parts per billion in air), and so high concentrations of the gas may be expected near to the electrical distribution system. Thus, if the damage was produced by about 20 000 miles car usage, then failure (deepest crack reaches tube bore) would be expected between 30 000 and 40 000 miles, assuming constant ozone production and a constant growth rate.

10.7.3 Mechanism of attack

Ozone is an allotrope of oxygen (O_2) and is highly reactive with many organic materials.[23–28] It reacts directly with double (olefinic) bonds and, because many rubbers exhibit such bonds in their main chains, it reacts with them and splits the chains:

$$-CH{=}CH- + O_3 \rightarrow \rightarrow -CHO + CO_2H-$$

The end groups are aldehydes, alcohols or carboxylic acids, which are also reactive, and aldehydes and alcohols oxidise further to form acids. Rubbers with double bonds include NR, NBR and butadiene rubber (BR) plus copolymers, which have repeat units:

NR $-[CH_2-CH{=}CHCH_3-CH_2]-$ or polyisoprene

NBR copolymer of isoprene and acrylonitrile repeat units

$-[CH_2-CH{=}CHCH_3-CH_2]-$ and $-[CH_2-CHCN]-$

BR $-[CH_2-CH{=}CH-CH_2]-$

SBR copolymer of butadiene and styrene units

$-[CH_2-CH{=}CH-CH_2]-$ and $-[CH_2-CH-C_6H_5]-$

Ozone cracking was formerly common on old car tyres, forming deep and long cracks aligned at right angles to the tensile strain, or radially on the side wall. However, tyres are now discarded well before cracking occurs, and the rubber is usually given protection against the effects of the gas. One simple remedy is to add a wax to the rubber compound so that it bleeds to the surface during tyre building where it forms a thin protective skin to prevent the gas approaching the surface.

The operating theatre tubing had been attacked by ozone produced by electrical equipment nearby, and was simply replaced by ozone-resistant tubing. Neoprene is more resistant, and Viton is even better at resisting ozone attack. However, the problem persists, especially in non-medical products, such as oil pipes and seals in low pressure air circuits, where tiny amounts of the gas can wreak havoc. Attack usually occurs from stress concentrators such as corners or even impressed lettering (Fig. 10.35), and is easy to distinguish from oxygen cracking, where a fine network of 'crazy paving' cracks is formed.

10.7.4 Condom failure

Rubber products are commonplace, and many are disposable items used just once and then discarded. Rubber bands and balloons are typical and show ozone cracks if left in a bent or strained state in most environments because they are unprotected single-use items. A less likely product is the

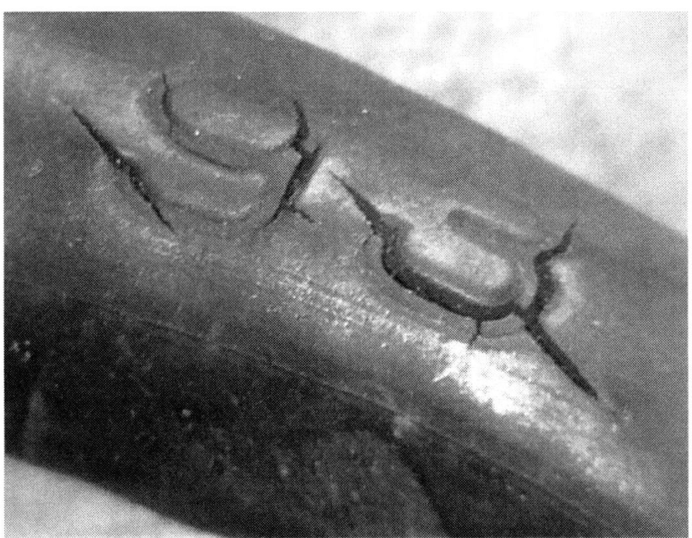

10.35 Ozone cracking from numerals in central heating diesel oil pipe.

condom made from natural rubber. It is made from a latex which is shaped over ceramic formers of the desired shape and size. A lubricant is added for other reasons, but means that all surfaces are, or should be, protected from the harmful effects of oxygen and ozone.

In a case which came before the High Court in the 1990s, a woman claimed that a condom she had been using with her partner failed at a critical point during use and she became pregnant as a result. The failed condom had suffered a brittle fracture at the tip, the crack completely encircling the device (Fig. 10.36). The woman claimed that she had found the damaged condom after intercourse, and she then stored the device under airtight conditions in a refrigerator. Such measures should protect the rubber, now with its lubricant absent, from any harmful gases.

10.7.5 Crack microscopy

When the device was examined in the scanning electron microscope, evidence for ozone cracking was found at several zones near to the fracture edge (Fig. 10.37). The size and distribution varied, and the long cracks appeared oriented generally at right angles to the edge. The area at left in Fig. 10.37 shows many small holes and cracks indicative of high ozone exposure, whereas the longer cracks indicate low exposure, so there may have been at least two separate and independent attacks by ozone after formation of the condom. It implied that attack may have occurred shortly after manufacture, when it was exposed to the gas. The woman had sued the manufacturer on the basis of this evidence. However, there was a problem in explaining how the final failure had been caused by the cracking because none of the cracks

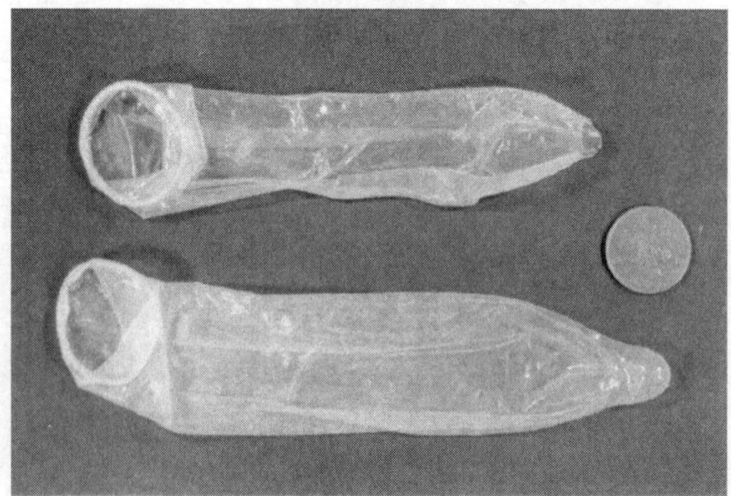

10.36 Failed and intact condoms.

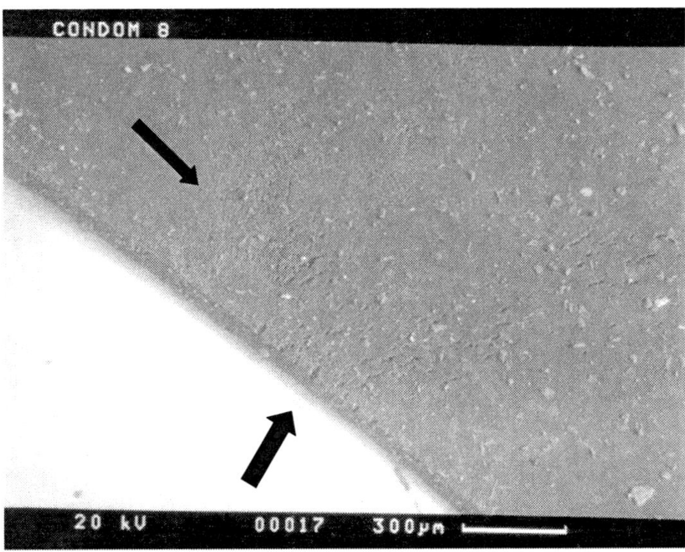

10.37 Ozone cracking near fracture edge.

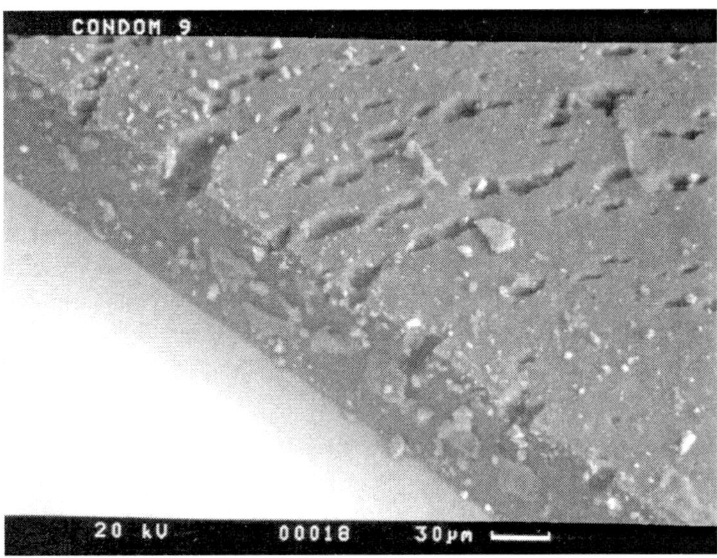

10.38 Close-up of ozone cracks near fracture edge.

appeared to be the origin of the fracture, although many had been bisected by the final failure edge (Fig. 10.38). Another close-up (Fig. 10.39) of the edge also revealed the significant porosity within the 60 μm thick wall caused by air entrapment during manufacture. When the point came up during cross-examination, the response was that any defects which lower wall thickness

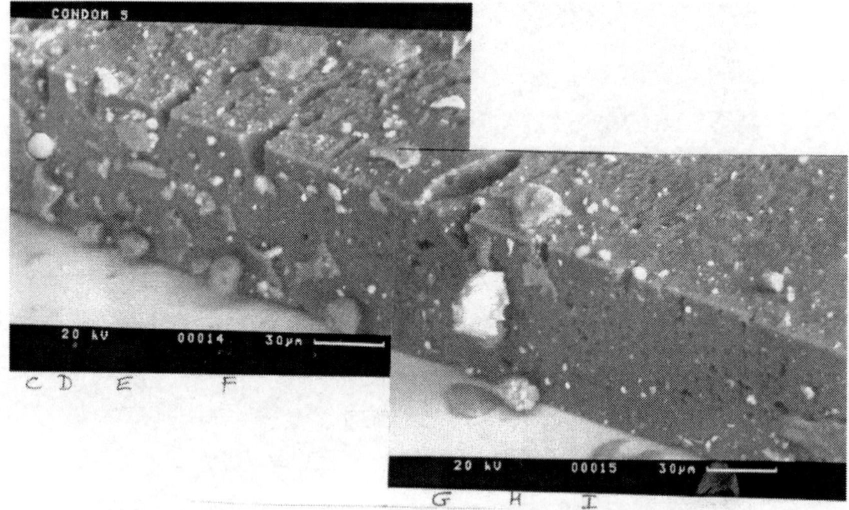

10.39 Oblique close-up of fracture showing inner porosity of rubber and cracks above.

can lower strength, but the expert had to admit that he had not traced the origin of the final fracture.

10.7.6 Aftermath

Whatever the cause of the problem, the judge was not convinced that the failure was caused by a manufacturing defect and the claimant lost her case. Disclosure of the manufacturer's complaints records did show that there were many complaints of premature failure, and the company had researched and introduced a synthetic rubber condom based on polyurethan into the market. This elastomer was much more resistant to ozone attack, but was ultimately withdrawn owing to the greater expense of the product.

10.8 Conclusions

The design of polymeric components in medical equipment is vital to their performance in demanding environments, and design for manufacture is an important subsidiary task. The mechanical strength is improved both by ensuring stress concentrators are ameliorated as far as possible, and that high molecular weight polymer is used for the components concerned. In addition, the product must be made under optimum conditions during injection moulding. The method requires careful setting of machine conditions combined with testing of the various components produced to a standard test, or set of tests. The catheter connector mouldings showed that extra care is needed for polycarbonate fittings, especially when warnings have already been reported in published studies. If necessary, a new test must be devised, as the security cap case illustrated. Once full production occurs, any moulding must be checked for quality to prevent defective parts entering products, which can then fail in service, as the crutch failure showed. Some engineering polymers are difficult to mould correctly, and care is needed to ensure a high quality end product such as a sight tube. Injection moulding defects must be found as soon as possible after manufacture, and setting conditions adjusted to eliminate them in the regular production process.

To the mechanical problem of optimising product strength must be added the effects of exposure to different fluids in many different environments. They include liquids used for disinfection of hospital surfaces (strong detergents, bleach and alcohols) as well as drug carrier fluids, and anaesthetics such as ether. The implant is exposed to many different body fluids and active enzymes, and must be tested against all expected environments before use in humans. Polymers are susceptible to many fluids, especially if products are made with significant degrees of residual strain, such as those produced by cold moulding. Brittle cracking may follow contact with active agents, often initially as hairline cracks, but which then grow along the path of greatest residual strain or chain orientation, as the catheter connection study showed. Such cracks are very difficult to spot by medical staff, who naturally have more important jobs to perform. When those cracks grow to completion, a product may leak internal fluids or simply fall apart, and it is usually then that staff notice the problem. If the device failure is a serious threat to the patient, then emergency action is needed, and the failure reported. Manufacturers must take those reports seriously to avert further failures, and not simply blame staff for product abuse. Similar comments apply to ozone cracks in elastomeric products. All such failures need investigation by qualified forensic engineers to locate the fault or defects, and recommendations must be accepted if medical device design is to improve in the future. The alternative is further accidents, and patient injury, or worse.

10.9 Acknowledgements

The author would like to thank Gordon Imlach for scanning microscopy, DSC, and FTIR spectroscopic analyses, and Stan Hiller for optical microsocopy. He also thanks Dr Patrick A Lewis of the Institute of Neurology, UCL for assistance in the literature searches related to medical products.

10.10 References

1. Cracknell, P and Dyson, R, *Handbook of thermoplastic injection mould design*, Chapman and Hall (1993).
2. Maier, C, *Advances in injection moulding*, RAPRA Review Report 72, (1994).

3. Crawford, RJ, *Plastics engineering*, Butterworth–Heinemann, 3rd Ed (1998).
4. Scheirs, J, *Compositional and failure analysis of polymers: a practical approach*, John Wiley & Sons Ltd, p. 352 (2000).
5. ISO 594/1 (1986) Conical fittings with a 6% (Luer) taper for syringes, needles and certain other medical equipment; EN 20594-1 (1993).
6. Lewis, PR, Environmental stress cracking of polycarbonate catheter connectors, *Engineering Failure Analysis*, **16**(6), 1816–1824 (2009).
7. Stubstad, J, *Female Luers – the frequent failers*, *ANTEC Proceedings*, 291–293 (1992).
8. Stubstad, J, *Troubleshooting plastics*, *Medical Device and Diagnostic Industry*, 100–103 April (1992).
9. Vilardi, J, Franck, LS and Powers, R, ECMO Accidents: a survey of the incidence of mechanical failure and user error, *Neonatal Network*, **11**, 25–32 (1992).
10. Niles, SC, Ploessl, J, Sutton, RGT and Steinberg, JB, Oxygenator failure due to contact with bathing alcohol, *Journal of Extra-corporeal Technology*, **24**, 69–71 (1992).
11. Kwan, ESK, Stich, RAH and Shrem, LA, Salvage of a flow-directed microcatheter after hub failure, *American Journal of Neuroradiology*, **17**, 868–869 (1996).
12. Lewis, PR and Ward RJ, Polishing, thinning and etching of polycarbonate, *Journal of Colloid and Interface Science*, **47**, 661 (1974).
13. Kambour, RP, A review of crazing and fracture in thermoplastics, *Macromolecular Review*, **7**, 1 (1973).
14. Moskala, EJ and Jones, M, Evaluating ESC of medical plastics, *Medical Plastics and Biomaterials* (May 1996).
15. McElwee, D and Snyder, EJ, The use of tapered plastic luer connectors in neonatal extracorporeal membrane oxygenation, *Heart and Lung*, **25**, 324–249 (1996).
16. Drury, CG, Handles for manual materials handling, *Applied Ergonomics*, **11**(1), 35 (1980).
17. Pheasant, S, *Body space – anthropometry, ergonomics and design*, Taylor and Francis, ch. 16, p. 231 (1986).
18. Union Carbide technical brochure, *Moulding of Udel polysulphones* (1995).
19. Potter, BE and Wallace, WA, Crutches, *British Medical Journal*, **301**, 1037–1039 (1990).
20. British Standards, Specification for elbow crutches, BS 4988: 1990.
21. MHRA, Medical Device Alert, MDEA(NI)2005/36.
22. MHRA, Medical Device Alert, MDA/2009/067.
23. Rugg, JS, Ozone crack depth analysis for rubber, *Analytical Chemistry*, 1952, 24 (5), 818–821.
24. Andrews, EH, *Fracture in polymers*, Oliver and Boyd (1968).
25. Andrews, EH, Barnard D, and Braden, M, Ozone attack on rubbers, ch. 12 in Bateman, L, *The chemistry and physics of rubber-like substances*, Maclaren (1963).
26. Lake, GJ, Ozone protection of rubber, *Rubber Chemistry and Technology*, **43**, 1230, (1970).
27. Anachkov, MP, Rakovsky, SK, Stefanova, RV and Shopov, DM, Kinetics and mechanism of the ozone degradation of nitrile rubbers in solution, *Polymer Degradation and Stability*, **19**, 293–305 (1987).
28. Solansky, SS and Singh, RP, Ozonolysis of natural rubber: a critical review, *Progress in Rubber and Plastics Technology*, **17**, 13–57 (2001).

Index